Pet medicine

Pet Medicine

health care and first aid for all household pets

BY ROGER CARAS / PAUL G. CAVANAGH, D.V.M. /
LESTER E. FISHER, D.V.M. / MICHAEL W. FOX, D.V.M., PH.D. /
FREDRIC L. FRYE, D.V.M. / JEAN HOLZWORTH, D.V.M. /
JAY D. HYMAN, D.V.M. / W. J. MATHEY, V.M.D. /
STEPHEN M. SCHUCHMAN, D.V.M.

WITH ILLUSTRATIONS BY SUZANNE CLEE /
DESIGNED BY BARBARA BELL PITNOF

AN INFORMATION HOUSE BOOK

MCGRAW-HILL BOOK COMPANY

NEW YORK ST. LOUIS SAN FRANCISCO LONDON DÜSSELDORF MEXICO
TORONTO SYDNEY

1234567890HAHA783210987

LIBRARY OF CONGRESS CATALOGING IN
PUBLICATION DATA

Main entry under title:
Pet medicine.
"An Information House book."
Includes indexes.
1. Pets—Diseases.   2.   First aid for
animals.
I.   Caras, Roger A.
SF981.P47   636.089'6'024   77-7958
ISBN 0-07-010294-5

Chart on page 40 modified from "Toxicities
in Exotic and Zoo Animals" by M. E. Fowler
in *Veterinary Clinics of North America*, vol.
5, no. 4 (November 1975), Philadelphia,
W. B. Saunders, pp. 690–691. Published
with permission.

Chart on page 62 published with the
permission of Ralston Purina Company.

Contents

Pet medicine

How to have a multipet family

MICHAEL W. FOX, D.V.M., PH.D.

How ordinary or extraordinary is a multipet family, comprised of, say, a dog, a cat, a parrot, gerbils, perhaps a skunk or boa constrictor — and people, too, children and adults of various ages?

In nature, of course, several different animal species live together and share the same habitat. Through evolution and natural selection, they all come to fit harmoniously into a balanced ecosystem. In a home environment, they may not fit together quite so well. There are many things you can do, however, to foster compatibility — and a number of hazards and pitfalls to look out for.

natural interspecies relationships

Some zoos today have mixed exhibits, compatibly and peacefully, ranging from elephants living with giraffes to penguins sharing space with seals. Watching different species interact is more interesting and entertaining for the public; and the different species provide each other more varied and often psychologically beneficial stimulation.

In the wild, naturalists have observed very different species playing with each other. It is a general misconception that members of a given species keep strictly together and interact only with their own kind. A young baboon was once seen riding a gazelle; when it fell off, the gazelle waited for it to jump back on again. Elephants and buffaloes have been seen to engage in playful fights, and wild and domestic species of deer, horse, antelope, sheep, goat, and cattle enjoy games of chasing and mock combat together.

Sometimes special associations develop: the badger and coyote that sometimes hunt together, or a rabbit or ground-nesting duck that may share its abode with a she-fox and her litter. Crows and ravens often follow behind coyotes and wolves that are out hunting, and these odd pairs have been seen playing together.

Foxes trapped live and tested with raccoons responded very differently to raccoons trapped near their own home than to those caught in a different locale. Even so-called solitary creatures like the nocturnal red fox have not only an intimate knowledge of the home range but also more than a passing acquaintance with other species living there. A blackbird's alarm calls are understood by other bird species — and also by squirrels, raccoons, skunks, deer, foxes, and other creatures; they alert each other to danger, though not necessarily consciously and cooperatively. Finally, different species of birds will flock together and mob a fox, owl, or hawk to drive it away.

There are four types of interspecies relationships identified in natural populations:

(1) Sympatric commensal: different species live together and share the same food source, often helping each other avoid predators. Crows and ravens, for instance, get scraps of food from a wolf or coyote kill — and their circling informs coyotes or wolves where food can be found.

(2) Symbiotic: more specific mutual benefits come from the association of two or more species. For instance, there are benefits to both the tick bird or cattle egret, and the buffalo or rhinoceros. The birds feed on the parasites that infest their companions and on the insects disturbed in the grass as the large animal moves around. They help their hosts by alerting them to possible danger — they fly up noisily when another animal approaches. Similarly, the surgeonfish keeps other larger fish free of external parasites, getting a meal from its "patients" — which sometimes line up in shoals to wait their turn to be cleaned. Another example is the remarkable association between the ratel, or honey badger, and a bird known as the honey guide. When the bird finds an active beehive, it will attract a ratel and lead it there. The ratel breaks open the hive, and both feast together — the ratel on the honey, and the bird on the bees.

(3) Parasitic: here the relationship is more one-sided, one species benefiting more than the other. Tapeworms and ticks are parasites — their association with other animals is to their own advantage only. Some would say that a cat has an essentially parasitic relationship with man, especially a fat and lazy cat that gives nothing in return for the food and shelter provided by its owner. The relationship, however, is commensalism, since owner and cat share the same roof — and, often, the same food. If the cat were a hunter and kept down vermin in the house or on the farm, the relationship would be symbiotic.

(4) Prey-predator: the final type of interspecies relationship, as between cat and mouse, wolf and deer, eagle and rabbit, fox and chicken.

These four major categories must be taken into account when one considers which species are most likely to fit together harmoniously in a multi-pet family. Naturally, the parasitic relationship is undesirable — and the prey-predator relationship could be a short-lived one, though animals can be trained to control aggression or be prevented from developing their natural predatory instincts. Commensal and symbiotic relationships are the most promising.

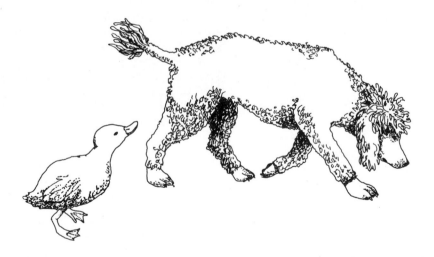

unnatural relationships

Different species raised together may develop relationships that, in the wild, occur almost exclusively between members of the same species. These relationships can be quite bizarre. A duckling has been known to attach itself to a dog, following the dog everywhere as it normally would its mother. Sexual and maternal relationships between different species may develop, and a peck order, or dominance hierarchy, may be established. One veterinarian has a rooster that lords it over all the cats. Jealousy within the social rank of the menagerie, where different species vie for human attention, may erupt. Worse, a low-ranking and defenseless member of the mixed social group may become the scapegoat for the frustration and anger of other animals at a superior they dare not attack. These problem relationships can be alleviated only by discipline from the owner or, in the case of jealousy, attention and indulgence, as with a child.

Genetic factors may subtly influence how an animal responds to another species. In one home, a hamster escaped from its cage and one dog in the house, a skipperkie (a breed developed to hunt down and kill vermin), tried to catch it, while the other dog, a sheltie (selectively bred to herd and protect livestock), opposed the skipperkie and defended its hamster ward.

CONTROL OF AGGRESSION

Playful interaction between two animals, one of which is more powerful physically and lacks restraint or awareness of the other's frailty or distress reactions, may lead to serious injury or death. A cat or a dog may get carried away, for instance, and play too roughly with a pet bird, rabbit, or tortoise. Even among animals brought up together, intense play may switch into play-with-prey, a natural prelude to prey killing. The reactions communicating distress, nipping, struggling, or passivity, inhibit rough play — but they may not be sufficient to prevent a highly aroused and playful predator like a cat or dog from suddenly — even accidentally — killing its companion. A quick escape movement can release an immediate, reflexlike bite, which kills.

Once, as I was playing tug-of-war with one of my young wolves, using a rag as "prey" for it to seize, it accidentally bit my hand. The wolf instantly knew from my reactions what it had done, and rolled over in a submissive apology. Rough play with a wolf or dog can result in accidental nips and scratches, but the animal quickly learns to control the intensity of its bites so as to cause no injury and to enjoy an unbroken play sequence. An owner who wears a protective glove while rough-playing with a puppy will raise a dog that bites hard later in play. "Soft mouth" and "soft paws" (sheathed claws) can be learned by dogs and cats respectively; they have the capacity to control precisely how far they go with a companion during playful fighting. Pups raised in isolation with no opportunity to play with others bite hard and hurt each other when first put together, but within hours, they learn to control the intensity of their play-bite. If one bites too hard, the injured companion, like me with my wolf, yelps and snaps and the play stops. Play is a rewarding activity, and the animals rapidly learn that they must bite each other gently or play will cease.

However, if the signals given by the injured party are inadequate — for example, if a young bird, rabbit, or fawn "freezes" passively when frightened or nipped too hard by an overexuberant cat or dog companion — it may be injured or killed. Human supervision is necessary when one animal is weaker and incapable of cutting off the other's playful but potentially injurious actions. Say "no" and "gently" to a dog, for instance, placing your hand in its mouth to be chewed instead of the kitten or skunk it has been harassing. Be careful not to move too fast, though, for the animal may think that you are going to steal its prey or toy, which may trigger a grab-bite reaction. Also, if it believes that you approve of its reactions and are joining in the hunt by rushing forward excitedly, it may kill or injure the other animal.

EARLY SOCIALIZATION: THE KEY TO PEACE

In the early 1930s a psychologist from Ceylon named Zing Yang Kuo experimented with various species that normally kill or are killed by each other. He successfully raised cats, dogs, rabbits, rats, and pigeons together, demonstrating that social experience early in life, presumably before prey-killing reactions develop, can lead to harmonious relationships between prey and predator. Some supervision was needed, however, when conflicts arose, especially over food.

Kinship bonds can be established between different species, early in life, during a critical period when they are open and receptive to developing attachment. After this period has passed, relationships with other species not encountered before are established with difficulty, if at all. The critical period ranges from five to twelve weeks after birth for a dog to twenty-four to forty-eight hours for a chicken.

Kinship bonds made early in life may be limiting: a crow, pigeon, or duck may be so attached to its human foster parent as to be indifferent to its own species. A dog or cat raised exclusively with people may be indifferent and even aggressive toward its own species and may even refuse to breed. Some animals so attached to an alien species subsequently develop a sexual preference for that species, or behave maternally toward it, or even regard some members of the species as sexual rivals or sibling rivals for the attentions of the leader of the household "pack," "flock," or "herd."

Just as these kinship bonds between species can be formed during an early time in a pet's life, there appears to be a similar critical period for learning to kill and eat prey, especially in cats. If a kitten has no experience with prey early in life, it may be friendly and playful toward a bird or small mammal and never injure it. But be careful! The behavior of the potential prey may eventually release killing reactions in *some* older cats anyway, independent of prior experience.

INTRODUCING DIFFERENT SPECIES

Whenever feasible, introducing animals as young as possible will enhance the establishment of harmonious interspecies relationships. Always assume, though, at first, that you will have to strictly supervise any play-fighting, to protect the weaker animal and to prevent the release of prey-catching and killing reactions. Avoid introducing two adults that have had no prior experience with each other's species.

Prior experience itself can be disastrous, since a cat, skunk, raccoon, or duck socialized to a dog at home, for example, may approach a strange dog and be injured or killed. The expectation of safety — of not being attacked by a potential predator — can place an animal in danger, an extreme example being a tame deer or fox that is shot by a hunter in the neighborhood.

It is often safer to introduce a young animal to an older one, because infant animals can evoke care-giving reactions and neutralize aggressive responses by virtue of their infantile actions and displays. Distress calls and care-soliciting actions are similar in the offspring of many different species. An animal acquired soon after birth or hatching will quickly imprint on, or become attached to, an older animal that is not inclined to attack. At a later age, it will have had some experience with and therefore developed some attachment to its own kind. This will block its propensity to become attached to an animal of another species. A fear (of the stranger) intervenes, which is not fully developed in most very young birds and mammals.

This fear response, when developed, may take one of three forms: escape (flight); "freezing," or immobility; defensive aggression (pecking, hissing, biting, and so on). These fear-motivated reactions may in turn evoke prey-chasing, uninhibited biting or mauling, and counteroffensive aggression in the other animals. Therefore, the introduction of alien species to each other must be carefully supervised. Gentle handling and gradual exposure may help the young animal to relax and overcome its fear.

You must also be alert to the possibility that the older animal, such as a cat or dog, may be possessive of its territory and resent the intrusion of a strange animal, no matter how young. It may react aggressively if the newcomer violates its own personal space, such as approaching too close or going near a favorite chair, basket, or feeding area and food bowls. I often advocate introducing animals for the first time on neutral territory. The resident animal is more likely to accept a new kitten or pup encountered off its property (in a park or neighbor's yard) than one placed immediately in its own home.

If the resident animal is closely attached to its owner, it may feel jealous and threatened by the presence of a newcomer (even a human infant), especially one that is given a lot of attention. The older resident animal should be reassured with attention and indulged in order to allay these reactions, analogous to sibling rivalry in human infants.

HORMONES AND INTERSPECIES RELATIONSHIPS

Hormonal changes can profoundly affect how one animal will respond to another. Sexual maturity increases aggression and status rivalry in both males and females of many species. In some species, there is a definite season when sexual hormones will drastically modify behavior and disrupt social bonds. Male dogs — and cats and roosters — are exceptions, lacking, like man, a breeding season per se and being, instead, constantly potent.

With sexual maturity of one member of a mixed family of animals, conflict and aggression may increase and bizarre sexual relations develop, especially between species that became attached early in life. A female cat in heat may solicit its owner, or a companion dog. A male dog, when aroused, may direct sexual actions toward any number of animals, including cats, skunks, chickens, ducks, and man.

Sex hormones may increase an animal's intolerance for the closeness of others, especially of the same sex, and make the animal difficult and even dangerous to handle. For many species, such as coyotes, this is the time when they set up their own territory and break ties with their parents and litter mates. In other species, such as raccoons and foxes, this intolerance develops before sexual maturity, but the effect is the same: aggression increases — in nature, this serves to disperse the family, an ecologically adaptive mechanism. In the confines of a home with a multipet family, this could be disastrous and is often the reason for people's getting rid of a pet fox or raccoon. Surgical sterilization prior to maturity may help in some species, but it is no guarantee. Many species are relatively solitary as adults and consequently do not make good pets, notably ocelots, margays, otters, and raccoons, although there are individual exceptions. In nature they undergo a natural separation from parents and peers; similarly, in captivity, the bond with the human foster parent may be broken, as well as any attachment to other species.

Other more gregarious species, which live in packs, like the wolf, or in flocks or herds, such as the duck and goat, do not go through this separation stage. Instead, the bonds with parent and peers persist throughout life, and the human foster parent will continue to be regarded as a parent/leader figure. This is why gregarious species are more easily domesticated than more solitary ones — one exception being the domestic cat.

Because so many wild animals mature to become independent, as well as for reasons of ecology and because they can carry disease, domesticated animals — born and raised in captivity — are best integrated into a multipet family.

Maternal hormones also affect behavior and may cause drastic changes in the social relations of a multipet family. In some cases, females become intolerant of proximity during pregnancy or brooding — they do not want other pets or any humans near them — and they aggressively defend their young when they are born. In other circumstances, another animal in the menagerie may be adopted, treated as a substitute offspring, and protected from other animals. One farm dog I know of enjoyed hunting baby rabbits, which it would kill and leave on its master's doorstep. When the dog became pseudo-pregnant, and its maternal hormones were active, it brought baby rabbits home alive instead, and attempted to nurse and guard them.

CROSS FOSTERING

A maternally motivated, lactating cat, dog, or goat can be enormously helpful in raising an orphan animal. A cat may accept an orphan pup, skunk, raccoon, or fox cub, and a dog will often accept a kitten, skunk, raccoon, or cubs of fox, coyote, or wolf. To facilitate acceptance, rub the orphan animal with a damp cloth that has been first rubbed over the body of the foster mother and, if she has her own young, over them as well. Odor is an important factor in the acceptance or rejection of another animal. Even a cat that is well known to a companion cat in the household may be attacked if it has been outdoors and in contact with other species.

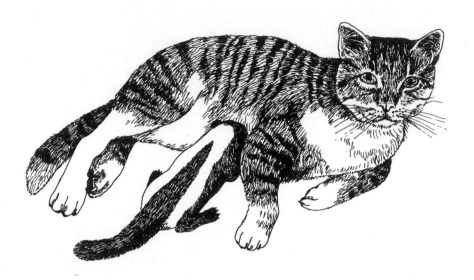

A PET FOR THE PET It may seem a little farfetched, but a pet may need a pet of its own and for this reason, mixed-species families are on the increase. I first realized this several years ago when a friend had a poodle that was a housewrecker. It did this out of boredom and loneliness since its mistress went out to work and left it alone all day. I suggested she get a kitten or another puppy for her dog, but this was put off since the dog was due to have pups. As soon as the pups were born, her dog was in seventh heaven, busy all day and night with her own growing family. Then the time came when the pups were all sold and the dog was again alone in the apartment. The dog became depressed, would not eat, began to mess in the house, and returned to destroying things as well. I happened to have a land turtle and decided to give it to my friend as a potential puppy-substitute and/or companion for her dog. The dog immediately responded to the bold turtle: she licked its hind parts, as she would a puppy, and followed it everywhere. The two became inseparable companions. The dog snapped out of its depression and never messed in the house or destroyed things again.

A kitten is often a good companion for a dog or cat that has to be left alone for extended periods, as when the owner or owners are at work all day. Follow the rules of introduction outlined earlier to restrain the resident animal from attacking the newcomer — and also reassure the original pet, so that it does not become jealous. If you have a cat and a dog, keep the cat food and litter tray behind a gate that gives the cat access but keeps out the dog, or on a high shelf out of the dog's reach. Most dogs will try to snitch the cat's food, and some enjoy eating or rolling in its stools.

An indirect way of providing entertainment if not companionship for cats is to have an aquarium that they can watch (but not get into). Another source of stimulation is an outdoor bird-feeder by a window where the cat can see it.

A multipet family can be a rewarding experience. Although it may never be an idyllic Garden of Eden where lion and lamb lie down together, you can help to foster some seemingly extraordinary animal relationships, and become part of a microcosm of relatedness that embodies the natural qualities of trust, kinship, and love in both animal and man alike.

How to choose a veterinarian

ROGER CARAS

Every animal owner must sooner or later face the problem of selecting a veterinarian. In every way it is as personal a decision as the selection of a family physician, dentist, or attorney. The veterinarian is not only the man or woman who will guide you in the day-by-day care of your pet but the person who will make that animal well in the event of an emergency, and who should at least be willing to attempt to ease the mind of the troubled owner. On the day a favorite pup gets hit by a car and the mother is rushing it to the hospital with two sobbing children in the back seat, the veterinarian becomes one of the most important people on earth. It is far better if the wise selection of a family veterinarian is made in advance, before an emergency arises.

Before you pick a veterinarian, it is a good idea to know what has gone into the making of this scientist. A veterinarian is a man or woman who has had a minimum of two years of undergraduate college and four years of veterinary training. In fact, though, very few students get into veterinary school after only two years in undergraduate school, and most veterinarians have had three, four, or more years. Students who, after four years of college, are not accepted for veterinary training may elect to go on to a master's and perhaps even a doctorate, usually in biology, applying to veterinary school each year until they are accepted. One young woman I know of was turned down for six straight years before being accepted and becoming, I am told, an outstanding practitioner. But many would-be veterinarians finally give up and become physicians instead, not the other way around, as some people seem to expect. The acceptance rate for medical school in this country is 37½ percent, while the acceptance rate for veterinary school is 12½ percent.

Thirty-two of our fifty states do not have veterinary schools. There is none at all in the heavily populated New England states, and Cornell — at Ithaca, New York, in a state of eighteen million people — can accept only seventy-two new students a year. They take fifty-seven from New York and fifteen from the rest of the world, including New England.

The schools in the western states (the University of California at Davis and the University of Colorado at Fort Collins, for example) will not even send a catalog to a student outside of their own region, much less seriously entertain an application. Most schools in Europe will no longer accept American students for veterinary training, figuring, quite rightly, that we should be able to educate our own. Their available openings go to students from developing nations.

There is, then, a critical shortage of schools and of new veterinarians. Cornell, the first university in the world to award the D.V.M. degree (in 1876), still can graduate only an average of 65 students a year. Recently, for the 65 graduating students, 360 jobs were posted. Some of these were critical, offerings from established veterinarians whose health was failing and who needed people to move in and take over their practices.

Once a student graduates as a D.V.M., he or she might get a residency in one of the small number of very highly desirable research hospitals or key clinics such as the Animal Medical Center in New York or the Angell Memorial in Boston. Few do. Others go right to work for other veterinarians (after passing boards that are at least as brutal as those faced by new M.D.'s). Sooner or later, though, the young veterinarian is likely to look to his or her own hospital.

Unlike the M.D., the D.V.M. can't go into practice with a desk, an examining table, and a blood pressure sleeve. A veterinary hospital needs cages, isolation facilities, outside and inside runs, an X-ray machine, medical and surgical equipment and supplies costing tens of thousands of dollars, and kennel help at least. The young D.V.M., unless from a wealthy family, starts out after perhaps eight years of college by going deeply into debt.

I have detailed all of this to explain if not justify the cost of veterinary care. It is a constant source of lament among relatively inexperienced animal owners, rarely among professionals or long-time animal lovers and fanciers. Those who set a veterinary career as a goal take great risks of failure, then work like the very devil for years after getting into a school, and start out their professional lives heavily in debt. It is no wonder that their expectations of reward are high. If they were lower, we would not be graduating even the 1,600 new veterinarians we now do each year. The risks and expense of the costliest and most strenuous of all careers to launch simply would not be worth it.

None of the foregoing justifies a poor veterinarian, however, or a dishonest one. There are perfectly dreadful practitioners of veterinary science just as there are of medicine, dentistry, law, or any other profession. Every pet owner should be able to spot these bad ones or, more importantly, the good ones.

Most people define a good veterinarian as the person who was apparently skilled enough to solve their pet's problem when it arose. But this does not take into account a lucky guess or an animal that has a self-limiting condition and would have gotten better anyway.

Since my family has six or more dogs, ten or more cats, and a horse or two as a normal population, I spend rather a lot of my time (and money) with veterinarians. Before finding our regular veterinarians, whom we count as close personal friends, we learned over the years that there are certain signs to look for. What are they?

A KIND OF PARTNERSHIP Are you comfortable with your veterinarian? If you do not feel that you can have meaningful communication or if you feel that he or she will not be even reasonably sympathetic to you as an individual and to your concerns, break it off. The relationship will be one of distrust, and you will end up in claims that you were overcharged and your animal killed. Successful pet raising is a kind of partnership between the animal's owner and doctor. Very often you have to go almost on blind faith, and the D.V.M. may have to depend on your superior knowledge of a pet's day-to-day patterns. If you two can't work things out together, the pet may suffer.

A FEELING OF CARING There are veterinarians — most, I like to believe — who care very much about animals. Some, however, are in the field because it can be a profitable business with a built-in position of prestige in the community. It is not very difficult to determine which category a person falls into. Veterinarians obviously cannot sit down and weep with owners when a decision or outcome is negative, any more than doctors can. But they should care because they *like* animals.

TWENTY-FOUR HOURS A DAY This point is controversial, and some veterinarians will disagree with me, though I consider it one of the most critical yardsticks. I do not deal with a veterinary installation on a regular basis (hit any port in a storm) unless there is a way of reaching the staff twenty-four hours a day, every day of the year. Disease and trauma do not follow schedules posted on clinic doors, and no pet or animal found injured by the road should have to die because of a golf tournament or a bridge game.

This is not to suggest that the privilege be abused. No pet owner has the right to call a doctor away from his or her Christmas dinner because a dog may possibly have ringworm. Everything but the real emergency should wait for normal office hours, but conditions like bleeding and convulsions and rat poison ingestion cannot. When I call a veterinary office and a machine tells me to call back after nine A.M. the next working day, I have called that number for the last time. On this point I am firm, and have terminated relationships with veterinarians over it. The team of four D.V.M's we use now and have for over a decade are always available, and on those one or two occasions every five years when we need them at some punishing hour of the night, they come or meet us at the hospital and never complain. They know the measure of our gratitude and they care about our animals. They also know we care about them as individuals with rights to be respected.

AMBIANCE: EFFICIENCY AND CLEANLINESS

A veterinary hospital should have the right *ambiance*. It should *feel* efficient and clean, and it should inspire a visitor with confidence that this is a place where things are done right and where things are likely to go well.

A place that is too dirty, too smelly, too casual — and where movements and decisions are not crisp, concerned, and designed to make you and your pet feel better, or at least safe, instantly — is probably not going to provide you with a positive experience. Everyone from the receptionist to the kennel boy to the reigning veterinarians themselves should inspire calm and confidence. Without that there may not be such good medicine either.

THE DETAILS

There are also fine details to look for, which make up the ambiance. I expect a waiting area and treatment room to be clean and orderly and I do not expect to find debris from previous patients. It should also be comfortable. I am impressed by the presence of humane society literature and a bulletin board for information about lost pets and pets up for adoption. I would like to see evidence that the veterinary staff is involved with some humane work.

I expect a veterinarian or technician to clean off the examining table with a disinfectant before putting my animal on it.

I expect a veterinarian's clothing and hands to be clean.

I am highly suspicious of veterinarians who are quick to suggest the hospitalization of cats for any longer than is absolutely essential. Cats are usually miserable in cages and they are highly susceptible to airborne viral infections. No cat should be caged near other cats any longer than can possibly be avoided.

I am, in fact, highly suspicious of veterinarians who call for what seems to be an unusual amount of hospitalization. Young friends recently called to say they were worried about their young bloodhound bitch. She had had a rash and they had taken her to a local veterinary hospital. The examining doctor said the animal would have to be hospitalized for at least a week and would need elaborate chemical baths every day. They left their pet but called us. Bloodhounds often do not do well when left like that, and when stressed *may be* more susceptible to a potentially deadly condition known as bloat. It all sounded suspicious. We told the couple to reclaim their animal immediately and go to our veterinarians instead. When they got there, they were given a tube of salve and sent on their way with their pet. Evidently the first veterinarian had had some empty cages and decided to put one of them to work earning revenue. Although this kind of thing unfortunately can happen, it is far more the exception than the rule.

I do not trust veterinary hospitals where boarding animals and sick animals are housed or exercised close to each other. If you have a pet you must board, there is no justification for its being put with animals that can infect it. If a hospital does not have boarding facilities, it should not take in boarders. Further, there must be adequate runs for large animals as well as small.

A word of qualification here: if you do board a dog you may get it back with a mild cough. This is called a kennel cough and is extremely difficult to avoid since it is caused by an airborne virus. It is a mild, self-limiting condition and is not fairly blamed on the veterinarian. He or she should be willing to treat it, though, if it was contracted while boarding. With new immunization it may soon be a thing of the past.

SEEING THE FACILITIES

In connection with the last two points, the ambiance and the details, because I am very much interested in animals, I expect a veterinarian early in our relationship to invite me to see the hospital, out back where most of the important things are done. A veterinarian who refuses me a tour when I request one (allowing for busy times, isolation problems, aseptic areas, and other reasonable considerations) is suspect. I want to see cleanliness, brightness, and I want to know where and how animals are maintained when they have to stay behind. I want to see how the staff handles animals. I want to see clean runs. A room full of animals has an inevitable smell, but it is neither stale nor rotten. There is a world of difference between the smell of animals and the smell of neglect.

REASONABLE RECOMPENSE — AND EARLY WARNING

Although veterinary bills are a major expense in my family's annual budget, I do not expect to waste money nor do I expect to be "taken." I expect to pay a veterinarian for his or her valuable time and I expect to pay for materials used in making the animals I bring in well. All of that within reason. But I also expect a veterinarian to warn me in advance if a situation, in his or her professional estimation, is going to assume the proportions of the national debt. Clients should be advised in advance of the expected price of surgery and special care and of procedures where the expense is likely to soar. Sometimes, unfortunately, we have to make decisions based on our ability to pay, and we should be provided in advance with the information necessary to make those decisions.

On the other hand, I do not expect a veterinarian to tell me that an animal is not "valuable enough" to warrant surgery or therapy. I will determine what an animal is worth to me, for that is a decision of the heart, not of the wallet. The animal's general condition and age will often be the basis for my decision, at least in part, and not its price tag. I also expect a veterinarian to tell me frankly how much an animal will suffer if we go forward, for that is usually the most important factor of all.

Exotic animals represent a whole new set of problems. I am opposed to the keeping of wild animals as common pets except under the most unusual circumstances, but the need can arise.

FRANK TALK ABOUT THE LIMITS

I am highly suspicious of any veterinarians (and I have known very few such) who are afraid to admit that they lack certain training and experience. When a serious zoo veterinarian faces a probable breech delivery in a gorilla or orangutan, he or she will seldom hesitate to yell for the help of a good obstetrician or perhaps an entire obstetrical emergency team. While obstetricians have had endless practice bringing animals very much like apes into this world, a D.V.M. is quite likely to have never seen this problem before.

Most serious veterinarians I know will call on a dentist for a peculiar or difficult mouth problem. Many zoo veterinarians, faced with a multitude of species they learned little or nothing about in school, will also do so. A

Texas zoo director, who also happens to be a veterinarian, recently used his own dentist to help him do root canal work on a leopard.

Small primates, particularly infant apes, are often as much pediatric as veterinary problems. A fine southern zoo uses a prominent pediatrician from the community to work with the veterinarian on the young primates. This is not unusual nor does it reflect badly on the D.V.M. It represents, instead, good common sense and real concern. It also works both ways. I know a medical school that has a veterinarian lecturing on dermatology because of his special skills and knowledge.

Unfortunately, there are some veterinarians who will not admit that they lack the skill to do a certain job. They may be from another era and not recognize that there are now veterinary neurologists, veterinary eye surgeons, and superb veterinary orthopedic surgeons. Good veterinarians, like good M.D.'s, use their own skill to maximum effect but will call upon anyone and everyone who will help fill the gap in their knowledge or experience. Wild dogs and cats are not much of a problem for veterinarians since their diseases (and anatomy) are the same as those of our domestic varieties. Skunks are susceptible to feline diseases and a veterinarian will know what immunization regimen they require.

The one area where the pet owner is most likely to get into trouble finding veterinary expertise is with reptiles. Most veterinarians will have information at their disposal on the weasels (skunks) and on birds, but the literature on the care (and certainly surgery) of captive reptiles is sparse and on relatively few practitioners' shelves. Reptile owners, unless they are lucky, may have to turn to a large zoo for assistance with their snakes, lizards, and turtles. Amphibians will be even more trouble.

SMALL AND LARGE We are fortunate in that our family four-man veterinary team handles both large and small animals. They do care for our companion animals and our horses and the odd zoo orphan we are asked to raise. It should be recognized, though, that very often, perhaps most often, small animal and large animal practices do not go on under the same roof. It is no reflection on a veterinarian if he or she does not want to see to your horse, cow, or pig. In a very real sense, they are specialists who have focused their attention on small companion animals, domestic dogs and cats, and you may need two separate veterinary relationships if you have both kinds of animals. Since it isn't always easy to find an equine practitioner within a reasonable distance, this should be considered *before* you buy a horse or other large animal.

Among the small animals, fish are a very big problem and most veterinarians have relatively little experience with them. As suggested elsewhere in this book, you may have to seek help at a veterinary college, school of marine biology, or wildlife service. The small rodents, lagomorphs (rabbits), and the birds should be within the experience of almost any practitioner, with birds being their most likely weak spot. Zoo veterinarians, of course, will be able to fill in almost everywhere, and there are some practitioners who do specialize in birds almost exclusively. You may have to ask around, and professional breeders and zoos are the likely places to start.

Not to coin a phrase, some of my best friends are veterinarians. They are the veterinarians we use at home and many others I know in other parts of the country. In candor and disgust they have told me of charlatans and worse who have somehow managed to get into the field. I don't want that kind of man or woman near my animals, and you don't want them near yours. Fortunately, they are in the minority. Most veterinarians I have known have been skilled scientists, honorable and sensitive men and women with very strong humane feelings toward all animals. The hard shell of detached involvement they sometimes are forced to affect is for preserving their own sanity. I respect this profession more than I do most others, and I feel a strong sense of obligation to the many men and women who down through the years have saved my animals and all of the other animals, whoever they may have belonged to, who came under their care. I am very demanding, though, in the standards I expect from the practitioners of this great healing art. No fool and no fraud will ever touch an animal of mine if I can prevent it. Every animal lover owes his friends this same consideration.

In the house and the yard

Dogs

PAUL G. CAVANAGH, D.V.M.

No one needs to introduce "man's best friend." Thousands of years of close association between humans and canines have resulted in an entire literature praising the dog as a companion. So, rather than discussing the dog in *your* life, let's start by looking at the people in the life of the pet you have or are considering getting.

Far too many of us forget, when some funny little rascal in a shop window captures our hearts, that by taking it home we are making a commitment. That the pup is willing to do so is obvious, and this is the greatest part of its appeal. But what of our own, in a relationship that may continue as long as thirteen years and more?

To the first humans who formed bonds with dogs, they were undoubtedly a new form of tool — efficient working animals that demanded a minimum amount of care. Today's hunting dogs and watchdogs demand more attention; nevertheless, they earn their keep. The vast majority of dogs owned today, though, are kept as pets. They are popular because they are social animals, which in their native state live in packs. Instinctively, dogs look for companionship, want to belong, and are ready to freely invest their love.

To be loved is flattering, of course, and because we too are social animals, we respond. Many humans form attachments to dogs they would find difficult with their own species, for a dog's love is undemanding — on the surface. It *asks* little and is quite ready to accept us and love us for what we are.

In that first wave of excitement as it charms us, it is easy to overlook the fact that it *needs* much. In a modern civilization, dogs are far more dependent on us than they were on our ancestors. Only a century ago, when the majority of Americans lived in rural areas, the dog was still able to do a fairly efficient job of fending for itself. Though it was far more likely to become diseased than is today's pet, it was able to get much of its food by catching small game. And, at the same time, it got the exercise it needed.

In the city or the suburbs where most of us live today, it is impossible for a dog to get its food and exercise independent of us. That is why it is so important, in getting a dog, to think of the future. What happens when the fresh charm of the puppy wears off and we find ourselves with the adult dog? What do we do with the nonhuman member of the family when vacation time rolls around? These things must be considered and, if they are, you can do a great deal to minimize the problems at the time you select your pet.

PICKING SEX AND BREED

The basic decisions about what kind of dog you should get center around sex and breed. In both cases, the important things to consider are your present circumstances — life-style, if you will — and your future intentions. You might well be drawn toward a particular choice because of a pet remembered from your childhood, but the pet that was ideal in the conditions your family lived under then might be poorly suited to your life today.

Male versus female? The majority of pet owners have no intention of

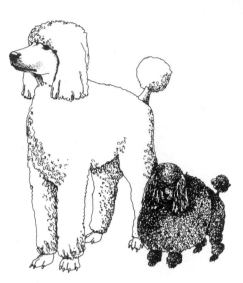

breeding their animals when they mature — and the sexuality of a mature dog is more inclined to pose problems than anything else. If you have a male and he can be allowed to run free where he will have sexual opportunities, there will be minimal problems; if he is confined, this is another matter entirely. Don't be so naive as to think a dog's sexual desires are stimulated only by the scent of a bitch in heat. A male kept confined is quite likely to become sexually aggressive with humans, which can be an annoyance if not an embarrassment.

Certainly, a female in heat is a stimulant to males in the neighborhood — and if you have a female, there can be unwanted pregnancies when she is allowed out, and there can be a pack of aroused males haunting your home. Fortunately, spaying can solve these problems simply and permanently — or, if you have ideas of breeding, the "pill" is available for dogs as well as humans.

There are too many breeds to allow any real examination of the merits of each, but some general rules are possible. First, there is the matter of size. Obviously, for an apartment dweller, one of the toy breeds is far more practical than a Saint Bernard or a Newfoundland. It isn't simply a matter of living space, either. Larger dogs require a proportionately greater amount of exercise space. Unless your dog will have an opportunity to run free, this means walks, in foul weather as well as fair.

This explains, to a great extent, the enormous popularity of dachshunds, chihuahuas, and miniature poodles and schnauzers today. But bear in mind that breeding for special characteristics usually means that when you make your selection, you are making a choice between problems. If you get a toy, for example, accept the fact that you're facing an uphill job in training it not to get on the sofa or easy chairs, something unlikely to interest a larger dog.

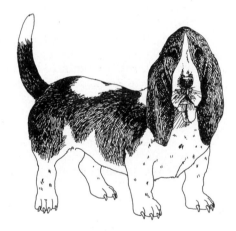

Then there's the matter of personality; here you must allow for individual differences, bearing in mind that the smaller breeds are likely to show greater variations in character than the larger. Generally, though, again, it is possible to arrive at some broad categories. A hound — whether Afghan, beagle, basset, or stretched-out dachshund — is always a hound. Let it spot a rabbit — or let your pet cat or bird make a sudden move — and instinct will probably override training. Dogs bred for guard duty, such as the dobermans, are not necessarily vicious by nature; but they will tend to settle their affections on either individuals or the members of a family group and not welcome the attentions of strangers. There are entire books on this subject, but any reputable dealer will be able to advise you in the choice of breeds.

The emphasis on breeding, testified to by papers showing American Kennel Club registration, obscures the fact that there *are* differences in quality among the purebreds no matter how pure a dog's ancestry might be. Everything hinges on the merits of the individual pup's ancestors. The pet shop owner might have the documentation but, no matter how well you have informed yourself, you cannot judge the perfection of form you will get in the mature animal by looking at the pup. And the papers, actually, tell you little beyond the fact that your pet is truly of its breed. To learn anything more than this involves a time-consuming, bothersome search through the A.K.C. record books to discover how well the pup's forebears did in competitive shows.

Purebreds, though, are more easily predicted than mixed-breed dogs; because of that, and because there is prestige attached to their ownership, purebreds are far more popular than the lowly mutt. But mutts have virtues of their own and, aside from the fact that there are so many without homes, don't deserve to be overlooked. Inbreeding, the very thing that produces the purebreds, also tends to produce congenital faults such as the German shepherd's inherent tendency to problems with its hindquarters. These are far less likely with the mutts, which are generally much hardier, healthier animals.

WHERE TO GET YOUR PUP   One good place to look for a dog is the local American Society for the Prevention of Cruelty to Animals, the ASPCA. Dogs you get there are, for the most part, disease-free — and there are money-back guarantees if the dog does become ill within a certain period of time. The ASPCA requires male dogs to be castrated, female dogs to be spayed (see Prevention of Pregnancy, page 26).

Generally, throughout the country, those in the business of selling purebred dogs must meet strict standards to get and keep their registration. Finding an honest dealer, then, is not a major problem — if you're given A.K.C. papers on a dog, there's little reason to doubt their authenticity. The fact remains, however, that they are in the business of marketing dogs, and the primary objective is to make a profit — which depends on volume, and on the ability to provide a wide variety of breeds for shoppers.

The pups they handle come from a number of sources, including kennels that may be thousands of miles away. After the strain of traveling, these young dogs are brought together in close quarters. Each could have contracted some infection at its point of origin and each, in a somewhat weakened condition, is likely to pick up another in the pet shop because its resistance has been lowered.

If, once you have settled on a breed you like, you are within reach of a kennel that specializes in this type, you could reduce the possibilities of contagion by going directly to the source. It's a good idea to have a look, yourself, at the conditions at the kennel — and if you have in mind showing or breeding your dog, the kennel is definitely a better bet: any kennel owner handling animals of show quality will have books showing the performances of the pup's ancestors.

This matter of lineage, by the way, is of importance only if you do have such plans for the future. You can expect every show point won by dogs in your pup's line to be reflected in its price. Unless you look forward to getting your money back through stud fees or selling litters, recognize that owning a member of the canine nobility can be an expensive proposition.

Ultimately, from the standpoint of assuring yourself that you are getting a healthy animal likely to have a good temperament, your best source is a personal friend. You will know that the possibilities of the pup's contracting an infectious disease are at a minimum — and you can get to know both the parents in advance, watching for traits that might show up in the next generation such as shyness, nervousness, or irritability.

In judging the individual pup out of a litter or a selection in a pet store, pick the one that appears healthiest and most alert. This is no guarantee that an infection is not incubating, and will emerge later, but it does reduce the odds. Shyness, again, is not a desirable characteristic, though it might to some have a certain wistful appeal in a pup. The more gregarious animal will give you the greater trust, I believe, and become the closer friend — though this is a matter of personal taste.

Many pet shops offer warranties allowing you to return a pup within one month if it has been inspected by a veterinarian and found to be diseased or suffering from congenital defects. While, in comparison shopping, it is desirable to consider this as a factor in your choice, you should understand that it is not any absolute assurance that all is well. The incubation period for many diseases extends beyond the warranty, and an apparently healthy pup may still become diseased. Many congenital defects will not become obvious until the dog has reached maturity. Putting off having the pup checked by the veterinarian until the last possible moment has its pitfalls, too. The longer you keep it, the tighter the hold it gains on your affections and it becomes increasingly difficult to return the pet you have come to love, knowing it will almost certainly be destroyed.

But love *is* what it's all about. The pup's willingness to give love is the source of its appeal. It is a commitment that deserves to be matched by your own, to make sure your pet lives a full and healthy life. This chapter is designed to help you do the best job possible.

rearing and preventive care
CAN A DOG AFFECT YOUR HEALTH?

Your health and your family's, of course, must be considered: if you suspect that someone in the family is allergic to dog hair, it's better to find out before you bring the dog home and then have to take it away, causing much sadness. Visit a family that has a dog, for several hours — if there are allergies, they'll probably show up.

It's obvious that if there were any serious danger of the transmission of canine diseases to humans the history of our relations with this closest of animal friends would have been quite different. Certainly, rabies can be contracted from the bite of an infected animal, but no owner is going to neglect having a pet immunized, not only as a standard precaution but because of legal requirements in order to obtain a license for the animal. Bites by strays or strange dogs must be brought to the attention of a physician, however.

The only other serious possibilities are fungal diseases, such as ringworm, and parasites. In both cases, prevention starts with the animal itself, and it is as vital that the pet be treated as the human to prevent reinfection. These problems are dealt with in the appropriate sections below. The most important thing to remember is that if you show proper consideration for your pet's health, you will be assuring that neither your nor your family's health will be affected by owning a dog.

TRAINING

For the safety and health of both pet and humans, a certain amount of training is essential. Just how much you give your dog will depend largely on your own tolerance — it's up to you whether you want to allow the animal on the furniture or not, for example. A completely undisciplined dog, though, will be impossible to live with.

Beating a dog to train it is not only unnecessary but poor practice. Who, after all, wants a pet that cowers? A firm scolding is equally effective. Dogs are sensitive animals and want your affection. You don't need to shout at them — they will understand the disapproval in your tone. You can reinforce your point by slapping a newspaper against your leg, but you need not strike your pet with it. Simply ignoring the dog is extremely effective, once it understands what it has done that is wrong.

The most important point is that when the dog has done something wrong, you should act immediately — it is most desirable to catch it in the act. Dogs are highly intelligent animals but, like young children, they have short attention spans.

Pups between six and eight weeks of age are quite ready to start learning the basics, such as housebreaking; more complex training, such as tricks, should be delayed until they are between eight and ten months old.

In spite of the old saw about old dogs and new tricks, it is, indeed, possible to train an older dog. It's harder — because it often entails *un*training from previous habits — but it can be done.

HOUSEBREAKING. Your housebreaking technique will depend on where you live — if you're in an apartment house, unless you're on the first floor, you'll have to paper-train a dog before it graduates to the outdoors. In any case, a puppy should not be taken out on the city streets until the age of twelve weeks, and until it has had its second distemper shot. Waiting until the series of distemper shots is completed is even better.

The first procedure, in outdoors housebreaking, is to select a designated spot outdoors. Prescent the area with a rag you've used to mop up the pup's earlier mistakes.

After a nap, meal, play, first thing in the morning and last thing at night, pick up the puppy and take it to its spot. The puppy should wear a leash to prevent it from escaping, both for safety and so that it will not be distracted from its lesson.

When it performs, lavish the puppy with praise and give it an occasional treat to underscore the point. Should it continue to make mistakes in the house, scold it firmly — and take it out immediately to the proper place. Soon it will get the idea and let you know when it wants to go out. As it becomes accustomed to walking on a leash, you can take it to other places than the spot originally used, and show, by your praise, that these too are acceptable. Contrary to common belief, male dogs can be trained to use the gutter rather than trees, flower beds, and stoops.

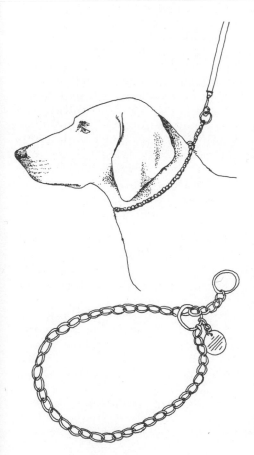

If you are training your puppy to go on paper, in a confined area, place newspapers over the entire floor. Choose the spot you ultimately want used and prescent it. Gradually remove portions of the newspaper around this, exposing areas of the floor, and encourage the puppy to use the remaining papered area following naps, meals, and so forth. With time, only a small area of paper will be needed, and the puppy will not make mistakes elsewhere in the house.

If or when the pup is to graduate and learn to go outside, remove the newspaper, prescent a spot outside with used newspaper, and follow the outdoors housebreaking technique described above.

LEASH TRAINING. Train the puppy to the leash as early as possible. Do not tug or yank at the leash, but call its name and give the command "come," gently pulling it toward you. This should be done simultaneously with training it to come on command without the leash. As it learns its name, the puppy will come spontaneously when called if you respond with praise and affection. But use the command "come" so that this will become associated with the act.

With or without a leash, the dog should be trained to walk at heel. This is not only a convenience (a lunging dog that tangles its leash around your legs is no fun to walk) but a safety precaution. Even in the country, when walking along roads with little traffic, you want sufficient control over your animal to be sure it will not be run down by a car. The training is relatively simple. Hold the leash in your left hand. Give the command "heel" and pull the puppy into position so that it is walking with its head beside your leg. When it tries to pull ahead or to lunge in some other direction, pull it back and repeat the command. When it has walked in position for a short while, praise it. Gradually give it more leash, command it to heel, and show your appreciation when it obeys.

Choke collars are excellent for large breeds to restrain them. Training choke collars are useful to teach the dog to walk with its head up. Holding the head up may help prevent nasal tumors, which have been postulated to be caused by inhaling carcinogenic pollutants from the ground. A dog with

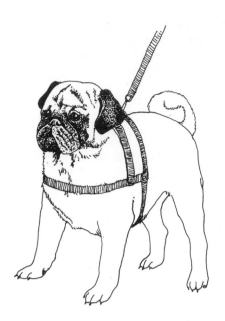

its head up will also avoid some of the contagion from worms (in feces) and dangerous food. Toy breeds such as poodles and pugs should wear harnesses rather than collars because of the risk of collapsed tracheas (see page 53).

BAD HABITS. Bad habits, such as jumping on people, getting on the furniture, biting, chewing, and begging for food, can be avoided *or* corrected early by gentle but persistent scolding. There is a strong connection between boredom and bad behavior — sometimes a high-spirited dog has such a tedious life, it develops bad habits to keep itself occupied, and in an effort to gain attention. Some variety, as well as scolding, would be the prescription.

Bear in mind that chewing has a function. It is virtually essential for a teething puppy and is important to the dental health of older animals. Chewable toys made of nylon or hard rubber are excellent. If the dog is given real bones, they should be removed before they have been whittled down to the point where they can be swallowed. Brittle, small bones, such as those of a chicken, should never be given to a dog. Heavier bones, such as beef or lamb, should be given the pet when raw (cooking destroys their resilence and there is the possibility of swallowing sharp fragments), after meat and fat have been trimmed off. Because of the risk of trichinosis when they have not been cooked, pork bones should be avoided.

HOUSING   A dog that lives outdoors must, first of all, be given enough space to allow it to run for exercise. Second, it should have a dry, draft-free house large enough for it to sleep in comfortably. In cooler climates, additional space is undesirable. Bedding should be well padded, dry, and warm.

Extremes of climate must be taken into consideration. In areas with harsh winters, only specialized breeds such as malemutes can be kept outdoors without risking frostbite. In the South, because of the risk of heat stroke, runs should be in the shade. (See Heat Stroke and Frostbite under Emergencies and First Aid, page 37.)

Indoors or outdoors, your pet's bedding should be changed once a week. Cloth bedding, which is excellent, should be washed before it is used again.

Exercise is as important for the house dog as for the pet that lives outside. Regardless of housebreaking requirements, which become less frequent as the animal matures, your dog should be taken out for a walk at least twice a day. The more exercise the better — and bear in mind that these outings are good for your health too. If you go in for jogging, your dog will thoroughly enjoy it and will make an excellent companion. In any case, once around the block is *not* enough. And don't let your dog persuade you to duck out and right back in again just because the weather is nasty. Owners who bundle their pets up in little coats during the winter fail to realize just how hardy these animals actually are, and that their natural coats actually become thicker through exposure to the cold. (One must be more careful of a clipped poodle, of course — but still a coat is unnecessary.)

As an example, for quite a few years New Yorkers enjoyed the early morning sight of one scottie who insisted on having his daily swim in Central Park's lake. As winter set in, he would jump up and down on the ice until he broke through. Even after it finally became too thick, he went right on trying, until spring finally brought the thaw.

If you have a puppy, there is one indoor danger of which you should be aware: watch to make sure it doesn't chew on electrical wiring. Chewing toys will help remove the temptation, but alertness is also necessary. The pup will not risk electrocution with the first nibble (see Electrical Shock, page 41), and if you keep your eyes open, you can train it to leave the wiring alone and to stick to its toys — or your favorite slippers.

Plants are another problem. Dogs, and particularly puppies, will chew them. In some cases, this can be a danger (see Poisoning, page 39), and, at best, it is bound to affect your interior decoration.

What about other animal residents? Forget all the myths about natural enemies. Certainly, a dog in the wild is a predator and behaves as such, but with an assured diet it will make a good companion to and enjoy the company of virtually any other animal. Bear in mind the domesticated breeds that defend sheep against their wild cousins, the wolves. The problem of bringing different animals together in the household has less to do with species than with concepts of territory. It is no easier to bring in another dog than a cat. The easiest way around any jealousy that might arise is to introduce the animals while they are young. The relationships can become quite close; and many a family dog has been seen to challenge larger animals of his own species in defense of his cat companion. (See "How to Have a Multipet Family.")

FEEDING

There is really nothing mysterious about the proper diet for a dog. Their nutritional requirements are quite similar to those of humans, and you would do much better to think of a dog as being like a child rather than belonging to an alien species.

Because of their high metabolisms, puppies have special feeding requirements (see Mothers and Puppies, pages 6off.), but for a dog over eight months of age, any of the commercial canned, dry, or semimoist diets are good, and the choice will depend largely on your dog's personal preference. At this age the dog should be receiving two meals a day. As it becomes an adult, depending on how active the animal is, this may be cut to one. The proper amount must be determined by trial and error and will depend on both the dog's size and, again, how active it is. If it appears to be ravenous, let it eat. If it seems to be gaining weight after it has reached its full growth, cut back.

Table scraps should not be the main staple of the diet — but they do have their uses. Vegetables, for instance, are excellent in the dog's diet and should be included frequently. Leftovers are fine for this purpose, and there is no need for any fixed schedule; simply make them available, and leave it to the dog whether they are accepted or not. Starchy foods, on the other hand — such as bread, potatoes, and rice — pose the same problems for dogs that they do for humans. They are fattening and, since they are not necessary from the standpoint of nutrition, can be considered undesirable.

All-meat diets are too high in phosphorus and too low in calcium and, fed over a long period, will result in very serious bone diseases. They should not be relied on as the main source of your dog's diet.

The best assurance of a healthy pet is to provide it with variety, using any of the available foods at any one time but constantly changing around, guided by your dog's own taste. Following this general guideline, no rigid formula diet is necessary. Bones, while they are desirable for other reasons (see under Bad Habits, page 22), should not be considered a factor in nutrition.

Fresh water should always be available, and should be changed daily. This is especially important for older animals. If you have an older dog whose thirst and, perhaps, frequency of urination have noticeably increased over a few months, or a dog that drinks so much that it vomits afterward, do not deprive it of water — instead, give it ice cubes to lick. This could indicate a disease, too, and the animal should be checked by a veterinarian.

Bowls for food and water should not have sharp edges. Plastic and steel are best because they are easily cleaned. The bowl should have a heavy, flat base so that it cannot be turned over. The proper size will depend on how large the animal is.

GROOMING

BATHS. A dog should receive a bath only when absolutely needed *or* when treating a specific skin disorder requiring medicated shampoos.

Since the majority of commercial dog shampoos are too harsh for the dog's skin, it is better to use baby shampoo. The water should be lukewarm; keep shampoo out of your pet's eyes. Various ophthalmic ointments or a drop of mineral oil can be put in each eye for protection. As with most shampoos, the most important step is to thoroughly rinse all the shampoo from the body. This is particularly important in long-haired dogs. Once the shampoo dries on the skin, it can become extremely itchy and uncomfortable.

When the bath is complete, either towel-dry *or* blow-dry the dog's hair with a hand hair dryer. Keep it confined indoors for the next eight or ten hours to prevent its catching a cold.

BRUSHING. Brushing your dog daily or several times a week can be an enjoyable experience and can minimize the number of baths needed. Remove all large hair mats before brushing. Using a wire-bristle brush and a wide-toothed comb, smoothly brush out all the snarls and additional hair mats. Brush gently in both directions to remove the loose, thick, undercoat hairs that are responsible for shedding and mat formation. A final brushing with any commercial dog coat conditioner will add luster and make the coat glisten.

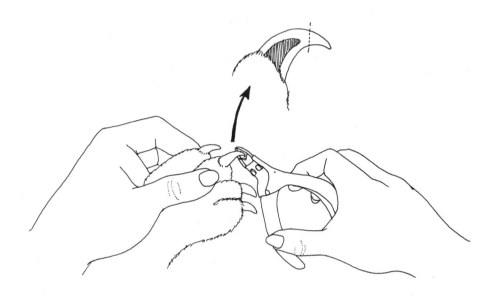

TOENAILS. Next, check the toenails. Using a Resco or White's nail trimmer, available in pet stores, cut just at the junction of the nail and its blood vessel. This can be seen easily in dogs with white, transparent nails. In dogs with black nails, cut the nail just beyond the point where it starts to curve downward. If unsure where to trim them, have your veterinarian demonstrate. The nails of house dogs should be checked; they will probably need trimming twice a year — unless the dog runs on rough pavement sufficiently.

EARS. Whenever you are grooming your dog, as a matter of routine inspect its ears and clean them gently with facial tissue and mineral oil. Avoid sticking Q-tips down deep into the ear. A good rule is to go down into the ear only as far as you can see.

At intervals, hair should be removed from the interior of the ear. Use the thumb and forefinger and pull out very small amounts of hair at a time. With schnauzers and poodles, this should be done four to six times a year, one to two times with floppy-eared breeds, and only once a year with dogs such as shepherds which have upright ears.

Signs of ear trouble to watch out for are pawing, redness, hot skin, and excessive dirt. Refer to the section Ears (page 51) for discussion of various ear conditions, and also Ear Mites (page 46) and their control.

PROTECTIVE INOCULATIONS

The nursing puppy, in the first eighteen to twenty-four hours of life, receives a large amount of protection against disease in the form of active antibodies in the colostrum of its mother's milk. This immunity is variable and short term, lasting anywhere from four to eight weeks.

Puppies are given a series of vaccinations starting around seven or eight weeks old, continuing every couple of weeks or so until the puppies are fourteen weeks old. Vaccination programs will vary from one veterinarian to another, but the same principles apply. After the initial series, there will be booster shots at intervals.

Most unfortunately, many pet owners, not understanding the technical questions in immunity, think their pets are immune when they are not. Owners who do not complete the series of shots — who stop after one shot, thinking it will protect their pets — are misinformed. They may lose their pets to unnecessary, preventable diseases; and endanger other pets and, in the case of rabies, humans.

The most common vaccinations are against distemper, hepatitis, leptospirosis, and rabies.

Distemper-hepatitis is a combined modified live virus vaccine to which leptospirosis bacterin is often added. The vaccine is given at two- or three-week intervals starting at around seven or eight weeks of age and continued until the puppy is thirteen or fourteen weeks old. Thereafter, it is a yearly booster. In areas endemic for leptospirosis, it is advised to receive the leptospira bacterin every six months. There are various forms of distemper or distemperlike vaccines available (measles virus, killed virus, and so on) that your veterinarian may use in establishing a sound program of protection for your pet.

Rabies vaccine is supplied either as killed virus or as modified live virus. Vaccinations are usually started at four to six months of age, and boosters are given at yearly intervals with the killed virus vaccine or else every two to three years with the modified live virus vaccine. If done properly, both types of vaccination series are totally effective; puppies under four months should not, however, receive the modified live virus.

DISTEMPER. Distemper is perhaps the most common viral infectious disease. The young, unvaccinated dog is most susceptible. The virus invades all the tissues of the body and may cause symptoms that include high fever, poor appetite, chronic nonresponsive diarrhea, weight loss, pneumonia, nasal and ocular discharge, muscle twitches, and convulsions. There is no absolute test to diagnose distemper. Diagnosis is made on the basis of no vaccination, a variety of symptoms, retinal changes, and conjunctival scrapings.

Not all distemper is fatal, but often it is. Treatment is combating the debilitating symptoms and preventing secondary bacterial infections. Prevention — provided the pet has the complete series of shots — is totally effective.

HEPATITIS. Infectious canine hepatitis (ICH) is a viral disease that can occur in dogs of all ages, but particularly in young dogs. It mainly affects the liver, intestinal tract, and eyes. Symptoms include very high fever, thirst, loss of appetite, bloody vomit and diarrhea, tense painful abdomen, and blue hazy cornea of the eye.

The treatment of ICH is prolonged supportive and intensive care. The disease usually ends in death. Prevention — hepatitis vaccine — is completely effective.

LEPTOSPIROSIS. Leptospirosis can affect both man and animal. The microorganisms are spread by infected animals in the urine. The disease is very rarely spread from a dog to a person, and it is not spread between people. Cattle are the most common source. Signs include fever, listlessness, depression, vomiting, and diarrhea. In more severe infections, kidney failure occurs.

Diagnosis is difficult and depends on finding rising leptospirosis antibody titers seven to ten days apart *or* finding the spirochaete organism in the urine during the acute phase under dark-field microscopy.

The favored treatment is penicillin and dihydrostreptomycin with supportive care. Prevention — by vaccine — is fully effective.

RABIES. Rabies is a viral disease that can infect people and animals. The virus is shed in the saliva during the active phase of the disease; if a rabid animal's mouth contacts an open wound — as through a bite wound, or licking cut skin — the disease can be spread. Depending on site of entry the incubation period varies between ten and forty days. Rabies is communicable only during the acute stage. Skunks and bats are perhaps the biggest reservoir of rabies infection. Rabies infection occurs in two distinct forms:

1. Dumb or paralytic, characterized by paralysis of muscles of the mouth and throat to the point the animal cannot drink water, becomes comatose, and dies within a few days.
2. Furious, a progressive deterioration of the central nervous system to the point where any noise or movement can provoke an attack.

Rabid animals die within ten days of the onset of the acute stage. Any suspected rabid dog should be quarantined under observation for a period of ten days. Any bite wound should be reported to local authorities.

There are shots available for people bitten by rabid animals; they are painful, and not totally effective, but are more effective the earlier they're begun.

optional operations
PREVENTION OF PREGNANCY

In pregnancy prevention both the male and female dog must be considered, especially if they live with one another.

The male dog can be altered by either a vasectomy (tying off the spermatic cord) or by castration (removing the testicles).

The female dog can be altered by complete ovariohysterectomy (removing both the ovaries and uterus), hysterectomy (removing the uterus but leaving the ovaries), which allows the dog to continue to cycle and still attract male dogs, or tubal ligation (tying off the junction between the ovaries and uterus), which prevents passage of the egg into the uterus, but still allows the bitch to cycle normally and attract male dogs. This may also predispose her to pyometras (see page 59), however. The complete ovariohysterectomy is still preferred.

Alternate methods include the use of the "pill," progesteronelike medication which is started at the first sign of heat. These products effectively bring the dog out of heat, but may increase the possibility of uterine infections.

An intravaginal device, like a diaphragm, recently on the market, which may be inserted by your veterinarian during the heat period, has shown some promise as an effective means of birth control.

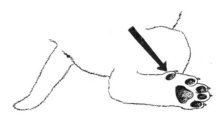

DEWCLAW REMOVAL

With the exception of certain show breeds, in which they are a factor in judging, dewclaws are strictly a liability and a source of injuries to the dog. Dewclaws get caught on furniture and fabrics, and the dewclaws are ripped. In certain states they are, in fact, required to be removed. In a puppy, the operation is harmless and painless and should definitely be considered desirable.

COSMETIC OPERATIONS While they have no practical value for the owner not interested in showing a dog, tail docking and ear cropping can give the pet a better appearance, a smartness it might otherwise lack. No suffering is caused if these operations are performed while the puppy is still young. Since the purpose is cosmetic rather than medical, a groomer might be better than a veterinarian to perform these operations.

DE-BARKING De-barking can be accomplished either temporarily or permanently. The former process is used primarily by people who are boarding animals, and recovery is swift and complete. Permanent de-barking, while not inhumane, should be considered in the light of the circumstances. There is simply no reason the average owner would find it desirable. But, for the apartment dweller with a nervous pet, it could become a necessity brought on by the threat of eviction with the only option being to have the dog destroyed.

the home clinic

It isn't necessary to go running to your veterinarian for help whenever a minor health problem crops up. Many of you are quite capable of handling yourself. You're in the best position to judge the state of your dog's health and to take action if something serious develops. All you need to know are a few basics.

Your first job is to know the different parts of your dog's body so that you can identify what is wrong and either treat it or report it accurately to your veterinarian. Try to become familiar with the diagrams on the following page and refer back to them as you read this chapter.

STOCKING A MEDICAL KIT When you need medical materials, you may need them fast. They should be kept where they are readily accessible in a container that will make it possible to take them quickly to an injured animal. Fish tackle boxes, toolboxes, or small cosmetic cases make excellent carriers. These contents are suggested as basic supplies:

rectal thermometer
bandage materials
 4 × 4 gauze pads
 3-inch cast padding
 3-inch kling gauze
 1-inch and 2-inch rolls of adhesive tape
12-inch wood splints (such as a ruler)
4- or 5-foot clothesline rope
bacitracin ointment
hydrogen peroxide (3 percent solution)
5 ml or 12 ml syringe (obtained from your local veterinarian)
bulb syringe or baster
mineral oil
bandage scissors
Betadine solution
Vaseline
hair clippers

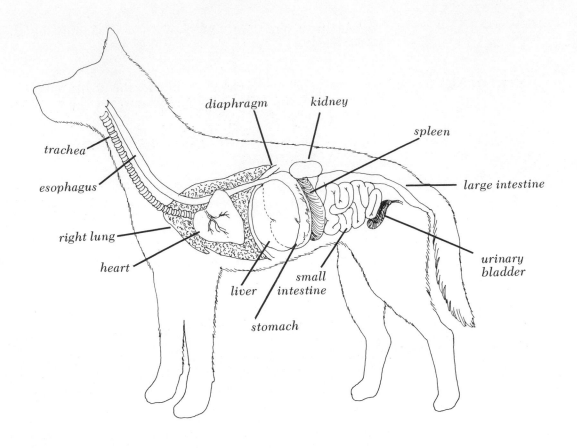

diaphragm   kidney

trachea

spleen

esophagus

large intestine

right lung

heart

urinary
bladder

liver   small
intestine

stomach

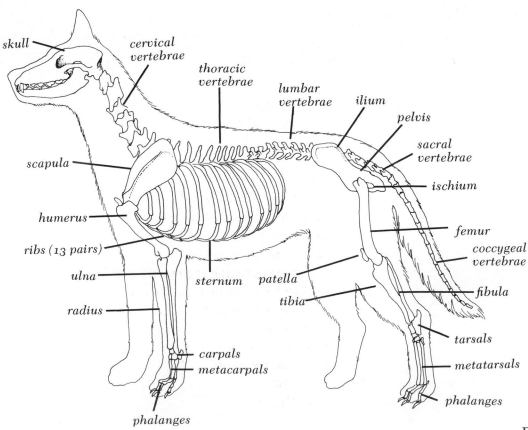

skull   cervical
vertebrae

thoracic
vertebrae

lumbar
vertebrae   ilium

pelvis

sacral
vertebrae

ischium

scapula

humerus

femur

ribs (13 pairs)

coccygeal
vertebrae

ulna

sternum   patella   fibula

radius   tibia

tarsals

carpals
metacarpals

metatarsals

phalanges

phalanges

HOW TO TAKE YOUR DOG'S TEMPERATURE

This is done most easily when the dog is standing, but the dog may also be sitting or lying down. Use a rectal thermometer and shake the mercury down below 95.0°F. Lubricate the bulb with Vaseline and, holding up the dog's tail with one hand, insert the thermometer until about half its length is in the rectum. After one to two minutes, remove the thermometer and read the temperature where the mercury stops. Normal temperatures for a dog range between 100.0° and 102.8°F.

IS YOUR DOG BREATHING PROPERLY

A dog's respiratory rate is one of the vital bodily signs, particularly, as we'll see, when you're checking for damage following a violent accident. So it is important that you be able to judge when things are not as they should be. A normal, healthy dog takes between twelve and twenty breaths a minute.

CHECKING YOUR DOG'S HEART

Certainly you're not equipped to detect subtle abnormalities such as a heart murmur, but you can read major signs of danger if you know how. Normally, a dog's heart will beat between 100 and 140 times a minute. The easiest means of checking this is to feel the beat through the chest wall on the left side, just behind the point of the elbow. In larger breeds, such as Saint Bernards and Newfoundlands, with massive chest walls, this may not be

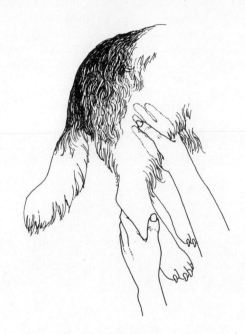

possible — the femoral pulse must be your guide. You can find this on the inside of the dog's hind leg, midway along the line where the thigh and pelvis are joined. You can feel the blood pulsing through the artery by placing your fingers over it and lightly pressing from the outside with your thumb. Normally, you will feel a strong, bounding pulse.

WHEN TO CALL YOUR VETERINARIAN

Any indication of a sudden, major change in your dog's health is a signal to get on the phone and seek professional advice. If you've learned your basics and use judgment, you needn't worry about being a bother to the veterinarian. (In an emergency, even though you have already decided to take the animal where it can get skilled help, this call will serve to alert the veterinarian.) As a rule, accept the fact that you will be making the trip, not the veterinarian — house calls are uncommon.

GIVING YOUR DOG MEDICATION

There are several relatively easy ways to administer the medicines your dog needs. One of these will suit your purposes:

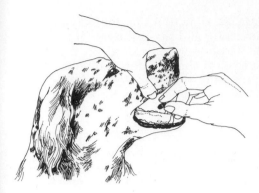

DIRECT PILLING. If you're right-handed, hold the dog's upper muzzle with your left hand, nose upward at about a 45-degree angle. Pry its lower jaw open with the third finger of your right hand, holding the pill between thumb and forefinger. As quickly as possible, place the pill as far back in the mouth as you can — on top of the tongue, not under it — remove your fingers and hold the mouth closed with one hand while you stroke the throat with the other to stimulate swallowing.

INDIRECT PILLING. As an alternative, if a dog gulps down its food, try hiding the pill in a piece of cheese or meat. You can also crush pills or open capsules to put the medicine in food, although sometimes they cause a bitter taste.

LIQUID MEDICATIONS. Most medicines currently available as pills and capsules also come in liquid form. Though these are usually a little more expensive, they can solve problems with giving your dog solid medicines. Holding the dog's mouth as you would to give it a pill (above), with a dropper squirt the medicine between the side molars or into the cheek pouch and the dog will swallow it reflexively. Give the medicine slowly so that the animal can catch its breath.

FORCE-FEEDING   Sometimes, in the case of a sick animal that refuses food, it is necessary to force-feed it. While in a veterinary hospital this might be done through a tube to the stomach, the owner must use another technique. Your veterinarian can provide you with a syringe for this purpose. Basically, you use the same principles as with administering pills or liquid medication in holding the dog. Using the syringe, you inject the food into the animal's throat. Beef or chicken baby food and soups may be used or a mixture of gruel with honey or Karo. To minimize the mess, make a bib out of a paper towel to put around the pet's neck. Even more than with liquid medicines, you need to take care that the dog has a chance to breathe during this process.

emergencies and first aid

A dog is an active animal. There is a good possibility that, as an owner, you will be faced with an emergency when your pet needs help before you can reach a veterinarian. If you prepare in advance by stocking a medical kit and learning the basics of what to do when danger arises, and if you remain cool in the face of crisis, you could be responsible for saving your animal's life.

HOW TO RESTRAIN YOUR DOG   Often, because of restlessness or pain, an animal will refuse to cooperate when you're treating an injury. It can easily be restrained by tying a loop of twine, rope, or cord around its muzzle and drawing the ends tight. Make a second loop beneath the muzzle and again cross or tie the ends and draw them tight. Then tie the loose ends behind the head to keep the loops from slipping off the nose.

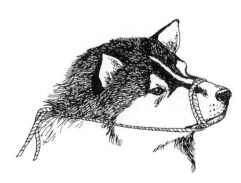

Restrain a dog's legs by approaching the dog from the side, grabbing the front and hind leg on the side away from you, and pulling the dog toward you so it is lying on its side. You are still holding the legs; this prevents the dog from gathering its legs under it and standing up. Carry a large dog from underneath, your arms around the top of all four legs. Hold a small dog with one hand under its chest; use the other hand to fold its legs underneath. If the dog is not cooperating, don't attempt to restrain the legs without muzzling the dog first.

While transporting an injured dog to the veterinarian, you want to keep it from injuring itself further, or causing itself greater pain, by struggling. If a limb has been injured, immobilize it with a makeshift splint (see page 38). Pick the animal up with the injured limb away from you, so that the limb

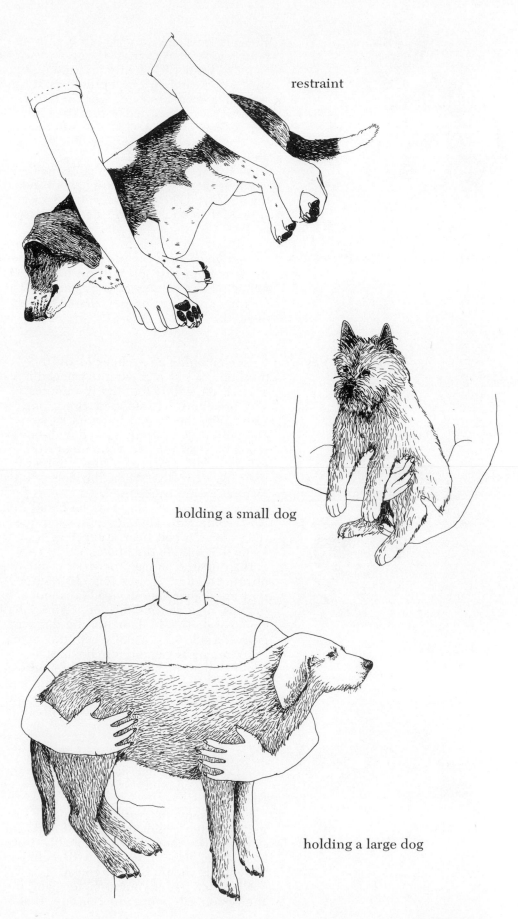

restraint

holding a small dog

holding a large dog

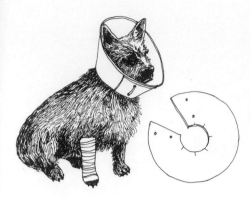

will not press against you. Lift it with one hand under the chest, cradling its hind legs with the other. If you are sure there are no internal injuries, you can also lift it very gently under the abdomen. This way you can support it and, if there are any chest problems, it can breathe easily.

If an animal has been very seriously injured, is in great pain, or has a broken back, use a makeshift stretcher such as an ironing board (see page 36). A blanket or towel is also an efficient stretcher and, because it confines the dog, prevents struggling. For this, you require two people, one to hold the corners at each end.

An Elizabethan or bucket collar made of cardboard is an effective means of keeping the dog from licking at wounds, biting its hindquarters, or scratching its face. This can be cut out of shirt boards or boxes. When you've slipped it around the dog's neck, tie, staple, or tape the ends together.

THE INITIAL EXAMINATION

Unless you actually witnessed the accident and know exactly what the injuries are, your first job will be to inspect your pet rapidly and thoroughly, following this step-by-step procedure. These priorities are vitally important, for they are based on degrees of danger, in terms of how quickly action is needed.

RESPIRATION

Before anything else, check to see that your animal is breathing normally. If the brain is not receiving oxygen, this can cause irreversible damage, and even death, within four to five minutes.

If breathing has stopped altogether, apply artificial respiration immediately. With the animal lying on its chest, cover its nostrils with your mouth and hold its jaws firmly closed with one hand. Blow steadily for two to three seconds, then remove your mouth for around three seconds to allow it to exhale before repeating. The volume of air should be enough to expand the rib cage normally. When the dog is breathing normally by itself, artificial respiration can be stopped.

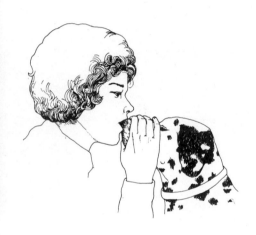

Even though the dog may be breathing, is respiration normal? Is it taking slow, shallow breaths or rapid, short ones as though it can't really expand its rib cage? Do you hear a gurgling sound when the dog inhales? This may mean free fluid in the lungs.

If an injured animal vomits or coughs up bubbly, frothy material, this may obstruct air flow. To prevent obstruction, raise the dog's hindquarters so that they are higher than its head (at about a 30-degree angle from the horizontal) to allow drainage and to keep it from inhaling the material into its lungs. You can also do this by hanging the dog's head over the edge of a table or the curb of a sidewalk, usually with the animal lying on its side.

If the dog is gagging or choking, move its tongue to one side and insert a small wedge, such as a roll of tape, between its jaws on one side. The wedge keeps the dog from biting its tongue and keeps the mouth open so air can move more freely. Take care not to put your fingers in its mouth, as an animal in pain will clamp down with all its strength.

HEART

Your second priority is to see whether your dog's heart is beating (see page 29). One possible and dangerous indicator would be blood spurting in pulses from a severed artery. If this *is* the case, go directly to the next step, External Bleeding.

Even though the heart has stopped, immediate external heart massage may get it started again, though if this doesn't succeed within twenty to thirty minutes the animal will probably never regain consciousness. The dog should be lying on its side, with its head toward you. If you're right-handed, its left side should be uppermost.

Place the flat of your stronger hand over the eighth rib, counting forward, the bottom rib being number one. It should be about two thirds down from the spine toward the center line of the chest. The flat of your other hand should be similarly placed under the dog's chest, beneath the ninth rib counting forward. Apply a pumping action downward with the topmost hand, using the other to stabilize the dog's body. The pace should be rapid, close to a pump every half-second, but use a steady pressure rather than beating or punching the chest.

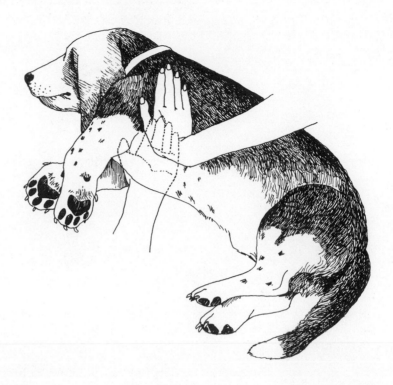

If you have someone to help you, artificial respiration (described above) should be given simultaneously, timed to the heart massage. After five massages, allow one breathing cycle (one breath in, one out), then resume the massage.

During the heart massage, the femoral pulse can be monitored to make sure the pressure is strong enough to eject a good flow of blood from the heart. After any accident severe enough to require heart massage, a veterinarian should be consulted.

EXTERNAL BLEEDING

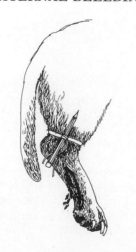

Your main concern here, from an emergency standpoint, is the possibility that major blood vessels may have been cut. If blood keeps soaking through the bandage as fast as you can apply it, a tourniquet will be necessary. Ropes, belts, stockings, or handkerchiefs can be used to make a loop around the limb. The tourniquet should be placed above the first joint of the limb, or at least four to five inches higher than the wound. Tighten the tourniquet by putting a stick, pencil, or a similar object through the loop and twisting it clockwise. Once the bleeding has been stopped, you will be able to get a dry bandage in place. If it is going to take time to reach a veterinarian, a tourniquet should be loosened, but not removed, for about a minute at intervals of ten to fifteen minutes.

If it is minor, a cut on a dog's limb can be easily controlled by a pressure bandage placed directly over the wound. Three or four gauze pads, facial tissues, or napkins should do the job. These are then wrapped gently but firmly with a meshed gauze or Ace bandage, or makeshifts such as a nylon stocking or strips of old linen sheets. The wrapping should not be tight enough to stop circulation.

The bandage should be wound from the top of the leg down to the toes. With serious wounds, don't waste time trying to clean them. All you want to do is to stop the bleeding until you can get the dog to a veterinarian.

When speed is not of the essence, the proper procedure for bandaging wounds is to first cleanse them with either hydrogen peroxide or Massengill's douching powder mixed with warm water, or Betadine solution, flushing to remove all pus and debris. Then apply an antibiotic ointment, such as bacitracin, and protect the wound with a clean gauze dressing.

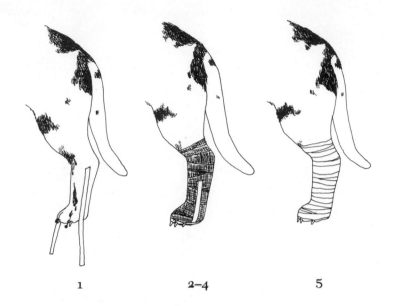

1   2–4   5

To apply a full bandage to a limb, follow these steps:

1. To prevent slippage, place two strips of 1-inch adhesive tape on the sides of the leg to act as stirrups.
2. Starting at the bottom of the leg, gently wrap thick, soft bandage until it is well above the wound, preferably as high as the next joint.
3. Cover this with gauze bandage. Wrapping the leg from the toe up will help prevent the toes swelling due to poor circulation, but the toes should be left exposed to be checked should any swelling develop and for signs of moisture accumulation.
4. Attach the two tape stirrups to the side of the bandage.
5. Wrap the final bandage with 2-inch adhesive tape to protect against soiling and to give added strength.

Wounds on the head, chest, or body are often difficult to bandage. The only solution may be to hold a pressure bandage in place with your hand.

INTERNAL BLEEDING Internal bleeding is a common result of car accidents or falls from high windows. You can detect it by examining the mucous membranes on the inside of the dog's upper lip: they will have a cold pale color rather than the normal warm pink. Also check the pulse to see if it feels weaker than usual, flowing threadily rather than with firm bounds. Breathing will usually be more rapid than normal.

The spleen, kidneys, and liver are the most common sources of internal bleeding following accidents. The most obvious sign of this will be a fuller abdomen than usual. Apply pressure with a body bandage wrapped snugly around the belly. Strips of sheets, gauze, or Ace bandages can be used.

If you suspect internal bleeding, the animal should be jostled no more than is absolutely necessary to get it to a veterinarian. The best means will be to move it carefully on a firm support, such as a stretcher of plywood.

SHOCK

Shock itself, while it might be the result of other injuries, requires treatment. The symptoms are weakness, physical collapse, subnormal rectal temperature, the pale cold appearance of the inside of the lips, listlessness, depression, fast but weak pulse, rapid, shallow breathing. There can be many causes, ranging from severe injury to electrocution.

If your animal shows symptoms of shock, wrap it in a blanket to keep it quiet and warm until a veterinarian can give it the care it must have for this condition.

The checklist above will assure you that you have done all you can, by yourself, to handle threats to your dog that require instant action to save its life. There are other situations, though, in which you can help your pet until it can receive the professional attention that is needed. Here are the things to watch for and what you can do.

THE UNCONSCIOUS DOG

Unconsciousness can be the result of a number of causes, from a blow to the head that causes concussion to a metabolic disturbance, such as hypoglycemia (decreased blood sugar), which often occurs when young puppies are unable to match their high energy demands with sufficient food to supply the necessary calories. The unconsciousness, a state of coma, may not be complete but will show up in a diminished response to a test such as a pinch on a toe.

Hypoglycemia occurs in puppies two to eight months old — it is an acute condition that can be prevented at an early stage if the puppy's owner is alert to the possibility. Signs of mental slowness or difficulties in walking (staggering) are danger signals and the puppy should be given a teaspoon or two of maple syrup, sugar water, or honey every two hours until the condition is corrected.

Unconsciousness (total or partial) should always be brought to the attention of a veterinarian, for there are metabolic diseases other than hypoglycemia that require a veterinarian's care. Among them are diabetes mellitus (high blood sugar), kidney diseases, severe uncontrollable vomiting, or congestive heart failure. (Do not worry about the sugar you gave your puppy for its temporary attack of hypoglycemia — diabetes does not occur in puppies.)

If your pet is in an unconscious condition, it should be kept as still as possible and, if it is going to take some time to get to a veterinarian, it should be turned over every twenty to thirty minutes to prevent congestion of the lungs on the lower side. Watch carefully for vomiting because the swallowing reflex may not be functioning and take the steps given above (under Respiration, in the section on the Initial Examination) to keep it breathing properly. Also, note the rate and depth of respiration in order to properly inform the veterinarian of the animal's condition.

SUDDEN PARALYSIS

This is usually a case in which a dog, with no apparent head injury and completely responsive to its owner, loses partial or complete control over one or more of its limbs. This is most often due to acute injuries affecting the spinal cord and peripheral nerves of the body and limbs. Spinal cord injuries as the result of a protrusion or rupture of an intervertebral disk are most common with dachshunds and poodles.

The intervertebral disks act as shock absorbers between the vertebrae of the spinal column. If one should rupture, this may place a direct pressure on the spinal cord that results in paralysis of the limbs to the rear of that point.

While they may be caused by an accident, ruptured disks are more usually the result of strenuous activity that places too much stress on a weakened disk. Spinal cord injuries may also be due to tumors. Unless they are the result of congenital abnormalities or severe accidents to the spine, the causes of paralysis sometimes can be corrected surgically.

If your dog suddenly becomes paralyzed, take the following steps:

1. Place it on a firm support, such as an ironing board or plywood.
2. Move it as little as possible to prevent further damage.
3. Get it to a veterinarian as soon as possible. While this is not a minute-by-minute crisis, time reduces the chances of reversing the condition.

Other causes of paralysis not due to violent injury are:

TICK PARALYSIS. While the poison of one variety of wood ticks can cause acute paralysis, this is fairly uncommon and the symptoms will usually disappear once the insect is removed.

FAMILIAL NECROTIZING MYELOPATHY. This is a progressive degeneration of the spinal cord apparently inherited in certain lines of Afghan hounds. It often results in respiratory problems and inevitably results in death.

GERMAN SHEPHERD MYELOPATHY. A slow degeneration of the lower spinal cord characterized by rear leg weakness and unsteadiness that usually leads to complete hind limb paralysis.

MYASTHENIA GRAVIS. A neuromuscular disorder, which results in acute but short-term paralysis following vigorous exercise. The dog's esophagus may swell and aspiration pneumonia is common, but the condition is sometimes controlled with the right medicine.

CONVULSIONS   The brain is surrounded by a certain level of electrical activity. Any interference can cause a "short circuit" with a discharge of impulses across the brain and throughout the central nervous system, resulting in a convulsion. There are many causes for seizures, among them distemper, viral encephalitis, lead poisoning, a scar defect resulting from past injury, and severe metabolic problems such as kidney failure and hypoglycemia. Epilepsy, probably the most common, usually occurs in dogs between three and five years old.

Regardless of the cause, a convulsive seizure will usually have three phases:

1. Preseizure — characterized by a dazed expression, sleepiness, unusual demands for the owner's attention, hiding, and confusion.
2. Seizure — symptoms vary according to the site of the discharges from the brain. The animal may have only chomping mouth fits, or may have a full-blown grand-mal seizure, falling on its side and thrashing its legs about wildly, losing control of its bowels and urine, frothing at the mouth, and yelping. This may seem to go on for hours, but in reality usually ends in less than three minutes, often only seconds.
3. Postseizure — this varies from dog to dog, but common signs are hiding, confusion, increased appetite, and sleepiness.

If your dog has a fit, you should immediately call the veterinarian and, while waiting, try to make your pet as comfortable as possible, keeping it out of harm, until the seizure subsides. Talking to the dog and stroking it gently will often have a soothing effect.

Do not try to prevent the dog's swallowing its tongue by putting your finger in its mouth. This is not a problem, as it is with humans.

Take some mental notes that will help the veterinarian in determining the cause of the seizure. How many seizures were there and how long did they last? On which side did the dog fall? Were there any preseizure signs? Has the dog forgotten any learned tricks, such as retrieving a ball, or has it been less responsive to commands lately? Has it shown any aggression to you, your family, or others recently?

If seizures continue to recur with increasing frequency, this "status epilepticus" can be fatal. The veterinarian uses a number of anticonvulsants — such as Valium, phenobarbital, and others — to control these seizures. While these don't remove the cause, they reduce the chance of an attack. But even the best-medicated epileptic will have one or two seizures a year.

BURNS There are three basic types of burns, caused by hot liquids (such as boiling water or coffee), chemicals (lye and sulfuric acid, for example), and direct fire or heat (perhaps from getting trapped under a car's muffler).

How serious these are will depend on the depth, location, and surface area covered. Most burns are minor and require little treatment. The hair in the burned area should be clipped clean, for lingering infections are common under matted coats. Wash the areas of chemical burns generously with water to dilute the irritant. Other burns should be rinsed superficially with cold water once the hair is removed. Then apply a protective ointment — without rubbing the burn — such as Vaseline, or one of the many products made especially for burns; keep the dog away from it by covering the burn with gauze bandage (cotton will stick and impede healing), or by using an Elizabethan cardboard collar (see page 32). This, and the bandage, can be removed when the dog is no longer bothered by the burn.

If the burns are extensive, covering more than one third of the body surface, it is essential to take the dog to a veterinarian for immediate treatment.

HEAT STROKE One of the most common problems, particularly in spring when the weather is changing, is heat stroke. Owners leave their dogs in the car while they shop, forgetting to roll down the windows, and apartments without air conditioning suddenly turn into infernos while the animal is home alone.

The dog's only real source of cooling (it has sweat glands only on its nose and the pads of its feet) is by respiration. With this handicap and a heavy hair coat, body temperatures can soar to as high as 110°F. The signs of heat stroke are rapid respiration and total collapse to coma, and often include vomiting blood and bloody stools. In such cases, take the following emergency measures:

1. Douse the dog in a tub of cold water or, if it is too large, spray it with a hose. In an emergency, rubbing alcohol can be used to lower the dog's body temperature, but only with care, for if the temperature drops below normal this can throw the animal into shock.
2. Apply an ice bag to the dog's head to prevent brain damage.
3. Cool the animal internally with cold water enemas or by placing ice cubes directly into the rectum.
4. Get to a veterinarian as rapidly as possible for fluid support and shock therapy.

FROSTBITE Frostbite in dogs invariably affects the ears. Until the pet can be taken to the veterinarian to receive antibiotics, the essential step is to lubricate the ears with Vaseline or any other soothing ointment in order to protect them from infection, drying out, sloughing. Do not apply heat.

FRACTURES If you believe your dog may have broken a bone, it should be taken to a veterinarian for an X-ray. Nevertheless, there are steps you can take to prevent further damage.

Once you suspect a bone in a limb has been broken, you should do your best to immobilize it. Until you can get veterinary assistance apply a splint — a wooden stick, yardstick, newspaper, or cardboard. It should be long enough to hold the entire limb still. Keeping the leg as straight as possible, secure it from above to below the point of the break with bandages. Using the same sequence as with the bandage (see page 34), add the splint between steps (2) and (3).

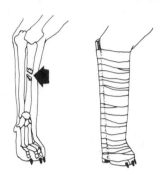

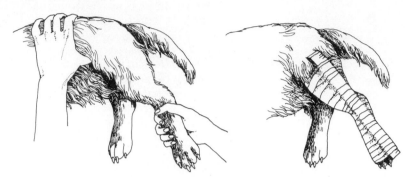

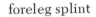

foreleg splint

hind leg splint

A fracture of the ribs, skull, spinal column, or pelvis is difficult to immobilize. In these cases, restraint is the best you can manage. The danger is a puncture of the lungs by a rib or a urethra lacerated by sharp pelvic bones. Use a temporary stretcher to take your dog to the veterinarian. In mature dogs, most fractures will mend in four to six weeks. The time is much less in young puppies.

DISLOCATIONS

The most common dislocation in dogs occurs in the hip joint. The ball, or head of the femur, in this "ball-and-socket" joint fits snugly into a depressed indentation of the pelvis called the acetabulum, which serves as a socket. Violent activity, whether in an accident or roughhousing, can pop this ball out of the socket.

Often the only way you can tell this has happened is when the dog starts to limp, trying not to put weight on the limb. Usually the toes will touch the floor; only rarely will the dog carry the leg off the ground. It should be taken to a veterinarian right away.

After X-rays eliminate the possibility of a fracture, the veterinarian may anesthetize the dog and try to relocate the joint manually. After more than twelve hours, muscle contraction makes this difficult and sometimes impossible.

Minor dislocations are quite common in poodles and Yorkies, and in these small animals are easily corrected. Shoulder, wrist, and hock dislocations are less common and can be detected by swelling and sensitivity.

BITE WOUNDS

How bad these are will depend on the sizes of the dogs involved, location of the wounds, and whether they are punctures or rips. Most are small and need nothing more than cleansing with a mild iodine or Betadine solution and application of a mild broad-spectrum antibiotic ointment such as bacitracin. Hot compresses placed on the wound for twenty minutes to half an hour, two or three times a day, will speed healing and lower possibilities of infection. The open wounds allow adequate drainage and promote healing from the inside out.

Small puncture wounds over which the skin has sealed can develop into painful abscesses because of the lack of drainage and the introduction of bacteria that infect underlying tissues. Extensive wounds may require suturing, drains, and antibiotics, which should be administered by a veterinarian.

SNAKEBITES   Nonpoisonous snakebites require little or no attention. The dog will show no more serious symptoms than mild localized swellings, a few hours of listlessness, lack of appetite, and lameness.

The pit vipers, such as rattlesnakes, water moccasins, copperheads, and coral snakes, which are found in some parts of the country, are another story. A commercial snake kit and sharp knife or straight-edged razor blade should always be available when traveling through areas where there are venomous snakes. Wounds inflicted by these snakes cause rapid, hot swellings, extremely tender and painful. If a bite is suspected, use the following procedure:

1. Apply a tourniquet (see page 33) between the wound and the heart if the wound is on a limb; this will slow the spread of the venom. Loosen the tourniquet every ten minutes for short intervals. Most bites are around the face; a tourniquet, obviously, can't be used then.
2. Apply an ice pack or cold water pack over the wound to minimize local tissue reaction, if possible. In addition to the swellings mentioned, there will be discoloration and tissue death. The toxin may also produce serious shock.
3. Phone a veterinarian immediately for advice.

As a last resort, if it is impossible to reach a veterinarian, use a sharp knife or razor blade to make a linear cut over each fang mark deep enough to cause free bleeding. If the puncture sites are not clearly visible, assume the wound is at the point of maximum swelling. Use a suction device, if you have one, to draw out the venom with the blood. Otherwise, do not use your mouth, but try to milk the venom out by pressing your hand down firmly on the leg below the tourniquet, stroking toward the wound.

INSECT BITES   Most often on the face, these can cause an acute generalized swelling of the muzzle, or a localized swelling at the site of the bite, which will usually subside completely within eight to twenty-four hours regardless of therapy. The best treatment is cold packs and ice placed over the wound for one hour. This is also true for bites and stings from black widow spiders, scorpions, and bees, which can be fatal. Deaths are usually due to acute allergic reactions. If a dog shows signs of weakness, difficulty in breathing, and pale mucous membranes in the mouth, a veterinarian should be called immediately.

POISONING   Consuming toxic plants or chemical intoxicants, or even physical contact with the latter, are the two major sources of poisoning in dogs. The effects vary widely, depending on the nature of the poison, the amount consumed, and the individual animal.

CHEMICAL POISONING. Almost every chemical has a toxic level in any living organism. The most common symptoms of poisoning include vomiting, diarrhea, drooling, shock, coma, convulsions, whining, and restlessness.

The basic approach to any poisoning should be the following:

1. Prevent further absorption of the poison.
2. Treat the poison specifically to aid its removal from the body.
3. Counteract the effects on the body with supportive care.

Many cities have poison control centers that can be called for specific information on potentially hazardous household products and their antidotes. Your Department of Health can give you their telephone numbers.

The specific steps to take when your dog has come in contact with or swallows poison are as follows:

COMMON CHEMICAL POISONINGS IN DOGS

POISON	SOURCE	TREATMENT
Amphetamines	Diet pills	Chlorpromazine
Arsenic	Herbicides	Dimercaprol (BAL)
Barbiturates	Sleeping pills, sedatives	CNS stimulant: Doxapram and Bemegride
Ethylene glycol	Antifreeze	Ethyl alcohol
Lead	Lead-based paints, linoleum, bird shot	Calcium EDTA
Organophosphates	Flea, ant, roach, and tick sprays	Pyridine-2-aldoxime (2-PAM) and atropine
Metaldehyde	Snail bait	Pentobarbital
Strychnine	Rodenticide	Pentobarbital
Thallium	Rodenticide	Prussian blue
Warfarin (D-Con)	Rodenticide	Whole blood transfusions, vitamin K

A FEW OF THE COMMON PLANTS POTENTIALLY POISONOUS FOR DOGS

COMMON NAME	SCIENTIFIC NAME	DANGEROUS PART OF THE PLANT	SIGNS OF POISONING
Dumbcane	Dieffenbachia sequine	Stems	Salivation, laryngitis
Philodendron	Philodendron spp.	Stems, leaves	Salivation
English ivy	Hedera helix	Leaves, berries	Vomiting, diarrhea
Privet	Ligustrum vulgare	Leaves, berries	Vomiting, diarrhea
Tobacco	Nicotiana spp.	Leaves	CNS stimulation
Oleander	Nerium oleander	All parts	Heart irregularities
Foxglove	Digitalis purpurea	Leaves	Heart irregularities
Lily of the valley	Convallaria majalis	Leaves, flowers	Heart irregularities
Poinsettia	Euphorbia spp.	Leaves	Heart irregularities
Rhododendron	Rhododendron spp.	Leaves	Vomiting, diarrhea
Castor bean	Ricinus communis	Leaves, beans	Diarrhea, shock
Daffodil	Narcissus spp.	Bulbs	Vomiting, diarrhea
Golden chain	Laburnum vulgare	Leaves, seeds	CNS stimulation
Larkspur	Delphinium spp.	Leaves, seeds	Paralysis, CNS depression
Autumn crocus	Colchicum autumnale	Leaves	Vomiting, CNS stimulation
Daphne	Daphne spp.	Bark, leaves, fruit	Vomiting, CNS stimulation

Adapted from "Toxicities in Exotic and Zoo Animals" by M. E. Fowler in *Veterinary Clinics of North America*, vol. 5, no. 4 (November 1975), Philadelphia, W. B. Saunders, pp. 690–691.

Induce vomiting. 1 to 2 teaspoons (5 to 10 ml) of hydrogen peroxide should work within three to ten minutes. Another less reliable method is to place a teaspoon of salt in the back of the dog's mouth. CAUTION: *Do not* induce vomiting in the case of corrosive poisons such as kerosene, strong acids, or lye.

Protect the intestinal tract. When the dog has vomited, protect the stomach and intestines with 1 teaspoon (5 ml) per 5 pounds of body weight of Pepto-Bismol, aluminum hydroxide, Methigel, Maalox, or Magwol. Kaopectate should be avoided because it slows the intestinal tract.

Skin that is inflamed or irritated because of corrosive materials such as kerosene, gasoline, excessive use of mange dips, flea or tick baths should be rinsed with large amounts of water to dilute the irritant. Afterward, you may lather the animal gently with a mild detergent such as Ivory soap and rinse. Do not scrub.

If the dog shows hyperirritability and convulsions, quiet the dog and keep it from further injuring itself until a veterinarian can be reached.

Call your veterinarian about any poisoning. Get advice by phone and, if the veterinarian thinks it necessary, preparations can be made for receiving a poisoned animal. Take a sample with you, if you go, of the poison or the dog's vomit. The best thing is the container with its label.

PLANT POISONING. The list of potentially poisonous plants is extremely long. Most are only in part toxic and symptoms will depend on how the poison works as well as the amount consumed. The commonest are copious salivations, vomiting, and diarrhea. Those affecting the central nervous system may cause hyperexcitability, convulsions, paralysis, shock, and in some cases death. If you have pets that chew on house plants, it would be wise to find out which are potentially dangerous. In cases of plant poisoning, all you can do is induce vomiting (see above) and rush the dog to your veterinarian.

SMOKE INHALATION

This usually results from an animal being trapped in the vicinity of a fire. In severe cases, follow the procedures listed for artificial respiration (page 32) and external heart massage (page 32). Then take your pet to a veterinarian.

Smoke inhalation can damage the epithelial lining of the respiratory system and cause severe bronchitis or pneumonia. Even though the animal responds well to initial treatment, it may later suffer serious effects as a result of permanent damage to its lungs.

ELECTRICAL SHOCK

Teething puppies are frequently injured by chewing through electrical cords. Burns at the corners of the mouth are the obvious damage, but a puppy that has suffered electrical shock can also develop an abnormally rapid heart rate (atrial tachycardia) and there may be a very heavy buildup of fluid in the lungs (pulmonary edema), so it should be examined by a veterinarian. Both these conditions, if untreated, can be fatal. Once these possibilities have been dealt with, the pup may need to go on a diet of liquids and soft foods because of its painful mouth. Ointments should be applied to the burns.

EYE INJURIES

Eye injuries are common in dogs. Foreign material, such as a splinter, may become lodged in the eye's surface. Interior damage as the result of a blow or puncture can result in a loss of the fluid of the cornea or the appearance of blood within the eye. The eye might even be torn entirely out of its socket. The first objective must be to get the dog to a veterinarian as soon as possible. Every moment is important. To minimize damage:

1. Place a wet paper towel or rag over the eye for protection and to keep it moist.
2. Comfort the animal to relieve its fear.
3. Get to the veterinarian immediately.

NOSEBLEEDS

Nosebleeds can be the result of injuries, but they may also be symptomatic of other problems, such as a nasal infection that has eroded the blood vessels, blood disorders, a foreign object in the nasal passages, or tumors. A dog with a nosebleed should therefore be taken to a veterinarian immediately, once the following steps have been taken:

1. Keep the dog as quiet as possible.
2. Apply an ice pack to the nose to reduce the bleeding.

Your veterinarian will administer hypotensive agents to lower the dog's blood pressure and nasal packing soaked in epinephrine to constrict the blood vessels in the nose. These will usually bring the bleeding under control so that the problem can be diagnosed and any necessary further treatment prescribed.

FOREIGN BODIES

A variety of accidents can result in foreign bodies becoming embedded in one part or another of the dog's anatomy. In most cases, so long as these are on the surface, no serious injury will result. An object under the skin will work its way to the surface, causing an ulceration as the body rejects it. Inasmuch as ulcerations can be indicative of other problems, these should be brought to the attention of a veterinarian. If there is nothing more serious, the ulceration will be treated for itself.

Objects embedded in the outer ear will follow the pattern above. If something reaches the inner ear, though, this is far too delicate an area for home treatment and should be treated as a medical emergency.

Symptoms indicating a dog may have swallowed a foreign object are vomiting right after eating, abdominal discomfort, restlessness, fever, and lack of appetite. The dog with any of these symptoms should be seen by a veterinarian.

The primary threat to the mouth and throat is bones. Even a needle, if it passes *down* the throat, is not necessarily cause for alarm. It can go through the dog's digestive tract without causing harm. But bones and even sometimes balls may become lodged in the throat. This constitutes a full-scale emergency and the animal must be rushed to the veterinarian immediately. Any attempts at first aid may well result in even further damage. Speed is the only answer.

INABILITY TO URINATE

Inability to urinate is a medical emergency and the dog should be taken to the veterinarian immediately. This is rarely a problem with females but is not uncommon in males and is usually the result of objects that have become lodged behind the os penis, the bone in the male organ. Dalmatians are particularly suceptible to this as a result of uric acid stones.

The symptoms of urinary obstruction are an increased urgency to urinate, straining while doing so, and short, repeated squirts rather than a steady stream. The owners of males should be alert to these signs.

parasites

Parasites are animals that live on or in another at its expense, steal nutrients, hold down weight gain, and may cause chronic diarrhea, blood in the stool, anemia, skin diseases, and heart disease as well as spreading bacterial, viral, or protozoan diseases. Most have life cycles that carry them through a series of hosts. The object of treatment is not only to destroy the adult parasite but, whenever possible, to break the life cycle.

The parasites of domestic animals fall into two clear-cut groups, internal (endoparasites) and external (ectoparasites). Those most frequently found in or on dogs are:

TAPEWORMS

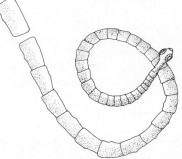

Tapeworms are fairly common but rarely cause any significant problem. Infections can occur when the dog eats uncooked meat, raw freshwater fish, or swallows fleas or lice, all of which may be intermediary hosts. Diagnosis is sometimes made by examining feces microscopically for eggs, but is more frequently the result of finding wriggling segments of the mature worm on top of stools — they look like cut pieces of white ribbon. These can be squashed, releasing packets of eggs for microscopic identification. After an overnight fast, the dog should be given an appropriate medication. Medication for worming is available in pet stores, but it is general — it does not distinguish the different kinds of worms — so a veterinarian's prescription is much better. Animals can be protected from infection by controlling fleas and lice, and cooking all meat and fish products fed them.

ASCARIDS

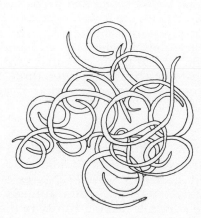

Ascarids are probably the most common internal parasites found in young puppies. A pregnant dog can be treated for ascarids; if infected, she should be. Piperazine is the generic name of the medicine. It is not toxic to the fetus — and infections can be transmitted prenatally, by way of the placenta, or postnatally in the mother's milk during the first twenty-four hours after birth. During its first month, the pup may also pick up the parasite by eating infected eggs. Lodged in the small intestine, the adult worms compete with the puppy for nutrition, releasing eggs that pass in the feces. In one to four weeks, these contain larval worms that, if the eggs are eaten, can infect a new host such as a rat. The rat too, if eaten, serves as a means of spreading the infection further.

When the larvae are released from the eggs, they spend from two to four weeks traveling through the host body tissues — the lungs and intestinal linings — until, at eight weeks, they reach maturity.

As a result of this migration through the lung tissues, puppies occasionally contract ascarid pneumonia. Emergencies sometimes arise when the worms have become so numerous that they form obstructions in the dog's system. While these are rare events, severely infected puppies nonetheless develop potbellies and chronic diarrhea, and appear dull.

Diagnosis can result either from spotting the long, spaghettilike worm in the puppy's stool or vomit, or by identifying the eggs under a microscope. Three or four treatments with prescribed medication, administered every two to three weeks, will destroy the adult worms, but the larvae are unaffected and must be treated later, when they have developed into adults.

Rarely, children will contract visceral larval migrans by putting their hands in their mouths after having played in the area of dog excrement. The ascarid larvae responsible, toxocara, do not come from dogs directly, however, but from the contaminated soil. Without displaying any symptoms directly connected with the worms themselves, infected children may develop pneumonia, liver disease, and even blindness in severe cases. Pets and sandboxes obviously do not go together.

HOOKWORMS

Hookworm infections in young puppies are quite similar to those due to ascarids. The adult worm, in the small bowel, passes its eggs out in the stool. From one to four weeks later, the larvae can gain entry to the host either when the eggs are eaten or by penetrating the skin. Prenatal and postnatal infections occur in the same manner as with the ascarids. Hookworm can be detected in the pregnant mother, but she should not be treated until after the puppies are born, since the treatment would be toxic to the fetus. Prenatal infection can result in blood loss anemias before birth, yet diagnosis through examining the stool is impossible until the dog is approximately eleven days old. The larvae migrate through the lungs before reaching maturity in the small bowel, occasionally causing pneumonia. In addition to competing for nutrition, hookworms feed directly on the dog's blood, invading the lining of the small bowel. The irritation and damage may result in a severe anemia, blackish diarrhea due to blood loss, and occasionally shock.

Hookworms are rarely passed in the stools, and most diagnoses are the result of microscopic examination of the eggs. Even without this evidence, progressive weakness in a puppy, pallor, and the characteristic diarrhea should cause suspicion, and treatment should be started immediately. Various products your veterinarian can prescribe are effective against the adult hookworm. In cases of severe anemia, blood transfusions, vitamins and other blood-building agents may be used.

WHIPWORMS
Whipworms (*Trichuris vulpis*), living in the cecum (appendix) and lower bowel, may cause chronic diarrhea containing red blood. The diagnosis can be confirmed by examining the eggs in the stool. Daily administration of prescribed medication for five days will destroy the adult whipworms, but it must be repeated after three months, when the new generation of larvae have reached adulthood.

PROTOZOANS
Protozoans most commonly found in dogs, *Giardi canis* and coccidia, infect the small bowel. These one-celled organisms cause a watery, mucoid diarrhea, which is plentiful. Identification and treatment must be by a veterinarian. Microscopic identification is necessary; then Kaopectate and bland diets may help in controlling the diarrhea. Giardia can be treated orally with prescribed medicines twice a day for three days, repeated after three more; antibiotics are used to treat coccidia, administered over a period of twenty-one days.

HEARTWORMS
Heartworm (*Dirofilaria imitis*) infection, once thought to be confined to the South, has now been identified in virtually every state. Immature microfilaria are taken with the blood of infected dogs by various species of mosquito. The mosquito then acts as a carrier, infecting other animals. After migrating within the body, the immature parasites reach maturity in the right side of the heart. Adult worms may range from 8 to 12 inches and a heavy infection can significantly slow circulations through the major blood vessels of the heart and lungs.

Symptoms include coughing, shortness of breath, loss of appetite and weight, and collapse. Diagnosis relies on microscopic identification of the immature parasites in a blood sample. When the disease has been identified, it is treated in the following manner:

(1) Adult heartworms are killed by four daily injections of medication for two successive days while the patient is hospitalized. The dog is then released but must rest and be confined, to prevent running, for six weeks. During this period the adult worms die and are trapped by the lungs, where they decompose.

(2) Immature microfilaria are killed when, at the end of the six-week confinement, the dog is started on oral medication. The circulating microfilaria cannot mature unless they develop within a mosquito, but they remain a source of infection. After five to seven days of treatment, the dog's blood is checked for microfilaria. If they are still present, medication is resumed at a higher dosage.

(3) Reinfection is prevented, once the blood is found free of microfilaria, by giving the dog either liquid medication or pills daily. This will destroy

any larvae transmitted by mosquitos. If you live in an area where heartworms are endemic, your dog should be checked for microfilaria every six months and placed on preventive medication throughout the year. If there are definite seasonal changes, checks should be made at the end of the winter or in the early spring. The animal should receive appropriate medication from spring to early fall.

FLEAS

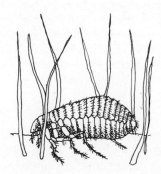

Fleas not only cause dermatitis with their bites, but carry elaborate allergenic toxins in their saliva that increase the reaction to subsequent bites. In severely infected puppies, fleas can cause blood-loss anemia. They also transmit other parasites, such as tapeworms.

The flea remains on the host animal only long enough to feed and mate, spending the rest of its life cycle — from one to six months, though they may live as long as a year — in household rugs and furniture, where its eggs are laid. Fleas are diagnosed by finding either the parasites themselves on your pet, or the black peppery specks called flea dirt lodged among its hairs. Treatment is designed to, first, rid the dog of fleas and, second, prevent reinfestation.

Various products are available to kill the adult fleas, including collars and medallions containing organophosphates; sprays such as Flyte, Norsect spray, and Para-S-Spray; powders; and shampoos. When using these products, watch carefully to see if the animal is sensitive to them, developing skin irritations. Frequent vacuuming, sprays, and professional exterminators can be used as means of ridding the home of fleas.

TICKS

Ticks infesting dogs are usually of two types. The wood tick requires an intermediary host in its life cycle, while the brown tick can spend its entire life on the dog. Ticks spread diseases such as babesiasis, a parasite-caused blood disorder; Rocky Mountain spotted fever; and tick paralysis.

Hardy parasites, ticks are capable of going months without a meal. The female can lay as many as 4,000 to 6,000 eggs at a time. As larvae, these feed on smaller animals, then drop off. After the nymph stage has developed in the soil, it finds a new host. It feeds for from five to seven days, drops off, and matures, finding yet another host.

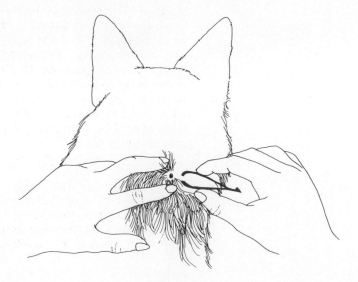

Diagnosis is simply a matter of finding a tick on the dog, usually in the area around the head, neck, and ears. It should be removed by gently pulling it away from the animal. If the head breaks off and remains embedded in the animal, try to remove it with tweezers. If this fails, place hot compresses on the site two or three times daily for a few days. A slight abscess will develop and the body will reject the foreign object. Do not use any caustic substances, such as kerosene or lighter fluid, or use burning matches — these can irritate the dog's skin. To prevent your dog's getting ticks, use one of the various tick shampoos during the summer months, as directed. If your house has become infested, an exterminator may be essential.

EAR MITES   Ear mites, a common parasite in young dogs, inflame and irritate the tissues of the ear canal. They feed upon the secretions caused by their own irritations. Dogs infected with ear mites will shake their heads and scratch at their ears frequently. Examination of the ears will usually reveal a black, waxy discharge. The tiny white mites can be extracted with a Q-tip and, if there is still doubt, examined under a microscope. A number of mite-killing preparations, if administered every other day for three weeks, will break the mite's life cycle.

MANGE   SARCOPTIC MANGE. This is caused by a microscopic parasite that infects humans as well as dogs. The mites burrow into the skin, causing irritation, and feed off the secretions that result. This causes intense itching. Young animals are most frequently infected, crusts forming around the ears, eyes, face, and limbs. The heavy chafing and oozing serum often lead to the development of a secondary bacterial pyoderma.

Mites lay from ten to twenty-five eggs, which hatch in three to four days and emerge on the skin surface as six-legged larvae. When they mature, in about fourteen days, the life cycle begins again. Mange mites, larvae, or eggs found on a skin scraping from the affected areas are used for diagnosis.

Applications of products such as lime sulfur and lindane — four to five treatments at intervals of from seven to ten days — are usually effective. These should be under the direction of your veterinarian. Antibiotics and corticosteroids are used to combat secondary bacterial infections and relieve itching until the mites die.

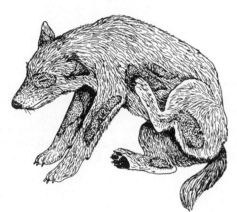

sarcoptic mange

DEMODECTIC MANGE. This is caused by a microscopic parasite that invades the hair follicles of almost all dogs while they are young. Young puppies may acquire demodex through contact with their mothers while they are still nursing. In its milder form, there are small, localized lesions around the face, ears, and legs. But there is no itching. A more severe generalized form is often accompanied by secondary bacterial infections and intense itching.

Skin scrapings from affected areas, containing the mites and their larvae, are the basis for diagnosis. Prescribed medication should be applied daily until the lesions disappear. Dogs with the more resistant generalized form should be treated in the same manner as those with deep skin pyoderma (see the following page), and given four to five weekly treatments with appropriate medication.

FLIES   Flies, biting the tips of dogs' ears, cause painful, crusty swellings and infect open wounds with their larvae (maggots). Vaseline applied to the ear tips helps to control the biting. Maggots can be removed by clipping away the hair and cleaning the wound with either hydrogen peroxide or Phisohex. Antibiotic ointments should then be applied to prevent secondary infections.

disease   The body is a series of systems, each performing specialized functions necessary to the animal's survival. When something goes wrong, we see it in terms of where the breakdown occurs. Only then can we diagnose the cause and arrive at the proper treatment. So, let's look at the dog from the standpoint of symptoms — where they might appear and what to watch for.

SKIN Itching, scratching, hair loss, or the appearance of reddened, inflamed patches on the skin are all symptoms of trouble. When they appear, you should try to determine the underlying cause — whether the dog has fleas or has come into direct contact with an irritating substance — and take the right steps to solve the problem. If the condition spreads, resists treatment, or appears to be more serious than a simple dermatitis, a veterinarian should be consulted.

The problem in diagnosing skin diseases is that there is an enormous overlap in the symptoms. Furthermore, you may be dealing with more than one condition simultaneously: dermatitis caused by a flea bite can result in the dog's tearing its skin in an attempt to relieve the itching, leading to a secondary bacterial infection.

DERMATITIS. Nonspecific inflammations of the skin may be caused by both allergies and direct contact with irritating substances. Both result in redness, intense itching, and breaks in the skin oozing serum, which forms scabs.

Allergic dermatitis can be due to an enormous variety of allergens, including pollen, fleas, grasses, rugs, foods, and the like. Once other common dermatological diseases have been ruled out, skin tests can be used to determine the specific agent. Internal medications, corticosteroids, and antibiotics can be used to treat the infection, and antihistamines to relieve the allergy. If these methods fail to yield results, a series of inoculations may reduce sensitivity to the allergen.

CONTACT DERMATITIS. This is frequently the result of bathing with harsh soaps or detergents, or of lying down on surfaces that have been sprayed with caustic agents and chemicals. In the latter case, the affected area may give a clue if the owner is unaware of the dog's exposure to the irritant. Any remaining caustic substance is removed and corticosteroids are applied. The dog should also wear an Elizabethan collar (see page 32) to protect the area from further irritation.

PYODERMA. This is a bacterial infection of the skin, which may be either superficial or deep. Among the superficial pyodermas are puppy impetigo and juvenile pyoderma, common in dogs less than a year old. Pustules (acne) are found on the chin, lips, ears, and the rear of the abdomen. Lip-fold pyoderma is frequently found on the lower lips of Saint Bernards and other breeds with drooping skin in back of the canine teeth. Vulvar-fold pyoderma is a problem with obese females. The vulva is recessed in excess skin folds, crevices that are moistened when the dog urinates, resulting in bacterial infection. In both lip-fold and vulvar-fold pyodermas, the physical defect must be corrected surgically. Treatment for the pyoderma will be discussed below.

Deep-skin pyodermas are the most difficult to cure — often, all that can be managed is to keep the infection under control. These are identified by location. Interdigital pyodermas, for example, often result from a benign cyst between the toes. To relieve the irritation caused by the cyst, the dog licks or nibbles the foot until a reddened dermatitis appears. The cysts eventually break and bacteria enter.

Generalized pyodermas, which are also deep, may affect from 60 to 70 percent of the dog's body and are among the most frustrating to treat. Infected animals are believed to lack the normal immunological defenses to fight infection, and bacteria can multiply without resistance by the body's mechanisms. These dogs suffer constant discomfort from sores and itching, in addition to having a bad odor.

Superficial pyodermas, if there are no complications, can be treated effectively at home in the following manner.

1. Clip all hair away from the affected areas.
2. Cleanse the skin around the lesion twice daily with a mild soap such as Ivory, Massengill's antiseptic douche powder (1 tablespoon of powder to 1 quart of warm water), diluted hydrogen peroxide (50 percent solution), or diluted Betadine solution (50 percent).
3. Apply bacitracin or the ointment prescribed two to three times daily.
4. If the infection is severe enough, oral antibiotics may be necessary. A prescription will be needed from your veterinarian.
5. If the inflammation is severe, oral corticosteroids may be necessary. Again, a prescription will be necessary.
6. Protect the areas from the dog by bandaging if it is feasible and using an Elizabethan collar (see page 32). Tranquilizers, if they are prescribed by your veterinarian, are also useful.
7. If pyodermas are deeply infected with bacteria, the dog should be taken to the veterinarian for skin cultures and to have dead tissue removed under anesthesia. Vaccines may also be necessary.
8. Interdigital pyodermas should be soaked for twenty to thirty minutes in Massengill's powder in solution (1 tablespoon powder to 1 quart warm water), or Epsom salts or Dum-Boro's solution, which will aid in drying up the oozing infection.

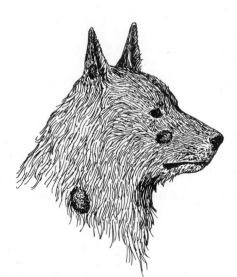

RINGWORM. A skin disease caused by a fungus, this affects both humans and animals and can be transmitted by coming into direct contact with either the infected dog or objects, such as bedding and furniture, which have become infected. The typical lesion is a circular, dry, crusty patch with short broken shafts of hair. These are most commonly found on the head, face, and ears, but may appear on other parts of the body. The lesions themselves are used in diagnosis, as well as ultraviolet light (Woods lamp), special fungal cultures, and microscopic examination of the hair shaft. Ringworm is treated with an oral fungicide and creams applied to the lesions. The dog's environment should be cleaned to avoid reinfection or exposure of others.

SEBORRHEA. Best known as dandruff, this is found most frequently in cocker spaniels, schnauzers, dachshunds, and German shepherds. While the cause is still not certain, hypothyroidism, in part, is strongly suspected. There are three known types of seborrhea:

Seborrhea sicca — a dry form with scales.

Seborrhea oleosa — an oily form.

Seborrhea dermatitis — similar in appearance to the other forms of dermatitis.

Rather than cure, because the cause is not known, the treatment is designed to control the disease. Antiseborrheic shampoos (Seleen, Fosteen, Sebafon, Thiomar, and Pragmatar) are helpful and should be used, depending on how severe the condition is, once to twice a week. If dry skin is a problem, either as a result of the disease or of bathing, fill a spray bottle of the type used for glass cleaners with diluted Alpha-keri bath oil (1 part to 9 parts of water). Spray a fine mist over the dog's coat. After working it into the coat for ten to fifteen minutes, wipe off the excess with a damp rag. This will act as a coat conditioner as well as helping to keep the dandruff under control. This can be used from one to three times a week, depending on the need.

If itching is a problem, short-term corticosteroids may be needed to keep the animal from injuring itself.

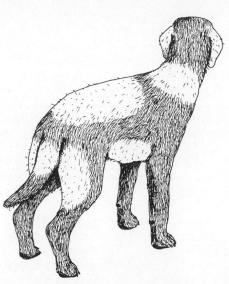

hormonal skin disease

HORMONAL SKIN DISEASES. These are characterized by symmetrical bald patches and changes in the thickness and pigmentation of the skin. There is no itching. The four most common of these skin disorders are:

1. Cushing's syndrome (hyperadrenocorticism) — which causes bald patches on the back and abdomen. The remaining hair in these areas is rough looking and can easily be picked off. The skin is frequently quite thin. This condition affects the adrenal glands and, as a secondary effect, increases the levels of corticosteroids. Medication can be used to destroy portions of the adrenal gland to reduce production of the corticosteroids, or both adrenal glands can be surgically removed. If this is done, deoxycorticosterone acetate must be administered orally or by implantation as a supplement.
2. Hypothyroidism — inadequate production of thyroxine and triiodothyronine hormones by the thyroid. This results in not only bald patches but thickened, darkly pigmented skin. Thyroid extract or synthetic thyroid is used as an oral supplement.
3. Sertoli cell tumor — a testicular tumor that produces excess estrogen. The results are bare patches along the neck and on the back of the thighs. The skin is even thicker and more heavily pigmented than in hypothyroidism. Castration is the only treatment.
4. Hypotestosteronism — quite rare, occurring in a few males castrated at an early age. The symptoms include both bald patches and darkened pigment. Diagnosis is usually based on the history of early castration and eliminating other possible causes. Synthetic testosterones, administered orally, can be used.

TUMOR. "Tumor" means any abnormal growth — and it should be pointed out that tumors may well be benign, localized and showing no tendency to spread, and definitely not cancerous. They can also be cancerous, malignant, and quite likely to spread. Tumors on the skin often include benign epidermal cysts, papillomas (warts), basal cell tumors, perianal gland adenoma, and lipomas — to name a few. Other potentially malignant skin growths are squamous cell carcinomas, malignant melanomas, mast cell sarcomas, and mammary gland adenocarcinomas.

Because of the possibility of malignancy, any growth on your dog's skin should be brought to your veterinarian's attention. Early diagnosis and removal may prevent spreading. No matter how insignificant it might seem, any growth removed should be sent to a lab for confirmation of the tumor type.

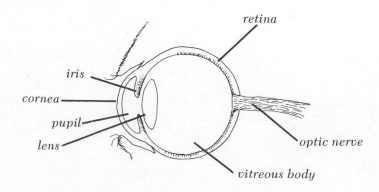

EYES The eye — a complex network of muscles, nerves, and blood vessels — is far too delicate an organ to be treated at home without the guidance of a veterinarian. Because there is always the possibility of a permanent loss of vision, any indication that your dog is having problems, regardless of the cause,

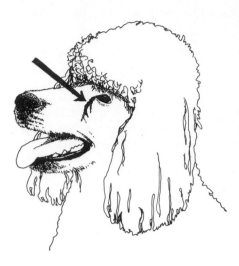

should receive professional attention as early as possible. Common symptoms include excessive tears, conjunctivitis or red eye, swelling, bluish haziness of the eye, pus discharge, aversion to sunlight, pawing at the eye, or rubbing the face on the ground. Some frequent causes include:

HEAVY TEARING (epiphora). In toy breeds, this may be the result of a congenital malformation of the "lacrimal lake." In poodles, stains on the fur that run down the muzzle from the inside of the eye are a common indication of this problem. Another possible cause may be extra eyelashes touching the sensitive cornea — these can be removed by the veterinarian. The problem may also be due to allergies, plugged tear ducts, corneal ulcers, entropion (the edges of the eyelids are curled in), and conjunctivitis.

Once the veterinarian has removed the underlying cause, the eye is usually flushed with a mild substance such as boric acid and applications of antibiotics or corticosteroids, which prevent formation of excess scar tissue.

CONJUNCTIVITIS (red eye). Inflamed eyelid membranes, this is usually accompanied by heavy tearing and a pus discharge. The causes may be physical irritation, bacterial or viral infection (often canine distemper), or allergies. Medication usually consists of flushing the eye with a mild boric acid solution, antibiotics, and/or corticosteroid solutions.

DRY EYE (keratoconjunctivitis sicca). This is most common in toy breeds, such as Pekingese and pugs, with bulging eyes. The surface of the cornea becomes dry because there is insufficient tearing. This can lead to ulceration, inflammation of the interior of the eye (iritis), darkening of the cornea, and conjunctivitis with pus discharges. Treatment is focused on relieving the symptoms by supplying artificial tears (0.5 to 1.0 percent methylcellulose) four to six times daily and medication for any ulcers (see Corneal Ulcers), and surgery if necessary. Pilocarpine can be added to the dog's food to stimulate tears but, because it has certain side effects, is used only under a veterinarian's supervision.

CORNEAL ULCERS. These breaks in the tissues lining the surface may be either superficial or deep. Indications of pain, squinting, and sensitivity to sunlight are frequent symptoms. Causes can vary widely, from exposure to chemicals in soaps and detergents or lye, wounds, and infections. Superficial ulcers can usually be healed quickly, in five to seven days, using pupil dilators (mydriatics) to reduce pain and antibiotics to control infections. Deeper ulcers are treated similarly unless there is reason to fear perforation to the interior of the eyeball, which would require surgery to support the cornea and prevent rupture while the ulcer healed.

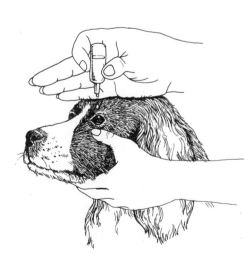

GLAUCOMA. An increase in the internal pressure of the eye due to excess fluids, this causes pain, swelling, and loss of vision. It can result from infections, displacement of the lens, tumors, accidental injury, or may be congenital. While the production of these fluids is a normal process, the pressure results from the fact that drainage is impaired. The affected eye has a hard, bulging appearance, the pupils are widely dilated, and the cornea turns blue. Eventually vision is impaired. Both drugs and surgery can be used to reduce the pressure temporarily, but there is no assurance that the problem will not recur.

CATARACTS. This condition, in which the lens becomes opaque, may be congenital. It can also be a result of the normal aging process or associated with a disease such as sugar diabetes. In the latter case, treatment would focus on curing the underlying cause. Generally, however, there is no way to control this problem medically. If the animal becomes blind, surgical techniques can be used to remove the cataracts if tests establish that the optic nerve and retina are functional.

MEDICATION. How to apply eye medication: when you administer either drops or ointment, the most important thing is to prevent accidental eye injuries if the dog moves suddenly. Using the proper technique, you can make sure that the hand holding the tube or bottle containing the medication will move with the dog's head. This should be the hand you normally favor. Place the fingers of your other hand under the dog's lower jaw and tilt its head upward at an angle of 45 degrees, halfway between the vertical and horizontal. Put the base of the hand with the medication, which should be held between the thumb and the first two fingers, on the dog's forehead. Holding the applicator between 1 and 2 inches away from the eye, gently drop or spread the medication over the surface.

EARS

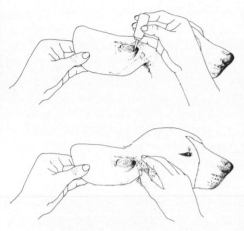

medicating the ears

The ears are the source of some of the pet owners' most frustrating problems, which can be both chronic and difficult to treat. Infections are not always the cause and treatments vary widely. Among the broader classifications of ear problems are:

Obstructive otitis, in which hair prevents air from reaching the deeper areas of the ear canal, is common in poodles. As a result, ear wax and moisture accumulate, creating a good environment for bacterial growth and infection.

Ceruminous otitis is an irritation of the ear tissues resulting from excessive production of ear wax.

Suppurative otitis, infections in which the ear canal becomes inflamed and pus accumulates, are caused by highly resistant organisms such as pseudomonas, proteus, and clostridial bacteria. These chronic infections are often complicated by the presence of yeast organisms, which are believed to be responsible for their resistance to treatment.

Proliferative otitis is a secondary effect of many of the conditions described above. As a result of chronic irritation, the folds of the inner ear thicken to as much as three to four times their normal size. Air cannot reach the inner ear, and material within it is prevented from draining.

Otitis media or interna, a nonspecific infection of the innermost portion of the ear, may affect a dog's sense of balance.

In general, the primary means of treating infections are designed to clean and flush out the ears. Antibiotics may be applied directly and taken orally. When infections prove resistant, cultures and solutions can be used to change the level of acidity in the ear. Occasionally, in severe cases, surgery is needed to provide drainage.

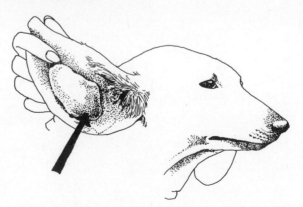

Ear hematomas, injuries to the small blood vessels within the ear caused by the dog's shaking its head and scratching the irritated area, are a common side effect of infections. Blood from the ruptured vessels forms soft, often painful clots between the cartilage of the ear and the skin. These can be relieved by draining the blood from the mass but, because of the likelihood of recurrences, surgery is often recommended.

MEDICATION. How to apply ear medication: with one hand hold the dog's ear so that it won't move its head. With the other hand, hold the tube or dropper one or two inches above the ear so that you won't accidentally poke deep inside if the dog does move. Once the medication is applied, still holding the ear, massage the base with the other hand.

NOSE   The commonest symptom of nose problems is sneezing. An occasional sneeze need be no cause for worry, but if the sneezing persists, this may be evidence of trouble, either acute or chronic. In diagnosing the cause, the veterinarian will consider a number of factors, including:

> The dog's environment — has it been exposed to grass lawns or other materials that might cause an allergic reaction?
>
> Where it may have traveled — funguses causing nose infections are prevalent in some areas.
>
> The dog's age — sneezing can indicate nasal tumors in their early stages.
>
> The dog's dental condition — a tooth abscess may have extended into the nasal sinuses.
>
> Nasal discharges — are they clear and watery, or thick and pussy?
>
> Whether the irritation is in one or both nostrils.

In most cases, sneezing problems can be treated with antibiotics, antihistamines, and nasal decongestants. If they are severe or resist these less complicated treatments, tests will be used to isolate the cause and arrive at a more effective solution.

MOUTH AND THROAT   Puppies have twenty-eight teeth. Each side of the upper and the lower jaw will include three incisors (which are the nibbling teeth toward the front of the mouth), one of the tusklike canines, and three premolars, or chewing teeth. Between its second and third month the puppy should be examined by a veterinarian for indications of any congenital abnormalities — such as an overshot or undershot jaw — that might cause future problems.

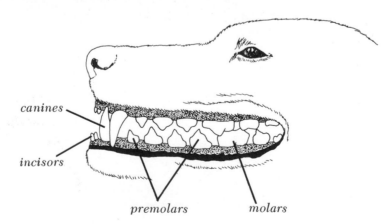

canines
incisors
premolars   molars

When the puppy is around six to seven months old, these baby teeth are shed and replaced. New teeth will also appear — another premolar on each side of the upper and lower jaws, two of the larger molars on each side of the upper and three on each side of the lower — bringing the total to forty-two. When the adult teeth have emerged, the dog should receive another dental examination so that any baby teeth that have not been shed, or any extra teeth, may be removed.

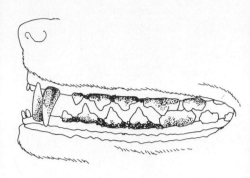

TARTAR AND CALCULI. These form on the dog's teeth and have become much more common problems for pet owners since the introduction of soft, canned dog foods. Feeding your dog large bones and hard biscuits will usually keep the accumulation under control, but your pet, especially if it is one of the smaller breeds, should receive periodic dental examinations in order to avoid abscessed teeth, periodontitis, or gingivitis. Periodontitis, an infection of the tissues around the tooth sockets, and gingivitis, gum infection, are common in cases of poor dental health. Both are capable of causing so much pain when the dog opens its mouth that it may refuse to eat.

In some cases, the infection of an abscessed tooth — most frequently the fourth upper premolar — may extend through a nasal sinus to drain beneath the eye. If a bad tooth infection is left untreated, it can also cause osteomyelitis (bone infection) in either the upper or lower jaw.

Treatment for severe dental diseases in dogs is similar to that given humans. The animal is anesthetized, the infected teeth are removed, and tartar and calculi removed from those that remain. Antibiotics, vitamin supplements, and oral flushes might be used to restore the animal to good health.

TRENCH MOUTH, OR STOMATITIS. This inflammation of the mucous membranes in the mouth may be caused by poor dental health but can be complicated by bacteria or fungi that are highly resistant to treatment. This infection may also result from advanced kidney disease or oral tumors. Treatment focuses on removing the underlying cause. Dead tissues are removed surgically, the area cauterized, and antibiotics or fungicides administered. Gentian violet, potassium permanganate, or B-complex vitamins may be applied to the surrounding areas. The pet owner's role is to make sure the dog receives a good, nutritious diet and plenty of water. Usually trench mouth can be cleared up in from three to eight weeks.

TONSILLITIS. This may be the result of either dental disease or simply too much barking — a problem the owner should be as anxious to solve for the sake of his own mental health as for the dog's physical health. The symptoms are difficulty in swallowing, loss of appetite, and, in some cases, evidence of pain when the inflamed tonsil is touched. The tonsils can also develop tumors that block the air passages and force the dog to strain for breath.

While recurring flare-ups or tumors might require removal of the tonsils, acute tonsillitis can usually be eliminated by correcting the underlying problem, administering antibiotics, and putting the dog on a semiliquid or soft diet until the symptoms disappear.

RESPIRATORY DISEASES

KENNEL COUGH. Kennel cough, or tracheobronchitis, is frequent among dogs that have been exposed to the stress of simultaneous confinement in a small space and exposure to other dogs — the type of situation encountered while boarded at a kennel, at a dog show, or in a grooming parlor. In itself, it is a mild disease that will eventually disappear, even without treatment, once the dog is in a more normal environment. The cause may be any of a number of viruses that infect the upper respiratory system.

The most obvious symptom is a repeated harsh, dry cough, which can easily be triggered by gently pressing on the dog's windpipe, or trachea. Other signs are mild fever and loss of appetite. These will normally vanish in a matter of a few days or weeks, and the only treatment necessary is antibiotics to prevent a secondary bacterial infection. If this does occur, however, matters can become more serious. A moist cough and discharges from the dog's nose and eyes are signals that complications may have developed, such as pneumonia, necessitating a chest X-ray or other tests.

TRACHEAS. Collapsed or narrowed tracheas are common in many of the toy breeds, especially poodles and Pomeranians. The characteristic symptom is a dry, repeated cough when the dog, as owners frequently describe it, "acts as though it's trying to get something out of its throat." The only yield, however, is sometimes a white, foamy phlegm. This condition is apparently congenital and results either from a narrowing of the tracheal rings, the stiffened "ribs" of the windpipe, or weakened membranes at the back of the trachea. In more severe cases both conditions exist, and the dog will sound like a honking duck. Excitement or straining at the leash will worsen the cough.

The history of the breed is an important factor in diagnosis. Medication may be given to dilate the bronchial tubes, increasing air flow to the lungs, as well as cough suppressants and sedatives for occasions when the dog might become excited. These are usually sufficient and surgery is required in less than 1 percent of the cases.

PNEUMONIA. This is a condition in which pus and debris accumulate in the air sacs and tissues of the lungs; it can usually be treated successfully if diagnosed early. Possible causes include bacteria, viruses, fungi, parasites, and foreign matter that has been inhaled. The usual symptoms are moist coughs, which yield matter, lack of appetite, depression, and high fevers. Physical examinations, chest X-rays, and blood tests are used in diagnosing this condition. Bronchodilators, vaporization, and expectorants are used to relieve the dog's breathing problem and antibiotics to check any secondary infection. The actual cure, however, is based on determining and removing the initial cause. Treatment may be necessary for weeks or even months. Massive, overwhelming infection, lung abscesses, and even the loss of a lobe of the lung are common results if complications develop.

CHRONIC OBSTRUCTIVE PULMONARY DISEASES. A broad category, these diseases share the common symptoms of a hacking cough and wheezing. And, as a group, they are resistant to antibiotics. The subdivisions used in describing these conditions are asthmatics, allergic pneumonitis, chronic bronchitis, bronchiectasis (narrowing of the bronchi, the large air passages in the lungs), and emphysema.

When other chest conditions have been ruled out, diagnosis is based primarily on the dog's history, examination of chest X-rays, and blood tests. Treatment is largely designed to relieve the symptoms and may include bronchodilators, vaporization, antibiotics, and corticosteroids.

CHEST TUMORS. These are often the result of cancer cells that have migrated from a primary tumor, in the breast, for example, and been trapped by the lung's efficient filtration system. Isolated tumors can sometimes be removed surgically, and cancer drugs have successfully prolonged the lives of dogs with certain forms of cancer, but the picture in such cases is not generally hopeful.

It is important that older dogs with a history of respiratory problems — such as rapid breathing or a chronic cough — or that show an increasingly poor ability to tolerate exercise receive a checkup to see if a chest disease is the cause.

SKELETAL DISEASES   While dogs are subject to a number of skeletal diseases, such as rickets, hypertrophic osteodystrophy in the larger breeds, and panosteitis, there is no means by which the layman can distinguish among them or attempt any form of treatment. The essential symptom is the same: reluctance to walk. A dog evidencing this should be taken to the veterinarian for diagnosis and appropriate treatment.

DIGESTIVE SYSTEM   VOMITING. This forceful, explosive expulsion of the stomach's contents must be distinguished from regurgitation, when undigested food and water are eliminated without violence. A dog that frequently regurgitates should be examined by a veterinarian for pharyngeal or esophageal problems or parasites (see above), but this cannot be considered an emergency.

Vomiting, on the other hand, can indicate immediate and serious problems, particularly if there are signs of blood. While it may result from nothing more than simple "garbage hound" gastritis, it could be symptomatic of an obstruction in the digestive system due to a swallowed foreign object, kidney failure, pancreatitis, or cancers of the stomach and bowels.

The first step is to eliminate the possibility of gastritis. To control it:

1. Withhold all solid food for twelve to twenty-four hours.
2. To coat the stomach, give the dog orally Pepto-Bismol or Maalox, 1 teaspoon (5 ml) per 10 pounds body weight.
3. *Do not withhold water* particularly if the dog is suffering from aging conditions that make it advisable. If the water is vomited, substitute ice cubes that can be licked, or try giving the animal frequent but small amounts of water.
4. In addition the dog should be started on a bland diet such as strained chicken or beef baby foods or chopped boiled meat and rice. Continue this for the next three to five days before slowly weaning the animal back to its normal diet.
5. If the vomiting continues twenty-four to forty-eight hours after you have begun these steps, or if there are signs of marked depression, fever, or vomited blood, the dog should be taken to a veterinarian.

DIARRHEA. This can be caused by many things. In young dogs, intestinal parasites are the most common problem. Other possibilities are too rich a diet, excessive nervousness, intestinal irritants such as plants or spoiled food from the garbage, bowel diseases such as salmonella, pancreatic and other diseases that make it impossible for the dog's system to absorb the food, or intestinal cancers.

Most diarrheas can be treated by following the same procedure outlined above for vomiting, with the addition of 1 teaspoon (5 ml) of Kaopectate per each 10 pounds of body weight, administered orally, to firm up the stools and protect the intestinal lining. If the diarrhea continues or there is depression or fever or signs of blood in the stools, the dog should be taken to a veterinarian immediately.

CONSTIPATION. This can result in a dog straining so hard to relieve itself that delicate tissues become injured. Common causes include a constricted colon due to a fractured pelvis; perineal hernia; a rectal diverticulum, which is a saclike structure resulting from a defect in the mucosal tissues of the rectum, which accumulates stool and causes an obstruction; masses in the rectum or colon, such as tumors or polyps; scar tissue in the rectum or colon; and nerve damage that inhibits colonic movements and causes a large, functionless colon.

Treatment, then, must aim at eliminating the cause, if possible. This is properly the job of the veterinarian, but the pet's owner can aid by giving symptomatic relief. This can include manually removing excess stool, disposable or suppository enemas, mineral oil or Laxatone lubricants, stool softeners such as sodium dioctyl sulfosuccinate, bulk laxatives, and, if approved by your veterinarian, intestinal stimulants.

COPROPHAGY. This condition, in which a dog eats its own or other animals' stool, may be due either to bad puppy habits or, as a few veterinarians suggest, to an attempt to make up for an insufficient supply of digestive enzymes. Discipline and time will often succeed in breaking a puppy of this habit, but you might add some papain — found in most meat tenderizers — to the pet's diet, to aid in breaking down keratin and other proteins.

A related problem is the licking up of other dogs' urine. This is caused by bad habits learned as a puppy, too.

FLATULENCE. Passing excessive gas is often related to diet, though no one precisely understands either the causes or the mechanism. If your dog has a problem, try changing its diet. If this fails, consult your veterinarian regarding products that might help.

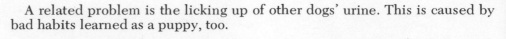

ANAL GLANDS. These glands, which open into the anus at angles of about 45 degrees, produce a thick, foul-smelling substance, which enters the rectum through a tiny duct. These secretions are believed to be a lubricant and the scent to serve as a means of marking off the animal's territory. Normally, the pressure of stool passing is sufficient to drain the two glands but the soft foods so many dogs receive today create a problem in some breeds. The glands are not sufficiently drained and start to fill up. The discomfort causes the dog to scoot along rubbing its anal area on the floor, or to lick it. The pet's owner should then apply pressure to the glands manually to drain them. This simple operation should be performed with a rubber glove. Lubricate either the thumb or forefinger, which will be inserted slightly into the anus. Pinching down gently will locate the swollen gland, which, once found, should be squeezed until the swelling disappears. If this is not done, they will become impacted and infected, breaking through the skin as abscesses. If this happens, the abscess must be cleaned, flushed with an antibiotic solution, and hot compresses applied two to three times a day. The dog should also receive oral antibiotics.

OBESITY. This is a growing problem with pets and cannot always be blamed on the owner's excessive generosity. Other factors include hormonal abnormalities such as hypothyroidism, metabolic rate, activity, the type of diet, and environment. Overweight dogs are prone to arthritic and back ailments and heart and respiratory problems. More serious, should the need arise, they are poor risks for anesthesia and surgery.

The answer lies in a strict diet, and you should make sure your friends and neighbors are aware of it and cooperate. Commercial (Cycle-4) and prescription (R/d, "O") diets are available and may help. If the diet is followed carefully and the weight problem remains, a veterinarian should examine the dog for indications of a hormonal problem.

UNDERWEIGHT. Weight loss, or a failure to gain weight at the normal rate, can be very disturbing to an owner. The subject is far too broad to discuss in depth in this book, but the possible causes can be lumped into several general categories:

Insufficient calories to keep up with the dog's metabolic demands — bluntly, starvation.

Inability to break down and absorb nutrients, possibly caused by a pancreatic problem.

Competition for nutrients by parasites.

Excessive loss of nutrients, due to diarrhea.

Disease of the heart or kidney, or diabetes mellitus.

Psychological — nervousness due to stress.

Neoplasia — tumors or other abnormal growths.

Obviously, this problem requires the advice of your veterinarian.

GENITOURINARY   CYSTITIS. Inflammation of the bladder may be caused by bladder stones, growths (polyps or tumors), bacterial infections, or congenital developmental abnormalities (diverticula). The first step in treatment is to determine which is the source of the problem and to eliminate it. Bladder stones, which injure the walls of the organ, can be diagnosed by X-ray. A bladder dye study (cystogram-pneumocystogram) can detect growths or diverticula. Urinalysis and urine cultures are used in diagnosing bacterial cystitis and determining the proper treatment. The symptoms of cystitis include increased frequency and urgency of urination, a result of irritation; blood in the urine (hematuria); or cloudy, foul-smelling urine due to pus (pyuria). Bladder stones, growths, and defects require surgery. Bacterial infections can be treated with antibiotics, regulation of urinary pH, and follow-up urine cultures.

PENIS AND PREPUCE. Balanoposthitis is an inflammation of the tissues lining the penis and the prepuce, which shields it. Foreign matter accumulated between the two irritates the mucous membranes and pus is discharged from the tip. By continually licking and bothering this, the dog usually alerts the owner to the problem. Various solutions — Massengill's (1 tablespoon in 1 quart warm water), or a mild boric acid solution — can be introduced into the prepuce, and a mild bacterial ointment worked in one to two times daily and massaged back and forth within the sheath. Bacitracin ointment could be used; Panalog would be better, because it's thinner.

PROSTATE. Prostate disease is common in dogs over six years old. The organ, which secretes the fluid carrying the sperm, may become enlarged (hypertrophy), inflamed (prostatitis), or develop abscesses, cysts, or tumors. Symptoms vary, depending on the type and severity of the condition, but they may include difficulty with bowel movements because of pressure on the colon by the enlarged organ, discharge from the penis containing pus or blood, stiff movement of the hindquarters caused by pain, and difficulty urinating. Abscesses may cause fever, loss of appetite, and listlessness. History is important in diagnosis, and physical examination will reveal an enlarged prostate. Other techniques include radiographs, possibly with dye studies, and flushes for cultures and cytological examination. Enlarged prostates may be due to a hormonal imbalance and require castration and/or the administration of estrogenlike compounds to induce shrinkage. Prostatitis, if there are no abscesses, can be treated by castration and the use of antibiotics. Abscesses, cysts, and tumors require surgery on the prostate itself.

TESTES AND SCROTUM. Problems in this area are likely to arise first when the dog is around six months old. One or both testicles may fail to descend into the scrotum, as they normally should at this age. This may require surgical removal, since retained testicles have a tendency to become tumorous as the dog grows older.

Scrotal dermatitis occasionally results when a dog has been lying on a surface that irritates the scrotum. The sac becomes inflamed, swollen, and painful; the skin may become discolored and peel. The scrotum should be generously rinsed with water to remove any caustic substances and a steroid-antibiotic ointment applied to soothe and keep it lubricated. For best results, the ointment should be prescribed by a veterinarian. The dog should wear an Elizabethan collar (see illustration, page 32) or muzzle so that he will not be able to lick the area.

Orchitis, inflammation of the testes, usually involves only one testicle. It may be a secondary effect of an injury or an infection such as *Brucella canis*. Another cause could be twisting of the testicle (torsion), which prevents blood from reaching the tissues. Antibiotics and hot compresses can be attempted but are not usually successful, and castration may be necessary.

Testicular tumors of three types — seminoma, interstitial cell, and Sertoli cell — are occasional problems. All can be identified by an asymmetry in size, with the tumorous teste becoming large and irregular, while the normal opposite teste becomes small and soft. The Sertoli cell tumor, however, is much more spectacular in its effects. It produces estrogen, and may result in

FEMALE GENITOURINARY SYSTEM

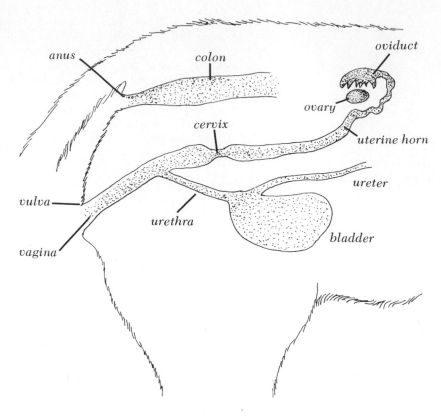

anus

colon

oviduct

ovary

cervix

uterine horn

ureter

vulva

urethra

bladder

vagina

MALE GENITOURINARY SYSTEM

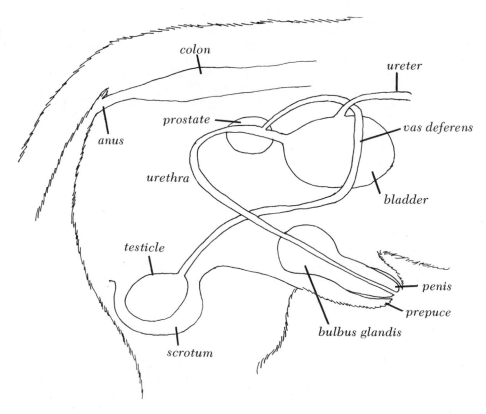

colon

ureter

prostate

anus

vas deferens

urethra

bladder

testicle

penis

prepuce

scrotum

bulbus glandis

the loss of hair in identical lateral strips on both the dog's sides, and thickening of the skin. He may also develop female traits, breast development and a tendency to squat while urinating, and attract other males. The prepuce will droop. When the possibility of cancer of the testes has been eliminated, castration is the proper treatment for testicular tumors.

VAGINA AND UTERUS. Vaginitis is common in young females prior to their first heat. The inflammation causes a yellowish green discharge from the vagina that the dog may continually lick and bother. Cystitis is a frequent side effect and may result in increasingly frequent and more urgent urination. While the cause may be in part hormonal, bacterial infections, especially *Streptococcus spp.* and *E. coli,* are frequently involved. Antibiotics taken internally, mild astringent douches such as Massengill's powder in solution (1 tablespoon in 1 quart warm water), occasional hormonal supplements, and ovariohysterectomies are used in treatment.

Pyometra is an infection of the uterus, occurring three to eight weeks after the dog has been in heat. Hormonal stimulation creates an environment favorable to bacterial growth. *E. coli,* the most common organism involved, causes the organ to swell with pus from its normal pencil size to that of a salami. Toxins in the bloodstream cause excessive thirst and frequent urination. Other symptoms include listlessness, vomiting, and loss of appetite. In severe cases, kidney function may be impaired, leading to endotoxic shock. If the cervix is open, a vaginal discharge containing pus and blood may be seen. If it is closed, the dog's belly will swell because of the lack of drainage and she may become seriously ill. Pyometra is an emergency condition and the animal should be taken to the veterinarian as soon as any symptoms are noted.

In the case of bitches with a valuable breeding potential, antibiotics and douches to irrigate the uterus may be attempted, but the favored treatment is ovariohysterectomy to remove the source of the infection.

HEART DISEASE   Heart disease can be the result of a congenital defect or may develop as part of the aging process. The commonest, and most dangerous, condition is congestive heart failure, most frequently caused by chronic fibrosis of the heart valves.

The heart is a complex pump, an organ divided into four chambers. Valves close the chambers off from one another when the heart contracts. If a valve fails, there is a backflow of blood into the chamber it has just left. The characteristic symptom of this condition is a heart murmur, a sound caused by the turbulence as the blood reenters the chamber from which it has been ejected.

A heart murmur does not automatically signal the onset of heart failure — it is merely a danger signal. The heart, a remarkable organ, compensates for a defective valve by increasing its size; there is a limit, however, to how large it can grow. When this is reached, the heart begins to fail.

A secondary effect of this is that fluid backs up into the lungs (pulmonary edema), and the patient is quite literally in danger of drowning. The first symptoms of chronic heart failure are an increasing coughing of fluids, often in the middle of the night. Appetite decreases and the patient will sometimes faint. In severe cases, the tongue and the mucous membranes inside the mouth will have a bluish appearance. Breathing will be in rapid pants, with mouth open.

Any of these symptoms should be brought to the attention of your veterinarian, who can evaluate the dog's condition with X-rays, an electrocardiogram, and blood tests to check out other organs, particularly the kidneys and liver. An animal that collapses with a heart attack should be handled as little as possible and subjected to minimal stress. The veterinarian will give it oxygen, diuretics (water pills) to decrease the fluid in its lungs, and digitalis to stimulate the heart's muscle contractions so that it will slow down and do a more efficient job of pumping. Once its condition has been stabilized, the dog will continue to receive digitalis and diuretics. Because salt retains fluids in the body, a low-salt or salt-free diet will be prescribed.

mothers and puppies

MATING

While male dogs are sexually potent when they are from five to six months old, they are not capable of mating until they are around three months older. Sexual maturity in the female arrives between her sixth and twelfth months. Her sexual activity is determined by a "heat" cycle, which occurs approximately twice a year. The cycle can be divided into four stages:

1. Proestrus is often confused with heat. The vulva swells and shows the first signs of bleeding. This phase lasts from seven to nine days.
2. Estrus is heat — it is the five- to seven-day period during which the female will accept a male and breeding takes place.
3. Metestrus is the period immediately following heat when, unless pregnancy has occurred, the uterus and ovaries return to their normal state.
4. Anestrus is the period of roughly three months in which the uterus and ovaries are at rest and under no strong hormonal influence.

FALSE PREGNANCY

The first heat is often erratic — the female should not be allowed to mate until the second heat, to ensure sexual maturity.

False pregnancy (pseudocyesis) may occur approximately six to eight weeks following a period of heat. Psychological and hormonal influences have been suggested as explaining the physical and emotional changes, such as the enlargement of the breasts, which secrete a serumlike milky substance, and the restless state, in which the female may show excessive affection and mothering behavior toward toys, shoes, and the like. While this condition will sometimes end if estrogen or testosterone injections are given, this is not recommended. The false pregnancy usually ends naturally within one to three weeks without therapy.

MISMATING

The owner of a female that has been accidentally mated has three options available:

1. If mating is known to have occurred no more than twenty-four hours earlier, the dog can be given an estrogen shot that will delay implantation of the egg in the uterus. This will also prolong the heat period two to three more weeks, however. There is also the possibility that the shot might not work and she may still be pregnant.
2. An ovariohysterectomy can be performed as soon as she's out of heat.
3. You can wait and take the chance that she may not be pregnant. If she is and the pregnancy is allowed to reach term, the mother can either have the puppies naturally, or they can be removed through a Caesarean section (an incision in the uterus) if problems develop.

PRENATAL CARE

VACCINATIONS AND PARASITE CHECK. The prospective mother should receive boosters for distemper, hepatitis, leptospirosis, and rabies prior to breeding. This ensures the pups good protective antibody passage via the colostrum during the first twenty-four hours of nursing.

Since many intestinal parasites can cross the placenta in utero, the bitch should have two or three fecal examinations for parasites and be treated prior to breeding if any are found.

WHEN TO BREED. Most breeders agree that it is best to take the bitch to the male rather than vice versa. There are many psychological and social factors that come into play during mating, and if possible, the bitch should spend her entire heat cycle with him.

The dogs should be allowed to "tie" (copulation) at will or at forty-eight-hour intervals at the first sign of heat. The male will mount the female from the rear, holding her between his forelegs, while she lowers her hindquarters to allow him to insert his penis in her vagina. In inexperienced animals, there may be some fumbling before this is accomplished. Breeders will not attempt to mate dogs unless one has already had experience because of the likelihood that nothing will be accomplished if neither has learned what to do. They should not be separated until the tie, which may last as long as ten or twenty minutes, is complete.

GESTATION. The gestation or pregnancy period lasts between sixty and seventy days.

Around a week prior to delivery, make a clean nesting area in a familiar part of the house out of the way of people going in and out of the room. The area should be quiet, warm, and free of potential hazardous obstacles to roaming puppies (stairs, electrical cords, and so on).

DETERMINING PREGNANCY. Your veterinarian should be able to palpate (feel) the fetuses through the abdominal wall twenty-one to twenty-eight days after conception. An abdominal X-ray, which will not harm the fetuses, can confirm or deny a pregnancy forty-five days after conception. The fetal bones should be visible at that time.

LABOR SIGNS. The pregnant dog will generally start to nest five to six days prior to delivery. Approximately twenty-four to forty-eight hours prior to delivery, she may become restless and have a slightly decreased appetite. Her body temperature may fall below 100°F. around eighteen or twenty-four hours prior to delivery. During this same period, colostrum may ooze from her breasts. Panting and straining may begin.

WHELPING. During the forceful contractions of the uterus that push the fetus through the cervix you may see either a clear saclike structure called the amnion, which surrounds the fetus, emerging from the vulva, or the passage of clear fluid (breaking water) if the amnion ruptures.

The pups may emerge either headfirst (60 percent of the time) or feetfirst (40 percent of the time) and may be delivered in fifteen-minute to two-hour intervals. Once delivered, the puppies should be cleaned of excess amnionic tissues so they can breathe. The mother will normally bite and break the umbilical cord as she cleans and attends to each new puppy. If she doesn't, then tie a piece of thread firmly around the cord near the pup's belly and tear the cord, slightly away from the pup's belly.

Individual placentas (afterbirths) are usually passed with each puppy. Count the placentas to be sure none are retained — they may lead to uterine infections. It is not unusual for the mother to eat a portion of the afterbirth.

DYSTOCIA. Dystocias, or difficult births, may be a result of oversized puppies unable to pass through the pelvic canal, uterine inertia or lack of uterine contraction when the mother is exhausted by prolonged straining, a compromised pelvis due to old pelvic fractures, or mechanical obstruction due to maldelivery or malposition of the fetus or fetuses.

Your veterinarian will assess the difficulty and attempt to remedy the problem either by manual manipulation or with hormones (oxytocin) to stimulate uterine contractions, or a C-section if medical therapy fails to correct the problem.

Dystocias should be considered in the following situations: when no puppies are produced after two to four hours of labor; when only a portion of the puppy appears and cannot be delivered with assistance; when a puppy has not been delivered within an hour after the amnionic sac "breaks water"; when a bloody vaginal discharge occurs; or when the mother is in distress with exerted breathing.

Any of these conditions warrants veterinary evaluation. Waiting too long may jeopardize the lives of both the puppies and the mother.

POSTNATAL CARE

FIRST SIX HOURS. The puppies should be placed immediately on the mother for nursing since it is during this first eighteen to twenty-four hours that antibodies against disease and the highest amount of nutrition are passed in the colostrum of the milk.

This period is also quite important in that there are always one or two runts that have problems competing with the other puppies for food and may need special attention. If left unattended, isolated from the mother, they may fall prey to malnutrition and hypothermia (subnormal temperature) and die.

TWENTY-FOUR TO SEVENTY-TWO HOURS POSTPARTUM. The puppies and mother should be taken to the veterinarian for examination for any congenital defects (umbilical hernia, cleft palate, or congenital heart defects). The mother is examined for any retained puppies and may receive an injection of oxytocin to stimulate her release of milk and help her to pass any retained placenta and fluids.

Tail docking and dewclaw removal are usually done at three days of age. The eyes usually open somewhere between twelve to fourteen days.

A normal greenish black vaginal discharge may persist for five to ten days following birth. Should the discharge continue after this, or change in character, you should call your veterinarian.

FIVE TO SIX WEEKS OF AGE. The puppies should be weaned onto solid foods gradually at this time. Baby teeth start to appear at three to five weeks.

Puppies from six weeks to six months old should receive three meals daily; six months to one year, two meals daily; and over one year, one or two meals daily, depending on the dog's activity.

A puppy feeding chart developed by Ralston Purina follows; it may be helpful in determining how much your puppy should eat.

PUPPY FEEDING CHART

BREED SIZE	6–10 WEEKS OF AGE	11–16 WEEKS OF AGE	17–26 WEEKS OF AGE	27–52 WEEKS OF AGE
Small				
miniature poodle, dachshund, Pomeranian, Pekingese	1½ cups	2½ cups	3½ cups	4½ cups
Medium				
pointer, setter, springer spaniel, Siberian husky	2½ cups	4½ cups	6½ cups	8½ cups
Large				
Labrador retriever, boxer, German shepherd	3½ cups	6½ cups	8½ cups	12½ cups
Giant				
Great Dane, Irish wolfhound, Saint Bernard, Newfoundland	4½ cups	7½ cups	11½ cups	16½ cups

AFTER WEANING. After weaning, any of the commercial puppy chow formulas currently on the market are fine up until six to eight months of age. These products are well fortified with vitamins and minerals and rarely need supplementation. After eight months of age, the dog can be put on an adult diet (see page 23).

PROBLEMS ENCOUNTERED

MASTITIS. Mastitis is an inflammation of the mammary glands, or breasts. This condition often accompanies false pregnancies; the pseudo-milk accumulates and does not drain properly. It also occurs during or after nursing when one of the mammary ducts becomes obstructed due to injury or infection. Signs include hot, painful, hard, and frequently discolored breasts. There is usually a blood-tinged to brownish discharge when the affected nipple is milked out. The dog generally runs a high temperature, has a decreased appetite, and is reluctant to nurse. The puppies should be taken off the mother; milk out the glands gently two or three times daily, and apply warm compresses to the glands two or three times daily for twenty to thirty minutes. If abscesses develop, your veterinarian will promote adequate drainage and start the appropriate antibiotics.

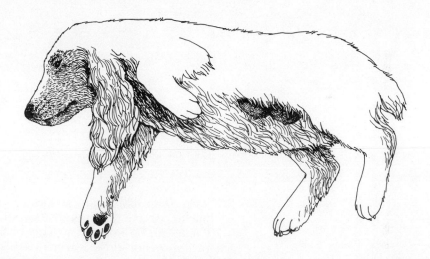

ECLAMPSIA. Eclampsia (low blood calcium), usually occurring two or three weeks after delivery, is a common problem among the smaller breeds of dogs. It has long been thought this is caused by an excessive drain of calcium by the puppies' taking the mother's milk. This condition occasionally occurs before delivery, however, suggesting a much more complex mechanism. Symptoms include restlessness, shaking, panting, high body temperature (often exceeding 104°F.), muscle twitching, and convulsions.

Mothers showing these signs should be cooled down by dousing in cold water and be taken to your veterinarian immediately, who will then administer calcium intravenously to bring her out of the crisis and dispense calcium–phosphorus–vitamin D supplementation for use at home. The puppies should be taken off the mother permanently and fed by hand, or kept off her for at least forty-eight hours.

HYPOGLYCEMIA. Hypoglycemia (low blood sugar) is a common problem among the toy breed puppies shortly after weaning. Their excess activity and high metabolic rates are often not met by the daily dietary caloric intake. The puppy becomes listless, lethargic, dull, wobbly, and, in more severe cases, comatose. Give a puppy with these symptoms 1 to 2 teaspoons of honey or maple syrup mixed with water (half and half) every two hours for the next six to eight hours. This will usually prevent the condition from worsening and will often bring the puppy dramatically out of its stupor.

Should you find your puppy flat out (comatose), with no sign of injury, wrap it in a warm blanket and take it immediately to your veterinarian for intravenous glucose and intensive care.

ORPHAN PUPPIES. In caring for puppies that have lost their mother several factors must be considered:

Warmth. For the first three weeks of life a puppy's body temperature is less than 100°F. and its heat-regulatory mechanisms are not fully developed. For this reason the environment of the pups should be kept in the range of 80° to 85°F. As they become older, this can be decreased to 70°F.

Isolation. Puppies should be handled as often as possible by members of the family during the course of the day to ensure emotional stability. At night a ticking clock or low-playing radio may prevent some of the loneliness resulting from the lack of body contact.

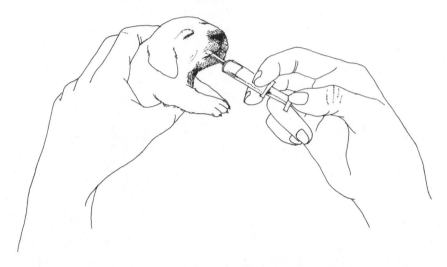

Feeding. There are a number of commercial formulas out on the market that approach the composition of normal bitches' milk (Esbilac, Orphalac). These can be bought at many of the pet stores or from your veterinarian. All formulas should be warmed to body temperature, and fed as directed on the label. Special puppy nursing bottles with special puppy nipples are generally available. If not, an empty syringe can be obtained from your veterinarian to administer the formula.

Puppies do not have well-developed swallowing reflexes — the formula should always be administered *slowly* at the side of the mouth. The puppy should be placed on its belly in approximately a 45-degree angle. *Never feed the puppy on its back.* One of the most serious problems in young puppies is aspiration pneumonia, caused by inhaling the formula down deep in its lungs.

old age
The life span of various breeds of dogs is variable, but as a general rule the giant breeds have shorter life spans than the smaller breeds. One expects the old dog to become less active, less playful, and somewhat altered in appearance.

Its sight may be altered by degeneration of the lens (a normal aging process), cataracts, or optic nerve damage. Loss of hearing is not uncommon. Arthritis of the hips, knees, and spinal column may cause significant discomfort, to the point where your pet may refuse to walk about. Medical problems such as heart and kidney disease, sugar diabetes, and cancer are frequently encountered and must be dealt with accordingly.

Senility is another symptom you can expect, with a decreased attention span and regressive behavior, such as increasing inability to obey earlier training, which includes housebreaking. Understandably, your affectionate pet of yesterday will also show some changes in temperament. The dog that once loved children may now find them irritating and snap at them when they want to play.

There isn't really a great deal that can be done to combat the symptoms of old age. The main thing to remember is that your dog is becoming increasingly susceptible to disease, and this means it should receive more frequent checkups. In approaching the treatment of geriatric patients, the aims should be to save, restore, or relieve the patient. The stress of unnecessary hospitalization should be avoided, and the most minimal therapeutic measures should be applied to produce the desired effect. Supportive care is of the utmost importance.

The subject of euthanasia is never pleasant, and it touches personal and moral issues in all of us. We all must face the question in our pet's life of whether, by treating the disease or condition, we are ultimately offering the dog a comfortable and decent future life. If the dog cannot live its life out without pain, deterioration as a result of disease (that is, cancer), or maintain itself adequately, then humane euthanasia, intravenously injecting an overdose of anestheticlike drug, will end its suffering quickly and painlessly.

further readings

ETTINGER, S. J. *Textbook of Veterinary Internal Medicine*, vols. 1 and 2. Philadelphia, W. B. Saunders, 1975.

FOX, M. W. *Canine Pediatrics*. Springfield, Illinois, Charles C Thomas, 1966.

————. *Understanding Your Dog*. New York, Coward, McCann and Geohegan, 1971, 1972.

GAINES DOG RESEARCH CENTER. *Basic Guide to Canine Nutrition*, 2nd. ed. New York, General Foods Corporation, 1968.

GILBRIDE, DR. ANNA P., ed. and pub. *Canine Practice*. Bimonthly. P.O. Box 4457, Santa Barbara, California, 93103.

KIRK, ROBERT. *Current Veterinary Therapy*, vol. 6. Philadelphia, W. B. Saunders, 1975.

MCGINNIS, T. *The Well Dog Book*. New York, Random House, 1974.

MCKEOWN, D., AND STRIMPLE, E. *Your Pet's Health from A to Z*. New York, Coward, McCann and Geohegan, 1973.

MILLER, M. E., CHRISTENSEN, G. C., AND EVANS, H. E. *Anatomy of the Dog*. Philadelphia, W. B. Saunders, 1964.

MORRIS, M. L. *Canine Dietetics — Nutritional Management in Health and Disease*. Denver, Mark Morris Associates, 1969.

MORRIS, M. L., AND COLLINS, D. R. *The Guide to Nuturitional Management of Small Animals*. Denver, Mark Morris Associates, 1968.

Cats

JEAN HOLZWORTH, D.V.M.

Cats have never had it so good. After centuries of playing second fiddle to dogs as "man's best friend," cats have now attained equal status. As the human population explodes, the cat becomes more highly valued. It takes up less space, it is quieter, it eats less, and its tidy habit of waste disposal makes it a nonpolluter. As an apartment dweller it is ideal: it does not have to be walked several times a day and it can be left alone over weekends with only a walk-in visitor desirable to make sure that all is well.

If your life-style meshes best with that of cats, if you are in tune with a creature that is independent, subtle, and low key in its relationships, a cat friend could be for you. It must *not* be regarded as merely one of the props in your *mise-en-scène* or as an educational item in the upbringing of your children.

The safest place to get a healthy cat, whether mixed breed or purebred, is probably from a home where there is but one mother cat and contact with other cats is minimal. Cats in groups — those in pet shops and shelters — even if together for only a few hours, may be exposed to a variety of feline infections: to panleukopenia (cat distemper), to several kinds of "cold" of which cats may then become carriers for life, and to ringworm, a fungus skin disease that is highly contagious among cats, dogs, and humans. If you acquire a cat from a shop or shelter, get a written guarantee that your pet will be replaced or your money refunded if the cat has or develops a problem for which the seller or shelter can reasonably be held liable. Breeders' catteries, especially large ones, are cursed with the same disease problems as pet shops and shelters, and because of continuity of breeding stock, diseases that persist in carriers are especially likely to be endemic.

Ideally a purebred cat should, before sale, have been vaccinated against panleukopenia and the upper respiratory infections, checked for parasites, and tested for feline leukemia virus. The purchase agreement should provide that the cat be examined either before or after sale by the buyer's veterinarian and also that the seller will make restitution of some sort if the animal eventually proves to have a defect or ailment for which the breeder can reasonably be held responsible.

Kittens develop best both physically and emotionally if they spend their first two months with a healthy mother and litter mates, being nourished principally on mother's milk, and playing and squabbling with other kittens their own age. Kittens that are orphaned or taken too young from a mother, so that they must be hand-fed or weaned early, are usually less sturdy and may develop neurotic habits that could be lifelong, such as suckling on their own or some other cat's toes, tail, or fur, or their owner's anatomy or clothing.

Cats are often acquired in pairs, either litter mates or cats close in age. An "only" cat will not consciously suffer, but may develop some neurotic traits and will be closer to its owner than if it had a cat companion.

If you already have a cat or cats, you should not add on indiscriminately. A new young cat may sometimes be accepted but is equally apt to be treated indefinitely as an interloper and subjected to various manifestations of jealousy and hostility. On the other hand, a young, exuberant cat may make existence wretched for a dignified and stodgy oldster. Two cats that like and enjoy each other should be the ideal. Lucky the owner who achieves this!

SELECTING A CAT Cats are above all individuals, and inheritance and upbringing may make them anything from sterling citizens to dyed-in-the-wool outlaws. You have a better chance of knowing what a cat is really like if you get it as a grown-up. Just about all kittens are appealing, but a grown cat that develops into, and continues through life as, a real personality is a rarity.

Males used to be preferred, mainly because the neutering of males is a less expensive operation. More and more, the balance of favor is tilting toward females. Because of anatomical differences, females are less gravely and expensively affected by the feline tendency to formation of urinary stones. They may be fed exclusively, if desired, on wholesome commercial dry foods, while this type of ration may be undesirable for males with a tendency to urinary problems. Neutered females, also, seem to be less apt to acquire excess weight than neutered males.

For some people, a certain breed has a particular appeal. For others, a purebred is an essential status symbol. Even more cat lovers have discovered that there are mixed-breed cats just as healthy, handsome, and personable as any purebred. In fact, some of the newer breeds have originated from chance crossings that produced cats so beautiful it was thought worthwhile to develop them as a recognized type. A currently popular example of such a cat is the lynx-point Siamese, a cross between domestic tabby and Siamese.

Shorthairs are currently the purebreds most in favor. They are easier to care for than the luxuriantly coated longhairs, which require much grooming, and as a rule are more spirited and active.

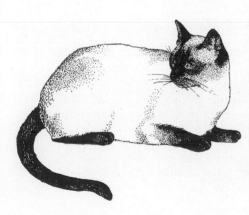

Among the shorthairs the most numerous are the Siamese, whose "points" come in fascinating variations of color. Owners of Siamese are probably right in claiming that they are in general the liveliest, most intelligent, and most responsive of all domestic cats. Their extraordinary voices are capable of an enormous range of expression: spine-chilling howls of menace, urgent mating calls, cosy conversational give and take, and soft little bleats of contentment and affection. The Siamese are said to have been the guardians of the temples in their native land, and a few still have such strong territorial instincts that they sometimes terrorize janitors and mailmen. All cats tend to be arboreal, but this instinct is especially strong in Siamese. They like to climb, perching on shoulders or proceeding around a room by way of draperies, bookcases, and mantelpiece rather than on the floor.

Certain faults characteristic of the breed have been largely eliminated from show specimens: crossed eyes and crooked or bobbed tails. Because of inbreeding, however, Siamese are subject to certain other defects. Structural abnormalities of the heart that lead to early death in kittens are the most common. Harelip, cleft palate, visual defects, malabsorption of food, and cloth-eating are disorders believed to be hereditary. A strange trouble — called variously causalgia or neurodermatitis — in which the cat manifests painful sensitivity of the tail, chasing and chewing it, occurs almost exclusively in Siamese (see page 104). Cancer of the small intestine and anal sac abscesses are rare except in Siamese cats; on the other hand, steatitis ("yellow fat" disease due to vitamin E deficiency) and meningiomas, tumors of nervous tissue common in cats in general, are virtually unknown in Siamese.

Cats that are part Siamese show to varying degree many of the characteristics of the purebred. Many first-generation crosses are black, but clearly betray their Siamese heritage by their svelte figures, smooth coats, loud voices, and personality traits. Some cats are also clearly part Siamese in eye or coat color.

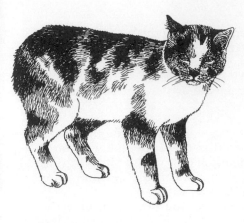

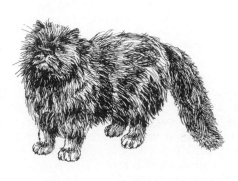

Owners of Burmese, Abyssinians, Russian Blues, and Manx consider that these breeds make unusually gentle and responsive pets.

As the Burmese and Abyssinians are becoming more numerous, certain congenital or inherited defects are beginning to appear. A troublesome problem in some lines of Burmese is a flattened rib cage that prevents normal functioning of the organs of the chest.

In Manx cats, an anatomical deficiency — absence of the tail — has become the prime breed criterion, it being considered desirable that there should be no coccygeal (tail) vertebrae at all. Unfortunately, there may be serious associated skeletal, muscular, and neural abnormalities. In some tailless or bobtailed cats the urinary bladder and anus do not contract normally, and the cat incurably dribbles urine or oozes stool. In some Manx there may be no anal opening at all; occasionally there is a common opening for the digestive and urogenital tracts. Such defects may pass unnoticed for a few weeks after birth but ultimately necessitate destroying the kitten.

Manx cats have smaller litters than other breeds. It is hypothesized that this may be because some of the fetuses are so abnormal that they die and are resorbed before birth.

The most popular of the longhaired breeds are the Persians. These heavy-set, magnificently furred cats tend to be more phlegmatic than other cats and, even according to their admirers, less intelligent, although usually gentle and affectionate. They may not come into heat as young as other cats, and sometimes they are so undemonstrative that you have difficulty knowing when this happens.

The short face of the Persians, so assiduously cultivated by breeders, creates problems, predisposing to nasal infections, blockage of the tear ducts, and malocclusion of the jaws. The jaws are so short sometimes, the cat cannot get its mouth into food but must put food into its mouth with a paw, and the male may have trouble getting a firm grasp on the female's neck in mating.

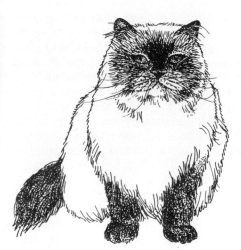

The Himalayan breed is not of Oriental origin as its name suggests, but was created in Boston by a deliberate cross of Siamese and Persians. In conformation and temperament the Himalayans are more Persian than Siamese.

Every cat has its own innate characteristics, but these will be modified by its environment and the amount of attention it receives. Most cats dislike loud sounds and rough handling and are happiest in a regular routine, but many adjust to large, noisy, and unpredictable households with numerous other pets. "Only" cats, which receive much human attention, companionship, and cuddling, become almost human themselves. Because of this pampering, thay have the hardest time adjusting to changes in routine, traveling, boarding, or hospitalization, and are often fearful of strange humans or animals.

There are no reliable statistics on the life span of cats. It is rare that unneutered males survive beyond ten years. By five years of age they usually have the look of battered veterans, with damaged ears, scarred jowls and legs, and broken fangs. Neutered cats with conscientious and observant owners, on the other hand, live well into their teens, and twenty-year-old cats are not rare. There are apparently a few well-substantiated instances of cats reaching thirty.

DISEASES TRANSMISSIBLE FROM CATS TO MAN

From time to time long and horrifying lists of diseases transmissible from cat to man appear in the public media. Upon calm investigation it appears that while many infectious or parasitic diseases common to man and cat may potentially or under unusual circumstances be passed between man and his pet cat, actual transmission has never or rarely been proven. Ringworm is probably the only infection that is clearly and commonly passed from cat to man.

Simple sanitary measures such as keeping cats off kitchen and dining surfaces and washing the hands after handling a cat or its litter box and before eating will eliminate most of the possible risks from other diseases.

"Cat scratch disease," an uncommon and usually mild infection of humans, in which lymph nodes draining the area of a cat scratch become painfully swollen, is not actually a disease of cats at all. It is believed to be due to some kind of soil organism which is transmitted on the claws of cats and is inoculated into human skin by a scratch. In some cases there may even be no history of contact with a cat, the scratch being acquired from a rose thorn or similar source.

rearing and preventive care
TRAINING

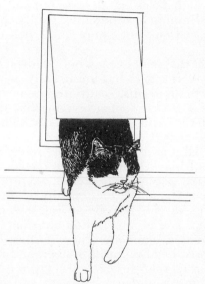

A new cat should be introduced to its surroundings with a minimum of noise and confusion. If there are other pets or lively children, the cat may need a day or two of adjustment in a room by itself. Cats are surprisingly patient with youngsters but should probably not be acquired for the very young. Because tiny children do not understand that they must treat an animal with gentleness and respect, a pet may be mauled and may get into the habit of retaliating in self-defense.

You may provide the new cat with a basket, box, or bed in a secluded corner, but it is very likely to make its own choice of a soft spot or hideaway. If the cat is to be allowed out-of-doors, this should usually not start till a kitten is three or four months old, and only briefly and under the owner's watchful eye. The cat will go only a few feet at first, and dart back at the first alarm or handclap. There should always be a safe retreat of some sort (trees, garage, roof, under the porch) where the cat can seek safety if threatened.

An outdoor cat that strays is more likely to be recovered if it wears a bell and identification tag. The collar should be at least partially elastic so it will pull off if it gets caught on anything.

Some owners provide for their cat to go in and out at will through a "cat port," an arrangement of overlapping flaps set into a door panel or window. Unfortunately other cats or wild visitors may also go in and out, and your own cat may surprise you by bringing in live prey, birds or rodents, that may be difficult to capture and remove.

Cats should not be confined for long periods in basements or garages unless these are clean and dry, with some daylight and with good ventilation.

HOUSEBREAKING

Housebreaking is a problem that must be dealt with from the moment the cat arrives. Practically all cats have a strong instinct for cleanliness and take readily to a litter pan from their first moment out of their nest. When a cat comes to a new home, the litter pan should be readily accessible but may eventually be moved to a closet, bathroom, utility room, basement, or some such semisecluded site. For young kittens the pan should be low enough to be climbed into easily. For adult cats the bigger and deeper the pan the better, in order to reduce the amount of litter that is inevitably scattered about when the cat digs. The plastic trays commonly available in pet shops are not large enough or deep enough for grown cats; enamel or plastic infant bathtubs are best.

Some owners remove stool daily but change litter only every week or so. Under certain circumstances, however, public health authorities recommend that litter should be changed daily and the pan washed with a mild soap solution and rinsed with scalding water (see pages 95ff.).

Unclean litter pans offend fastidious cats and may cause them to break their toilet training. The clay-type litters are acceptable to most cats, but occasionally the dust from this material causes chronic bronchitis and cough. Possible alternatives are the less dusty green litter, sawdust, wood shavings, sand, soil, or torn paper.

Ideally, cats that go out will use the litter pan only as an emergency convenience, but some become so habituated to it that they never avail themselves of the great outdoors. In this event the owner may try placing a litter pan outside. In emergencies, cats are very resourceful about using fireplaces, bathtubs, and showers.

The importance of maintaining training cannot be overemphasized. Once a cat has soiled any area, except perhaps glazed tile, it is marked once and for all as a possible toilet spot for any cat that sniffs it. The only cleaning procedure that may possibly remove the odor is thorough laundering with soap and hot water.

An occasional cat spontaneously learns to use the toilet — the best of all solutions. Cat magazines advertise methods for training cats in this activity. They must learn as kittens and may not cooperate if other cats in the household are using ordinary litter pans.

PLAY, COMPANIONSHIP, AND TOYS

Young cats are at the liveliest and most inquisitive stage of their lives. Simple objects such as a paper bag, Ping-Pong ball, spool (without the thread), pencil, or a wad of paper to chase and tear will give them as much fun as more costly and elaborate toys. Avoid toys that cats can dismember and swallow. Elaborate upholstered "trees" for climbing and perching can keep cats entertained for hours and are available from pet shops and mail-order houses.

The taste for catnip is an inherited trait that may or may not manifest itself as a cat matures. Catnip mice may be favorite toys but are usually made of such flimsy cloth that the cat soon tears them to bits, scattering the contents widely. Good quality, freshly dried catnip can be homegrown or obtained in pet shops. In many cats it acts much like marijuana, inducing a high that varies from blissful stupor to mad antics.

Cats, it is often said, are creatures of habit and like to be able to count on their owners for the routine pleasures of homecoming, feeding time, play, grooming, bedtime, and the like. A regular play period can be the brightest spot in a cat's day, and will cement your personal relationship. Hide-and-seek and tag are games some cats enjoy. Most like to be swung in a paper grocery bag. Roughhousing and boxing are fine in moderation but sometimes lead to undesirably aggressive behavior. Cats can sometimes be induced to learn standard dog tricks — shaking hands, begging, rolling over, and fetching — but are more apt to develop individual routines of their own.

Cats enjoy being talked to in both human and cat language and many, especially Siamese, carry on expressive conversations with their humans. After a dull day alone at home, they also seem to relish the sound of radio or television provided it's not too loud or frightening.

PUNISHMENT

When a cat behaves in an objectionable manner a loud, firm "No!" or "Bad!" perhaps accompanied by a smart smack on the behind is about the only discipline that is effective. The reprimand must be simultaneous with the misbehavior; the cat will not understand if punished for a misdeed committed some time previously. Severe spankings merely terrify a cat, and may cause it to strike back.

Try to understand that the objectionable things cats do are often natural cat behavior. Clawing furniture and walking on kitchen counters and dining tables should be discouraged if possible, but are accepted with resignation by most cat lovers. Hunting also comes naturally to cats, and punishment is neither fair nor effective. A few very civilized cats can be persuaded by gentle coaxing to relinquish their catch, which, if suffering only from shock, may be released at a safe distance. A bell on an outdoor cat may serve as a warning to potential victims.

FEEDING

Cats in the wild are strictly carnivores and devour the whole body of their prey — muscles, organs, bones, and contents of digestive tract — except that they may vomit or leave uneaten feathers or fur. Such fare obviously provides a large proportion of protein, considerable fat, minerals, and vitamins. Cats do not need starches (carbohydrates), vegetables, or fruits. Cellulose is poorly digested.

Domestic cats that hunt provide their own good diet. Since the food is fresh and uncooked, no vitamins or minerals are lost or destroyed. The only drawback to such raw fare is that a cat may acquire internal parasites (chiefly tapeworms and ascarids; see pages 93–94) or certain infectious diseases (see discussion of toxoplasma, page 95).

Many cats today have little or no chance to hunt but eat a varying combination of commercial cat foods, human foods, and table scraps. Ideally this diet should reflect the cat's high needs for protein and fat. That is, about 20 to 25 percent protein, 10 to 15 percent fat, plus a little carbohydrate, and about 2 percent mineral (ash). The remaining 60 percent — water — is important because many cats drink very little fluid as such (that is, little water or milk). In dry foods, the proportions would be about 25 to 50 percent protein, 15 to 40 percent fat, 5 percent ash, and only 10 percent water. Percentages in the moist foods fall somewhere between. These are figures for cat owners to keep in mind when reading cat food labels. In addition, since some cats relish sweet or starchy foods, vegetables, and even fruit, there is no reason why some of their energy needs cannot be supplied by these. A moderate taste for starches should be encouraged. If a cat develops kidney disease later in life, increasing starch and decreasing protein in the diet can be important in prolonging its life.

Dog foods rarely contain enough protein and fat for cats.

Many of today's commercial meat- and fish-based cat foods, particularly if produced by food companies that have extensively researched the nutritional needs of cats, provide well-balanced diets, especially if a cat is brought up as a kitten to accept a variety of the products — dry, "maintenance" in large cans, and "treats," usually higher in meat protein, in small cans — and is not permitted to become addicted to only one or two foods. The semidry and dry foods, although complete and well balanced nutritionally, have little moisture and cats eating them must eat them moistened or have additional fluid. Some veterinarians are convinced on the basis of practical experience that the dry foods may be a contributing factor to the urinary disorders (urolithiasis) to which male cats are prone if they do not consume sufficient water.

The commercial cat foods may be supplemented by well-cooked meat, fowl, and fish, and by table leftovers, especially those containing fat and bacon grease. Eggs (the white must be cooked to preserve biotin), yogurt, and cheeses are also sources of protein and fat that appeal to cats. Costly meats and fish should be only occasional treats, otherwise a cat may become exclusively addicted to them, so that the diet becomes unbalanced or deficient.

As examples: (1) A diet mostly or entirely of liver may contain such an excess of vitamin A that bone disease results. (2) Dark-meat tuna, either plain or mixed with other nutrients, is a favorite for palatability among cat foods, but should be fed only occasionally. Cats eating it exclusively, or as a substantial part of their diet, may develop a painful inflammation of the fatty tissues of the body due to chemical processes that destroy the vitamin E in the food. Although the tuna cat foods now contain extra supplements of vitamin E and the processors attempt to preserve this vitamin in canning, occasional cats still develop the typical signs of the deficiency (yellow fat disease, steatitis). (3) A diet of muscle meat only may provide an excess of phosphorus and inadequate calcium, resulting in soft and brittle bones (osteoporosis, secondary nutritional hyperparathyroidism). (4) A diet made up exclusively of several kinds of raw fish may result in nervous disorders due to destruction of vitamin B_1 (thiamine).

If a cat will eat only one or two foods such as meat or fish, your veterinarian will prescribe a supplement of vitamins and minerals.

Milk — fresh, canned, or powdered — is an excellent supplementary food, provided it does not cause diarrhea, as it unfortunately does in many cats that lack the enzyme for digesting milk sugar. It is an important source of calcium for breeding and nursing queens (females) and for formation of bone in kittens, which may otherwise need a calcium supplement.

For older cats prone to urinary stone formation or bladder inflammation, especially males, owners should look for cat foods that show the lower range of ash (mineral) content on their labels. Your veterinarian may even advise a specially formulated low-ash prescription diet.

Although few cats consume much fluid when in good health, fresh water should always be available. An increase from little or moderate to conspicuous water consumption may be a sign of serious illness and calls for veterinary attention.

Cats love to chew on bones, but small ones should be taboo, especially hollow bones of fowl, because they may become lodged in the mouth or throat, or splinter and irritate or puncture the wall of the digestive tract.

Cats often scavenge in the trash for string from fish or meat packages, or from scraps of roast. This can do serious or fatal damage if swallowed (see page 91).

Most cats, if fed a varied diet, do not require vitamin or mineral supplements. Exceptions may be breeding females, young kittens, and ill or old animals. Supplements should be given only on a veterinarian's advice because excessive amounts of certain vitamins and minerals are not simply harmless, but may actually produce disease.

In the wild, the big cats live on occasional large meals of prey, but most domestic cats prefer to snack frequently. There is no reason not to indulge this preference as long as the cat's total intake does not make it fat, and provided the weather is not so warm that the food spoils.

There are no rigid guidelines for how much to feed a cat. Follow the suggestions on the cat food labels if you like — you may even weigh portions and count calories if you have the time — but the fundamental principle is: enough to keep an adult cat in good flesh, but not fat. Cats that are growing, unusually active, pregnant, or nursing a litter require proportionally more than the average adult. (Diets for kittens are discussed on page 120.)

Dishes should be low, heavy, and cleaned after each use. If there is more than one cat, or dogs and cats, they may have to be fed separately so the less aggressive get their share.

Many cats like to chew grass. Some cat owners speculate that the cat is instinctively seeking vitamins — veterinarians, that there is an irritation of the digestive tract and the cat eats the grass to evoke vomiting.

GROOMING   Many cats that wash conscientiously with their spiny tongues and manicure their claws by nibbling and chewing manage for a lifetime to keep themselves immaculate without human help. Nonetheless, regular brushing with a suitable cat brush (such as wire bristles set in rubber) reduces shedding, the swallowing of fur, and in longhaired cats the formation of fur mats. If mats are present, these cannot be removed by brushing. One must first slide a coarse, strong, blunt-toothed comb under the mats and tug with repeated gentle pulls to dislodge them. If you are skillful and patient it will rarely be necessary for you to cut the mats away or, worse yet, to have the cat denuded by a mechanical clipper. Cats hate being clipped bare and may even act psychically traumatized. A rambunctious longhair must sometimes be anesthetized at a veterinarian's for grooming. Owners of longhaired show cats comb first with a coarse comb, then a fine comb, and give a final brushing forward to produce an impressive stand-up coat and thick ruff.

CLAWS   The superficial longest layer of the claw is shed periodically as the claw grows, but if a cat does not wear down its claws by outdoor activity or a scratching post indoors, the owner or his veterinarian should trim the tips of the claws. Since the cat's claw is usually unpigmented and almost transparent, it is easy to distinguish the underlying pink-colored "quick" and to avoid bleeding by clipping well ahead of this area. Clawing of rugs and furniture may also be somewhat reduced by clipping the claws or by providing a scratching post, board, or log. This may be bare wood, covered with bark, or upholstered.

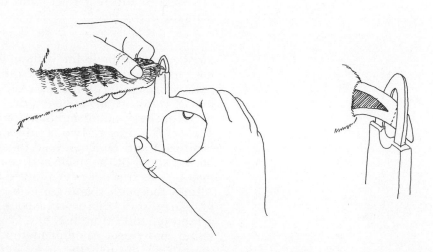

It is essential that cats with extra toes (polydactyl) should be regularly inspected for ingrown and infected claws — a condition that occurs if the extra claws are abnormally jointed to the paw and never get any wear.

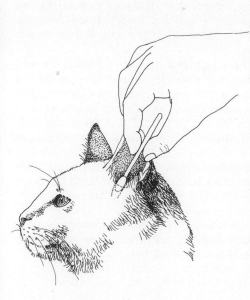

EARS Since as many as 50 percent of all kittens and cats may have ear mites, the ears are of prime concern in maintaining a cat's health. The inside of a healthy ear is pale pink and shiny. Accumulations of dry, dark brown, gritty material deep in the ear canal are usually a sign of mites, pale parasites about the size of the tip of a pin. By crawling about and sucking serum from the lining of the ear canal, mites cause the cat to shake its head and sometimes paw and scratch at its ears so violently that the skin is lacerated and bloody. A magnifying glass or microscope is usually needed for positive demonstration of the presence of mites.

Neglected mite infestations can lead to secondary infection, possible perforation of the eardrum, middle-ear infection, and even fatal meningitis. If one cat in a group is infected, other cats, and also dogs, are almost certainly infected as well.

If your veterinarian diagnoses ear mites, the ears will be given a thorough professional cleaning, and follow-up treatment can be carried out by the owner. A few drops of any bland oil (mineral, cooking) massaged into the ear twice a week for several weeks will suffocate and kill the mites. When the oil has softened and loosened the masses of brown debris, they may be removed by gentle probing with Q-tips. Preparations containing parasiticides are rarely necessary and may be irritating. Flea powder dusted lightly over the cat's body after cleaning destroys any mites that have been scattered from the ears into the fur.

Ear-cleaning stimulates a natural scratch reflex by the hind legs. If your cat is difficult to handle, wrap it tightly in a large bath towel with only its head exposed. Have a helper grasp it firmly, or immobilize it on your own lap between your knees. Taping the forefeet together and the hind feet together with adhesive is still another restraining method (see page 81).

Ear mites invariably parasitize both ears. If a cat has trouble of any sort in one ear only, there could be infection or a growth deep in the ear canal that requires prompt veterinary attention. A few cats suffer intermittently from an itchy bacterial infection characterized by a brown discharge similar to that caused by mites, but it requires quite different treatment.

EYES   Occasional wiping with tissue to remove the matter that accumulates at the inner angle of the eye is all the attention needed by the average cat. Persians often require constant cleaning because the flatness of their faces may cause blockage of the tear ducts into the nose and therefore constant oozing of tears down the face.

BATHING   Most cats go through life without ever having a bath. If a bath must be given, it should be done gently and quietly, and with a minimum of water. Two pails or dishpans, preferably plastic to eliminate frightening noise, filled half full of warm water and set side by side in the bottom of a bathtub can be used for shampooing and then for rinsing. First, protect the cat's eyes against soap with a drop or two of mineral oil or an ointment, such as boric acid or White's A and D. Then hold the cat in the shampooing pan, with one hand on the scruff of the neck, and gently wet and lather with the other. The cat may be less frightened if allowed to rest its forepaws on the edge of the pan. After a thorough soaping use the other receptacle for rinsing. If your cat is unmanageable, there are a couple of other approaches. Stand a window screen on end in the bathtub. Chances are the cat will cling to it while you lather and rinse. Another method is to put the cat in a pillowcase with a drawstring through the hem and tied loosely around the cat's neck, and bathe cat and pillowcase together. Towel the cat thoroughly at once and put it in a warm, draft-free place to dry.

If the cat is merely dirty, shampoo with something mild such as Ivory soap or baby shampoo. If a medicated or parasiticidal material is required, obtain from your veterinarian a preparation that is safe and recommended specifically for cats and use it exactly according to directions.

PROTECTIVE INOCULATIONS   Inoculations against infectious diseases are among the most important things that you do for your cat.

PANLEUKOPENIA. Under ordinary circumstances a healthy mother cat's first milk (colostrum) passes protective antibodies against panleukopenia (cat distemper, infectious enteritis) and perhaps some other diseases as well to her kittens. These antibodies give protection for about six weeks, but when the antibody level drops, the kitten must be inoculated with vaccine that stimulates it to manufacture its own antibodies.

In an environment or time of year when panleukopenia is prevalent, kittens may be vaccinated at six, ten, and sixteen weeks. Some kittens do not receive a vaccination till weaning, at about ten weeks, and may or may not receive another vaccination four to six weeks later, though this is a wise and desirable precaution in case the earlier vaccination did not take. All cats should be revaccinated annually since definitive information about duration of immunity is lacking.

Very rarely, a mother fails to pass antibodies in her colostrum and her kittens may contract panleukopenia soon after birth. Kittens of such mothers must be given antibody-containing antiserum at birth and at three- to four-week intervals till they are of suitable age for vaccination.

If your cat is exposed to another cat with active panleukopenia, consult your veterinarian at once. A booster vaccination or an injection of antiserum may have to be given. Antiserum, because it contains ready-made antibodies, provides immediate protection, whereas several days must elapse before vaccine stimulates production of a protective level of antibody.

UPPER RESPIRATORY INFECTIONS. Vaccines against three of the cold-type infections (upper respiratory infections, URI), are often advised for cats that are to be exhibited, boarded, or hospitalized. For the owner's convenience, they can be given at the same time as the panleukopenia inoculations. Many veterinarians use a combination vaccine that protects against the virus of rhinotracheitis and those of the calici (formerly picorna) group — these being the most widely distributed microbes of upper respiratory infection. Pneumonitis, caused by *Chlamydia psittaci* (alias *Miyagawanella felis*), seems to be a less prevalent infection; a vaccine is available, but it is given less often.

The other germs that may be involved in colds in some cats are of minor importance and no vaccines are available.

RABIES. Rabies vaccination is strongly urged (and in some places is required by law) for all cats that go outdoors. Rabies is endemic in a variety of wild creatures (foxes, skunks, raccoons, rodents, bats) throughout the United States. Since outdoor cats hunt and scrap on their own, an owner rarely knows the perpetrator of the scratches or bites the cat receives. There will be no cause for concern if a cat is vaccinated regularly. And if your cat should bite a human, it would not be considered a likely transmitter of the disease.

Cats should be vaccinated annually with a vaccine licensed specifically as appropriate for use in cats. Even if your cat does not wear its rabies vaccination tag, safeguard the certificate of vaccination in case you should ever need evidence of the fact and date of vaccination. Your veterinarian will advise you about the type and time of the first vaccination.

Be correctly informed, *in advance*, about requirements in any state or country to which you plan to travel with your pet.

optional operations

It has been estimated that as many as 80 million unwanted cats are destroyed each year. Except for breeders of purebreds, conscientious pet owners should not allow their cats to reproduce unless future homes for the kittens are assured.

FEMALE PREGNANCY PREVENTION METHODS

Spaying (ovariohysterectomy), which means removal of both ovaries and uterus, is still and probably will be for the foreseeable future the most dependable, least bothersome, and in the long run the least costly method for preventing reproduction in female cats.

It used to be thought, for no very sound reason, that it was good for a female cat to have one litter. It is now known definitely for dogs and presumptively for cats that even one heat period may greatly increase the risk of breast cancer later in life. A female should therefore be spayed before she ever comes into heat. The first heat is influenced by many factors — age, season of the year, climate, and whether she is an indoor or outdoor cat. Breed may also be a factor. Siamese, for instance, tend to be precocious, enthusiastic, and vocal in the pursuit of sex, while Persians are often low key, sluggish, and late breeders.

Most female cats come into heat between five and seven months of age, but they may not only come into heat but become pregnant as early as four months. For this reason four months might well be considered the best time for spaying. If your cat happens to come into heat and mates before the date set for the surgery, proceed with the spaying on schedule; many a cat is spayed in early pregnancy with absolute safety and no complications. It is preferable, however, not to do the surgery during a heat period because there are sometimes problems with hemorrhaging.

Spaying may also be safely performed at an advanced age, both in cats that have never had kittens and in those that have had many litters.

Far from having any adverse effect on a female's personality or health, spaying eliminates the periods of nervousness, meanness, and bad toilet habits often associated with repeated heats. Physically, the cat is in better condition because she is not worn down intermittently by nursing a litter. Autopsy records suggest that spayed females may well be the longest lived of cats.

Some veterinarians allow a reliable owner to take the cat home the same day; others prefer to keep her for a couple of days to make sure she has fully recovered from anesthesia and has no problem with the incision.

Other methods of pregnancy prevention, suitable only for breeders, include ovulation induced artificially by vaginal stimulation by a veterinarian, causing a cessation of heats for about two months; tubal ligation, which prevents conception but not the heat cycle; and the use of various hormonal drugs, which are of uncertain effect or still in the investigational stage.

MISMATING An unwanted pregnancy in a purebred cat can sometimes be aborted if a veterinarian gives an injection of estrogen on the second or third day and again on the seventh to tenth day after the mismating. This will of course prolong the manifestation of heat and may delay the next heat period. Unwanted pregnancy in mixed-breed cats should be solved by immediate spaying.

NEUTERING OF MALES Castration involves surgical removal of both testicles and is necessary to convert the typical male of the species into a contented and well-mannered house pet. Depending on species, climate, environment, and season, males mature at varying ages. Some male cats exhibit sexual behavior as early as six months, but most mature sexually at nine to twelve months. They are fertile and capable of mating throughout the year. Their active interest is aroused only by females in heat, but once mature their voices become capable of deep, loud masculine yowls, they pace restlessly, and hang about the door ready to dart out. If they succeed they will take their time about coming home, and often with scars of battle. Most obnoxious is the spraying of highly odorous urine on funiture, walls, and even people. Once this starts, castration should be performed at once, lest the spraying become a fixed habit.

Castration is less of an operation than spaying a female since the abdominal cavity does not have to be opened, except in the rare case of cryptorchidism, when only one testicle is in the scrotum and the veterinarian has to explore for the other. Nowadays, castration is always performed with a short-acting anesthetic, and most veterinarians ligate the spermatic cords instead of merely tearing them, to prevent possible postoperative hemorrhage. The cat is almost always discharged the same day.

It will be some days or even several weeks before the calming effect of castration is fully evident. Altered males do not suffer undesirable personality changes, but may tend to gain weight unless their food intake is somewhat reduced.

Vasectomy is of possible use to breeders who might need a male to stimulate female ovulation without conception, but is of little use to pet owners, for the cat pursues females as noisily and enthusiastically as ever and continues to wander, fight, and spray.

DECLAWING This operation (onychectomy) is a last resort if a cat's clawing becomes intolerably destructive to carpets, furniture, or wallpaper. It is often the only alternative to having a cat destroyed. It will not handicap a cat that lives strictly indoors and will not need the claws for climbing or protection.

Removing the claws from the forepaws only is usually sufficient. The brief operation is performed under a short-acting general anesthetic. A sterile toenail clipper or scalpel is used to remove the claw and the tissue from which the claw develops. The skin may or may not be sutured. Snug bandages control hemorrhaging and may often be removed as early as twenty-four hours after surgery. Once in a great while an owner reports that a cat apparently suffers some temporary psychic trauma when it discovers the loss of its claws, becoming anxious and withdrawn and hiding under furniture.

DEVOCALIZATION

Devocalization — ventriculocordectomy — is once in a while performed for the same reason as de-barking in a dog — to make a loudly yowling cat (almost always a Siamese) less disturbing to neighbors. The operation consists of removing a portion of the vocal cords, greatly lessening the sounds that the cat can make.

the home clinic

The safety and success of home pet care depends on the accuracy of observation and common sense with which an owner distinguishes between a problem he can handle — that is, the cause is clear and treatment within his ability — and a condition in which professional help is needed to determine cause and prescribe correct treatment.

If something is amiss with your cat, be sure that you don't just guess at but really know the cause before you think of giving treatment yourself. If you are in any doubt, telephone your veterinarian.

STOCKING
A MEDICINE CABINET

Keep your pet's paraphernalia and medicines in a separate box or chest from that of the human family.

- sturdy rectal thermometer (preferably one with a little glass ring for attaching a string)
- water-base lubricating jelly or Vaseline (the best material for lubricating a thermometer, although skin lotion or cream or any bland oil may be substituted)
- absorbent cotton
- Q-tips
- mineral oil
- curved, blunt-tipped surgical scissors (for trimming fur from wounds, cutting away fur mats, removing bandages)
- gauze sponges
- 2-inch gauze bandage
- 1-inch adhesive tape
- tongue depressors (for simple splinting)
- hydrogen peroxide
- boric acid and White's A and D eye ointments
- boric acid solution
- several plastic medicine droppers

TAKING TEMPERATURE,
HEARTBEAT, AND PULSE

You take a cat's temperature exactly as you would a human infant's. It helps if you have an assistant to immobilize the cat. Shake the thermometer down to its lowest point, then lubricate it well with Vaseline or a lubricating jelly. It should be inserted 2 inches into the cat's rectum and left for two minutes. Cats have a strong, tight circular muscle in the wall of the anus, and you may have to use gentle pressure and manipulation before the cat relaxes enough to allow the thermometer to slide in. Ask your veterinarian to show you how. If you suspect a cat of being ill, taking the temperature is the *first* thing you should do. The temperature normally ranges from about 100° to 102°F. Un-

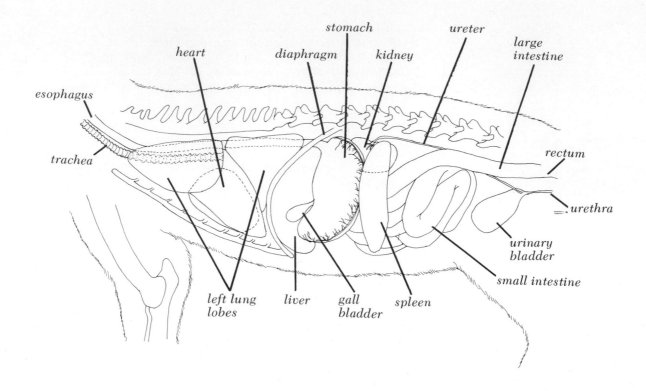

esophagus

trachea

heart

diaphragm

stomach

kidney

ureter

large intestine

rectum

urethra

urinary bladder

small intestine

left lung lobes

liver

gall bladder

spleen

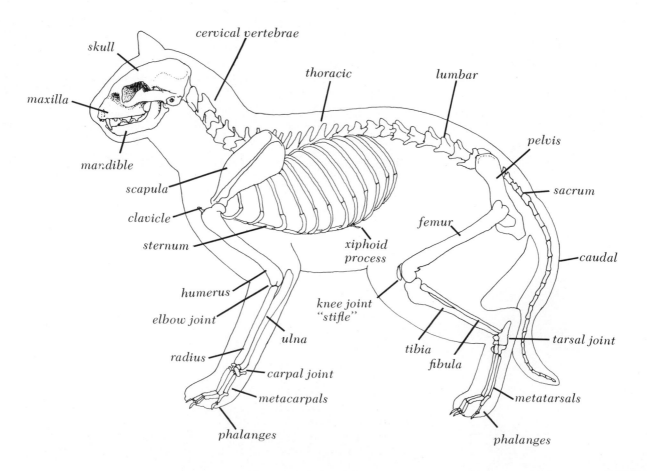

skull

maxilla

mandible

cervical vertebrae

thoracic

lumbar

pelvis

sacrum

caudal

scapula

clavicle

sternum

humerus

elbow joint

radius

ulna

carpal joint

metacarpals

phalanges

xiphoid process

knee joint "stifle"

femur

tibia

fibula

tarsal joint

metatarsals

phalanges

less a cat is very excited or overheated, a fever is a sure sign that it should visit its veterinarian promptly.

A freakish accident that once in a great while accompanies temperature-taking is that the thermometer vanishes completely into the cat! Don't panic. The cat will soon get rid of it. This may be prevented by having a thermometer with a ring, to which a string is attached. A much more serious accident is to have the thermometer break off. This is an emergency requiring your veterinarian's intervention.

Your cat's heartbeat can best be felt if you grasp its chest from below between your thumb and fingers. Move your fingers about until you feel the thump of the heart against the chest wall. In normal cats the heart rate may vary tremendously (100 to 200 beats per minute), depending on the environmental temperature and the mood and state of activity of the cat. During examination in strange surroundings, rates over 200 are common. There may also be certain irregularities in rhythm that are of no serious significance. While it is important to know that the heart of a seriously ill, injured, or comatose cat is actually beating, owners should rarely concern themselves with the heart rate.

The pulse is normally synchronous with the heartbeat and may be felt where the femoral artery on either side of the groin passes to the inner side of the thigh. Considerable experience is required to feel and evaluate the pulse.

GIVING PILLS AND LIQUID MEDICINE, AND FORCE-FEEDING

If you can become adept at medicating your cat, hospitalization for treatment or illness may often be avoided. When your veterinarian prescribes pills, capsules, or liquid medicine, ask for a demonstration of how to give them.

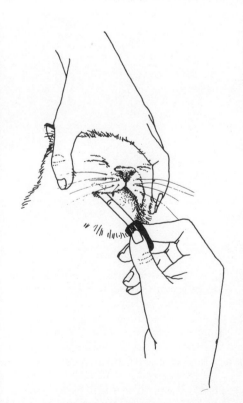

PILLS. Pilling a cat is easiest if the cat is in some kind of corner or on an assistant's lap where it cannot back away from you. If you must perform unassisted, try to time the deed when your cat is asleep in the corner of a sofa or armchair. Rouse it with an affectionate word, then quickly and gently grasp the top of its head with your left hand (if you are right-handed), pressing its mouth open from the sides with your thumb and index finger and keeping the skin of the cat's cheeks between your fingertips and its teeth. As the cat's mouth opens, tilt the head back a little, hold the lower jaw down with your right middle finger, and with your thumb and index finger drop the pill or capsule over the back of the cat's tongue into its throat. Sometimes you may have to give the pill a quick little push with the tip of your index finger or the eraser end of a pencil. Never use any instrument that could injure the cat's throat.

Once the pill is down behind the tongue, close the cat's mouth with your left hand and hold it closed till it swallows. Stay with your cat long enough to be sure it has really swallowed the pill and does not spit it out after your back is turned.

Cats often resist, choke on, or gag up a dry pill or capsule. Lubricating the pill with butter or tasty tuna or sardine oil may make it go down more easily, but it is also more apt to slip out of your grasp as you give it.

LIQUID MEDICINE. This is most safely given with a plastic medicine dropper. Immobilize the cat and hold its head with your left hand as for pilling, but don't force its jaws open or tilt its head back. Introduce the tip of the dropper into the side of the cat's mouth, in the space just behind the fang (canine tooth). Give no more than a few drops at a time and allow the cat to swallow this before giving more. Never give liquid medication with a spoon or bottle. There is danger that the cat may get more into its mouth than it can swallow, and inhale the material. This could lead to an ultimately fatal inhalation pneumonia.

Oral medication in the form of an ointment, jelly, or paste may be squeezed onto a paw to be licked down by the cat or squeezed into the side of the mouth. Most cats relish brewer's yeast powder, and tablets and preparations in which this is used as a base or flavoring may be eaten voluntarily. Sometimes if the taste of the medicine is not disagreeable to the cat, and the cat feels well enough to eat, a finely crushed pill or the powder or liquid content of a capsule can be mixed thoroughly with the cat's food; the owner must watch vigilantly to see that all is consumed.

Despite this range of possibilities, there are a certain few unmanageable cats which will not accept any method of oral medication. Fortunately, your veterinarian can give many medications by injection if necessary.

FORCE-FEEDING. Hand-feeding (force-feeding) is necessary if an ill cat being treated at home is not eating or drinking. In general, liquids or pureed foods are more easily given than solids and contribute to the cat's fluid requirement. Whatever nourishment of this type your veterinarian prescribes can be given in small, frequent feedings with a plastic medicine dropper just as you would administer liquid medicine. Give only as much as a cat can take at one swallow. If you try to get the cat to take a greater quantity than it wants, a fight may ensue and the cat may even vomit what you have worked so hard to get into it. If, as is likely, you are holding the cat in your lap, drape its front and your lap with a towel to keep both of you clean.

Strained baby foods diluted with warm water, milk, corn syrup, or vegetable oil, as well as commercial kitten feeding formulas, are easily given by dropper and provide both essential fluid and nutritious food. For a cat that resists hand-feeding, your veterinarian may give you a highly concentrated, well-balanced jelly-type food that comes in a tube and may be squeezed in small amounts onto your cat's lips or paws, for it to lick down itself.

PROTECTIVE RESTRAINTS　A cat being taken *anywhere* should be transported in a secure, roomy, and well-ventilated carrier that opens from the top for easy removal. A large, thick bath towel inside can provide the cat with "a bit of home" and the veterinarian with a means of restraint. A cloth bag or pillowcase with a drawstring top may also be used for carrying or restraining a cat.

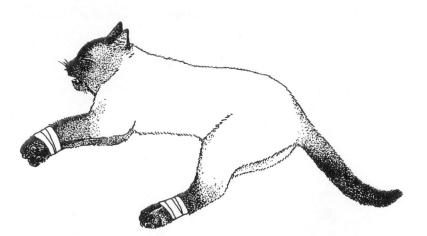

Many cats require a minimum of restraint if handled quietly and gently, but if a cat is nervous or bad-tempered, most parts of the body can be examined or treated while the rest of the cat is firmly swathed and immobilized in a large towel or piece of blanket. Even the head can be loosely covered without danger of suffocation, and a cat that cannot see what is going on tends to lose some of its aggressiveness. A cat that is frightened or angry may often be safely captured if a large towel or blanket is dropped over it before an attempt is made to grasp it.

If a cat is by nature ill-tempered or reacts badly with strangers, an owner

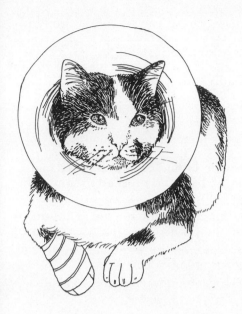

will do well to give warning, so that proper precautionary measures may be taken, including perhaps initial administration of a sedative or tranquilizer. Some cats that become nervous or nauseated when traveling are routinely given a sedative or tranquilizer before departure. Thick gauntlet gloves such as are available for heavy outdoor work may be helpful to an owner or veterinarian in restraining, examining, grooming, or treating a fractious cat.

Muzzling is a virtual impossibility in cats, because of their short faces, and an owner will rarely succeed in getting a muzzle on securely. The best that can be done is to drape the head loosely with something thick enough to protect against biting. To immobilize a cat so that it can be groomed or otherwise worked on, taping the forefeet and hind feet together with adhesive tape is often successful.

Sometimes it is necessary to keep a cat from licking or lacerating itself or from fussing with an incision, bandage, or splint. For this purpose there are many commercial or homemade versions of the so-called Elizabethan collar. The simplest is a circle of heavy cardboard with a hole cut out of the middle that just barely slides down over the cat's head. The width of the collar should be such that the cat can drink and eat without difficulty, but not get at the area of its anatomy that needs protection. Your veterinarian probably can supply you with such a collar, ready-made, of firm light plastic and adjustable in size and in contour from flat to partially cone-shaped. Many a perfectly satisfactory protective collar has been fashioned by cutting a hole in the bottom of a cardboard box.

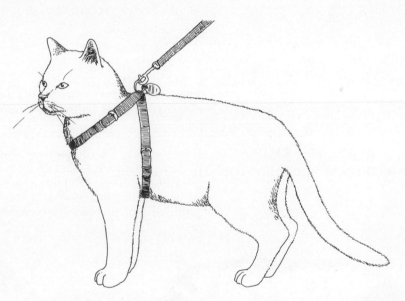

If a cat is allowed out of its carrier during travel, it should wear a harness. The best kind for a cat consists of two adjustable buckled leather straps, one passing around the body in front of the forelegs, the other passing around the body behind the forelegs, the two joined together at the back of the neck by a ring to which a leash and identification tag can be snapped. Such a harness could never result in accidental choking.

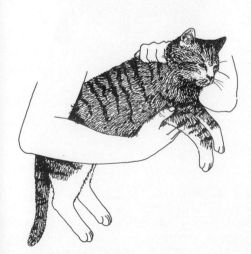

Collars, needed only for outdoor cats, should be as light and narrow as possible so as not to wear down the fur of a cat's neck and should be partially elastic at least. The most satisfactory of all are homemade from a piece of narrow flat or round elastic available by the yard from any sewing counter. A small, strong, metal key ring with identification tag and small bell is snapped around the elastic. The collar itself is usually invisible and inflicts no damage on the fur. (For flea collars, see page 97).

When you carry a cat, drape it over your forearm, with your hand and fingers turned up to support and restrain the foreparts and its body held gently between your arm and body. If the cat is frightened or trying to get away, grasp the skin of the back of the neck firmly with your other hand — but be careful not to pull on the cat's collar in such a way that it feels it's being choked. Never carry a cat by the skin of the back or the neck with the full weight of the body dangling. If necessary a cat can be rolled firmly in a towel or blanket to be carried.

No matter how you, or you and an assistant, are attempting to restrain a cat, if it should turn on you, frantic with rage, fright, or pain, let go of all of it simultaneously! Otherwise you may be badly bitten or clawed.

emergencies and first aid

Signs that an emergency exists and demands immediate action are:

Absent or failing heartbeat — this may be difficult for an alarmed and inexpert owner to detect, so hope for the best and proceed to some other life-saving step such as maintaining respiration

Choking or other severe respiratory difficulty — the tongue and lining of the mouth are likely to be bluish, and the cat may gasp for breath or pant

Massive bleeding — uncommon in cats, except for internal hemorrhage, which is suggested by blanched mucous membranes

Severe anemia, indicated by pale mucous membranes and weakness

Inability to urinate

Excessive vomiting and/or diarrhea

Convulsions

Unconsciousness

Shock

These emergency situations and other hazards to which cats are subject are discussed in the following sections.

HEART MASSAGE AND ARTIFICIAL RESPIRATION

Heart massage and artificial respiration are important emergency measures. Because of the cat's small, narrow chest and the heart's position roughly in the middle of the rib cage you can easily squeeze the area with your fingers (at one-second intervals). If you cannot detect a heartbeat, simply proceed to artificial respiration — which, because of the cat's small-scale anatomy, will

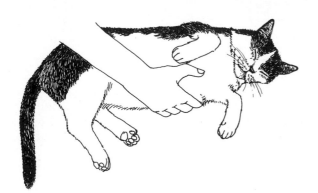

external heart massage

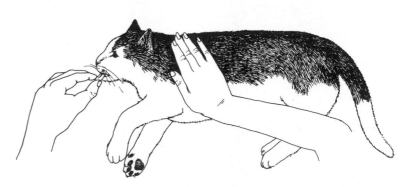

artificial respiration

also provide some stimulation to the heart. With the cat lying on its right side, hold the tip of the tongue out of the mouth with your left hand and press down intermittently and with moderate firmness on the cat's chest with the heel of your right hand — at three- or four-second intervals. The

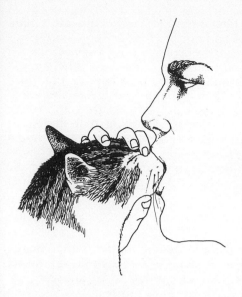

purpose of pulling out the cat's tongue is to assure an open airway. For this you must also swab out any obstructing fluid or blood. Swinging the cat gently by its hind legs two or three times may get rid of obstructing fluid and also stimulate breathing. This of course would be inadvisable if there were serious injuries.

Do not give up your routine of intermittent pressure on the chest until you are convinced that all is over.

Mouth-to-mouth resuscitation can even be attempted as a last resort. First look into the throat and remove any obstructing object or material. Then hold the cat's mouth closed, put your mouth over the muzzle, and breathe forcefully into the cat's nose. If you succeed in inflating the lungs, remove your mouth and allow them to deflate. Repeat the procedure half a dozen times a minute, meantime checking the heartbeat or, if necessary, massaging the heart.

If you see the color of the cat's mouth turning from gray or blue to pink, you will know that your efforts are being rewarded. You may then occasionally interrupt your effort at artificial respiration to see if the cat will breathe by itself.

Make every effort to get to a veterinarian at once.

CIRCULATORY EMERGENCIES

Acute heart attack and stroke are uncommon emergencies in cats, but embolisms of large arteries, originating in chronic heart disease, are among the most spectacular and frequent feline catastrophes. Owing to some abnormality or disease of the heart, which may often be asymptomatic, a clot forms in the heart and breaks loose into the circulation.

Most often the clot lodges at the rear end of the aorta (the main artery of the body), blocking the smaller arteries that branch to the hind legs. The resulting paralysis of the hind legs comes on so suddenly that an injury to the spine is often suspected. The hind feet become cold and the calf muscles hard and painful. The cat evinces great anxiety, restlessness, and distress. If clots lodge farther forward in the aorta, cutting off circulation to the intestine or kidneys, or wedge into major vessels of the lungs, death may come after a very short period of agonizing discomfort.

There is nothing that you can do in this emergency but to get your cat to a veterinarian immediately. The veterinarian's first concern will be to evaluate and treat the basic heart disease. Whether or not to attempt surgery to remove the embolism can be a very difficult decision. If the embolism appears to be blocking only the circulation to the legs, a conservative course of medical treatment is usually adopted.

ACUTE ASTHMA

Many cats are subject to a mild, chronic asthma, but a few suffer violent and acute flare-ups that can threaten them with asphyxiation. There is nothing an owner can do in such an attack but get the cat to a veterinarian for emergency treatment with oxygen and appropriate drugs at the first sign an attack may be starting.

Asthma is discussed in more detail among the Respiratory disorders (see page 108).

SEVERE ANEMIA

Cats are more prone to anemia of various kinds than any other animal. To the owner, a cat may merely seem to be vaguely apathetic, less active, and eating less than usual. Then suddenly it is prostrate, breathing with difficulty if it makes any effort to move. If its toe pads and nose are ordinarily pink, they may now be chalky white — as are the gums and tongue. With as little stress and delay as possible, get your cat to a veterinarian. Without a blood transfusion, the cat may not survive a day.

Anemia will be discussed more fully under Blood (pages 114ff.).

INABILITY TO URINATE

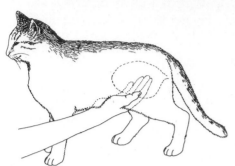

Inability to urinate is a grave and often fatal emergency affecting adult male cats. If your cat keeps licking at his penis and goes to his sanitary pan repeatedly, squatting and straining but producing no urine or only a few drops, he is almost certainly suffering from a urinary (urethral) blockage. Owners experienced with this condition can sometimes confirm it by feeling the tense and overfull urinary bladder like a large lemon in the posterior abdomen. Get your cat to a veterinarian *at once*; a delay can mean death from uremic poisoning. Do *not* make the common mistake of assuming that the cat is suffering from constipation and waste precious time plying him with home treatment for that! (See also Urolithiasis, page 111.)

After an injury, failure or inability to urinate may indicate rupture of the bladder or urethra. It is very important to report this to your veterinarian at once.

CONVULSIONS

Convulsions, or "fits," as they are often called, are a symptom rather than a disease. Causes vary from minor to fatal — to name a few: ear mites, internal parasites, excitement, overheating, unsuitable or spoiled food, injuries, poisoning, epilepsy, and a variety of infectious diseases or tumors.

There should be no attempt to handle or medicate a cat during a seizure, but the owner should note carefully the character of the attack and its duration. Afterward the cat should be kept by itself in a quiet place until it recovers, then taken to a veterinarian for examination as soon as possible. The more accurate descriptive details you can give your veterinarian, the more likely he will be to arrive at some conclusion as to the cause. Sometimes the convulsion is a one-time happening; sometimes they recur in a more or less definite pattern; sometimes they become increasingly frequent and severe.

If the cause is not readily determined and the convulsions continue, a thorough diagnostic study may involve a number of sophisticated and costly procedures, and even then the cause is not always discovered. Fortunately, treatment with an anticonvulsant drug may often be successful without exact determination of the cause.

SHOCK

Shock is most easily recognized by the layman when it is the result of a sudden catastrophe, but it may also be the end event in illness of some duration. The basic phenomena are lowered blood pressure and circulatory failure affecting all organs and tissues. A number of symptoms offer clues. Weakness occurs, progressing to prostration and coma. The temperature usually falls below normal and the extremities are cool. The membranes of the mouth are usually pale pink or grayish. If you press the gum with your finger firmly enough to cause blanching, color will be abnormally slow to return. If there has been severe hemorrhage, the mucous membranes will be white. The heartbeat is weak and rapid, and the femoral pulse is weak and thready, or perhaps cannot be detected at all. The pupils of the eyes are dilated. There may also be thirst, vomiting, and the passing of blood from the intestine. Among causes of shock are severe injury, hemorrhage, extensive burns, prolonged or severe vomiting or diarrhea, dehydration, heat stroke, poisoning, serious infectious diseases, and advanced disease due to a variety of other causes.

The cat should be handled as little as possible, and body heat conserved by some warm covering. Hot water bottles and heating pads are not recommended. In some cases of less severe shock, these conservative measures alone will permit the body's natural defenses to reverse the downhill course. Often, however, sophisticated emergency treatment — including administration of blood and oxygen — is required for survival. Telephone ahead to make sure your veterinarian is available for the emergency, and get there as quickly as possible.

AUTOMOBILE-RELATED
INJURIES

Automobiles present many hazards. In addition to the commonest — being hit or run over — a cat may investigate an open car door or trunk, curl up to nap, and awaken far from its frantic owners. Some cats like to perch invisibly on top of a tire under a fender. Others, seeking warmth in winter, climb up into the motor and are seriously mangled or killed by the fan belt when the car is started by its unknowing driver.

The ethylene glycol antifreeze, such as Prestone and Xerex, put into radiators each fall is a special hazard to cats, which relish its taste and will lap up the least little puddle on a driveway or garage floor. A small amount leads to almost certain death.

For antifreeze poisoning, ethyl alcohol is the only antidote — and it must be given, preferably intravenously, within a few hours of the swallowing of the poison. If your animal definitely has swallowed antifreeze and emergency veterinary attention is not available, give it repeated small amounts of vodka (preferred because tasteless) in milk (1 teaspoonful of 80 proof for an 8 to 10 pound cat) orally every six hours for two days or until you can reach your veterinarian.

Automobile injuries are the commonest emergency involving outdoor cats. Many cats are killed outright — sometimes with no marks on their bodies because the injury was to internal organs; but an apparently dead animal lying in the road is sometimes only temporarily stunned and could be saved.

While lacerations and broken bones are often the eye-catching and horribly apparent effects, less obvious internal injuries may be more serious. Any severe abnormality in breathing could indicate acute and life-threatening injury to the respiratory tract or a tear in the diaphragm, the muscular partition that separates the organs of the chest from those of the abdomen. Bleeding from the nose is a less grave sign than the coughing up of bloody foam that suggests damage to a lung.

Extreme weakness and paleness of the mucous membranes and unpigmented skin of ears or toes may indicate a rupture of the liver or spleen that could lead to death unless the animal receives a prompt blood transfusion.

Two types of automobile injury to which cats seem especially prone are injuries to the head and rump.

HEAD INJURIES. A blow to the head frequently forces an eye from its socket and damages it so greatly that removal is necessary. Fractures at the front center line of union between the two sides of the upper jaw (maxilla) or of the lower jaw (mandible) are frequent and, happily, can usually be easily repaired. Although there are few sights as pitiful as an animal that has been hit in the head, a cat may make a surprisingly rapid comeback, often with no more than a broken tooth or two as a reminder of the disaster.

RUMP INJURIES. Contusions to the rump can have less obvious but nonetheless serious consequences. Aside from extreme tenderness of the area, the two chief clues are a dangling, paralyzed tail and perhaps also a paralyzed urinary bladder. A radiograph may show damage to lumbar vertebrae or pelvis, but the crucial point is that there has been sufficient contusion to the spinal cord so that the nervous mechanism involved in emptying the bladder has been damaged.

Your veterinarian will be in no rush to amputate a paralyzed tail, because the paralysis may be gone within a few days — or, if not, the tail can be removed later. The important thing is catheterization or gentle manual pressure on the urinary bladder, to avoid permanent stretching while nature has time to attempt repair of the nervous tissue. This healing process may take weeks or months. Many owners have not the patience nor the very considerable financial resources for the care involved and may reluctantly decide to have the cat destroyed.

Other common injuries inflicted by a blow to the rump are fractures of the pelvis, and dislocations and fractures of the hip (see Bone and Joint Injuries, page 88).

For the tiny, inexperienced kitten, the greatest danger is of being accidentally stepped on and suffering crush injuries.

Owners often confuse the effects of any injury to a limb with the swelling arising from an infected bite wound. Since the two conditions should be treated quite differently, a veterinarian's opinion should be sought.

If an injured animal is unable to move its hind legs, or worse yet, lies on its side with all four legs either rigidly or limply paralyzed, it may have suffered a fracture of the spinal column or a vertebral dislocation so severe that the spinal cord has been seriously damaged or even severed. (See Bone and Joint Injuries, page 88.)

WOUNDS AND BANDAGING

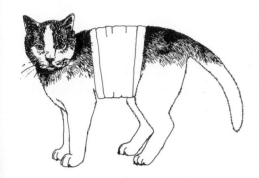

Wounds may be slight or major. Among the more serious injuries are those inflicted when a cat is mauled by a dog. The dog often grasps the cat on either side of the spinal column, puncturing the lungs or lacerating the kidneys. Despite the seriousness of these internal injuries, the skin is sometimes not even broken. Whether or not injuries are obvious, a cat should be examined at once by a veterinarian.

The skin of the cat lends itself well to repair of extensive wounds, because it can be easily moved and stretched to cover large defects or to form flaps and grafts.

The cat owner will only occasionally need to apply bandages to halt bleeding and prevent further exposure to infection until veterinary treatment can be obtained.

Cats can be difficult to bandage. Except for a very few points of firm attachment, they seem to be "walking around loose in their skin," and they shake off or wriggle out of most amateur bandages with the ease of Houdini.

With good assistance and a cooperative cat, a dressing of gauze pad, a layer of cotton, and 2-inch gauze bandage can usually be successfully applied around the neck or body. Care must be taken that it is not so tight that it interferes with comfortable breathing. Final strips of adhesive tape applied partly to the bandage and partly to adjacent fur will usually keep the dressing in place.

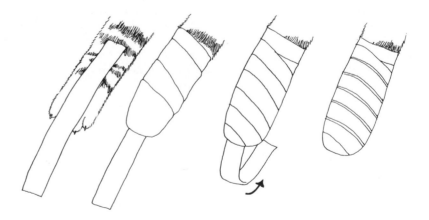

Bandaging of limbs or tail requires resourcefulness with an adhesive tape anchor. Suppose the back of a cat's left forepaw has been lacerated. The cat is held down on its right side by an assistant, only the left foreleg being left free. After the proper treatment of the wound (see below), a strip of 1-inch tape twice as long as the foreleg is applied to the fur of the front of the leg, the rest being left for the moment to dangle. Whatever dressing is required is then applied on a gauze sponge to the wounded area on the back of the leg, and a thin layer of cotton is wrapped around the leg over the strip of tape. Spiral bandaging with gauze is then started from the foot up, not so

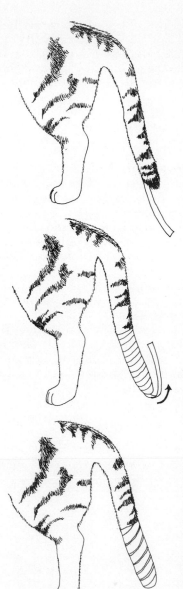

tightly as to impair circulation. After one layer of bandage has been applied, the dangling free end of adhesive tape is folded back up on the gauze bandage along the back of the leg and pressed on firmly so that it adheres to the gauze. Bandaging is then continued back down around the leg over the tape.

If the procedure has been done correctly, the strip of tape has secured the dressing to the fur of the leg so that it will not come off even though the bandage is not dangerously tight. The outside of the dressing is protected by a single layer of 1-inch adhesive tape applied in spiral fashion from the paw up and overlapping about half an inch onto the fur at the top.

The dressing will "breathe" better if an ⅛-inch space is left between the edges of the spiraled tape. Resist the temptation to keep adding layers of tape.

The same technique of first anchoring a strip of tape to fur may be used for bandaging the hind leg. An extra advantage in bandaging the hind leg is the angle formed by the heel (hock) joint. Bandage extended above this angle helps in keeping the dressing in place but must not be too tightly applied.

Bandaging a tail involves the same procedures as the bandaging of a limb — adhesive tape anchor, then gauze bandage wound around, folding the adhesive up onto the bandage, winding the bandage back down the tail.

Because of the cat's thick coat, you will be unaware of many wounds — especially tiny punctures, which may be the most serious — until some secondary effect brings them to your attention. Unless a wound is so obviously serious that it requires immediate professional attention, do some preliminary investigation yourself. This takes the form of scissoring away the fur from the area to see what has happened and how extensive the damage is.

Many a wound is so small that it does not require suturing. What is more, if the wound is more than a few hours old, it has been subjected to abundant bacterial contamination and may heal better as an open wound. Remove all fur, wash the wound with mild soap and water, and apply an antiseptic, such as hydrogen peroxide. Keep the wound clean, and apply the antiseptic daily till a scab forms.

BITE WOUNDS. The puncture wounds inflicted by the bites of other cats can have many possible complications. If your previously intact cat returns limping from an evening stroll or night on the town, your first move should be to take its temperature. If the temperature is elevated, start looking for a bite wound. If you run your fingers through the fur over the ailing part, you may find some loose tufts of fur or dried blood. Feel also for tenderness and swelling. If you find any such clues, scissor the fur away and look for puncture marks. Keep searching; you will often find four or more.

Cat bites are puncture wounds that seal over rapidly, trapping bacteria from the assailant's teeth. Almost invariably these wounds become infected. The result may be a diffuse, ill-defined swelling known as "cellulitis," or may be concentrated into an abscess, which in two or three days will "point up" into a soft-centered, thin-skinned swelling.

Either type of infection will ultimately break down spontaneously and discharge pus. With a cat's licking, such an area sometimes heals itself. Often, however, infection recurs at the site, and bacteria circulating in the blood may disseminate infection to other parts of the body — heart, liver, lungs, kidneys, brain. Bite wounds should therefore have prompt veterinary attention — liberal surgical drainage, together with administration of a broad-spectrum antibiotic. Stubborn, recurring infections may even require bacterial culturing of the pus and sensitivity testing to identify the organisms and determine the most effective antibiotic.

For wounds that are caused by foreign bodies — a splinter of wood or glass, or a fishhook — detection and removal of the foreign object usually require a veterinarian's attention. The damage done by gunshot varies greatly. Lodging in the spinal cord, it may cause paralysis, but in soft tissues may do little harm and is sometimes discovered only accidentally when a cat is radiographed for some other reason.

BONE AND JOINT INJURIES

Sprains and dislocations of joints or fractures of bones can rarely be differentiated by the owner. Careful palpation and radiographs, often under anesthesia, are required. Because cats naturally favor an injured part and because their small size puts less stress on a damaged bone or joint, repair is often easier and faster than in the dog. They also tolerate splinting and immobilization more patiently.

Only when there is severe deformity, displacement, mobility, or laceration at the fracture site, may splinting be necessary at home. Otherwise, the cat itself will carefully protect the injured leg until it can be treated by a veterinarian.

Fractures of the pelvis vary in severity. If they are of a severe, crushing type, and knit without proper realignment, a cat could later have difficulty in passing stool or giving birth to kittens. Some pelvic fractures heal simply with rest; others require orthopedic procedures.

Dislocations and fractures of the hip are also frequent and may be difficult to differentiate without a radiograph. Many a cat, with only cage rest, and by keeping weight off the leg on the affected side, has formed a "false" joint that eventually functions without even a limp.

Do not attempt to handle or move an animal that is unable to move its hind legs, or that lies on its side with all four legs unable to move — it may have a spine fracture or dislocation, endangering the spinal cord — until you can move it without aggravating the damage already done. Some rigid, thin, flat object (thick cardboard, screen, plywood, cookie sheet) should be laid down behind the cat's back, and the animal then pulled gently onto the flat surface by the loose skin over its backbone. If nothing better is available, a folded newspaper or coat may serve as a stretcher.

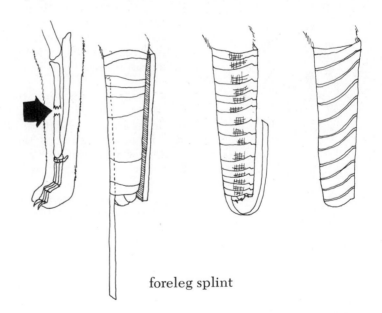

foreleg splint

SPLINTS. Splinting forelegs and hind legs requires the same type of adhesive tape anchoring and bandaging described above, but a thicker layer of cotton padding before the splint is applied. A splint for a fracture below the elbow or heel could be a tongue depressor trimmed to toe-to-elbow or toe-to-heel length, bandaged firmly with the splint between the cotton and gauze layers. For a fracture above the heel (that is, a fracture of the tibia) an angled splint can be cut from heavy cardboard or fashioned by taping together two suitable lengths of tongue depressor. A splint of this type is applied to the outer side of the leg.

For fractures higher in the limbs (humerus, femur) than those just mentioned, amateur attempts at temporary splinting could do more harm than good, and a veterinarian's help should be sought as soon as possible.

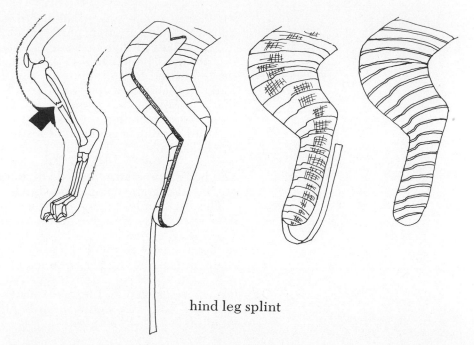

hind leg splint

In general, it can't be overemphasized that a bandage or splint ineptly applied can easily do more harm than good. Many an amateur splint is laboriously applied to a supposed fracture site, only to have the veterinarian discover that the site of trouble is actually elsewhere and may not even be a fracture at all. Very often an owner mistakenly diagnoses a painful swollen area of limb as a fracture site, when there is actually an infected and abscessed bite wound. For this, bandaging and splinting could conceivably end in gangrene and death, when what is actually needed is open drainage of the abscessed area and an antibiotic.

BURNS

Burns that are severe and extensive result when grease or some other hot material is accidentally spilled or overturned on a cat. The cat's thick coat is to some extent a protection, and the owner may not actually be aware of the extent of the damage until the surface of the skin sloughs off together with the fur.

Only a very small burn should be treated by the owner — with immediate cutting away of the fur and application of cold water or ice. This may be followed with a soothing preparation such as White's A and D ointment or Vaseline. Occasionally a cat jumps onto a hot surface or material. Such burns to the foot pads are first treated for twenty minutes with cold water or ice compresses, than gently bandaged with Vaseline or an antibiotic ointment.

Burns involving 10 or 15 percent of the body surface may have such a poor prognosis that it is kinder to destroy the animal at once than to attempt treatment.

Severe burns that are very slow to heal may be inflicted on the mouth from the chewing of electric wires and may even result in electric shock. If breathing ceases altogether, give artificial respiration. Respiratory difficulty may develop from accumulated fluid in the lungs. In any case, veterinary attention is needed.

EXTREME HEAT AND COLD

HEAT STROKE. Cats instinctively move out of the sun as soon as they become uncomfortably warm, and in hot weather rest quietly in the coolest place they can find.

Practically all cases of heat stroke in cats result from confinement in hot weather in a poorly ventilated carrier or automobile. Unless in an air-conditioned vehicle, any transportation of cats should be avoided in hot weather.

There must always be some circulation of air in an un-air-conditioned car. If a pet must be left in a parked car, the windows should be slightly down, shade assured for the duration of the driver's absence, and a drink of fresh water available. Owners who have forgotten that when the sun moves, the shade moves too, have returned to find a dead pet. Cats have relatively less tongue area than dogs for evaporation, so gain less relief from panting.

Rapid panting, gasping, and restlessness are the warning signs of impending heat stroke. As the cat's temperature rises above normal, the mucous membranes turn bluish, and the cat becomes prostrate and then comatose. The body temperature may go higher than the thermometer can read (107° to 109°F.), doing grave damage to the heart and brain.

The cat should be moved to a cool place and soaked continuously with cold water. The skin and limbs should be rubbed to stimulate circulation. The rectal temperature must be checked frequently, the objective being to reduce it below 103°F. Even after being brought down to normal, it may rise again, unless cooling has been maintained.

An episode of severe heat prostration is best treated at a veterinary hospital, where oxygen and intravenous fluids may be administered if necessary, and the body temperature and other vital signs can be continuously monitored.

FROSTBITE. Cats can withstand cold to an extraordinary degree. If accidentally left out in bitter weather, they huddle down or take whatever cover they can find, and are usually no worse for the experience. Rarely, the tips of the ears are frostbitten: the edges slough, leaving a thickened, rounded rim of scar tissue. Treatment is neither required nor effective.

BITES   Cat bites are discussed under Bite Wounds (page 87).

FROM INSECTS. Insect bites are not infrequent in cats, because they are attracted to, capture, play with, and swallow any bug that moves, and sooner or later receive a bee or wasp sting. Usually you will know or suspect this when your cat appears pawing at an impressively swollen face, mouth, or eyelid. The swelling usually subsides without treatment in a few hours. If the reaction is severe enough to cause difficulty in breathing, owing to swelling around the throat, get the cat to a veterinarian at once.

SNAKEBITES. If you see your cat bitten by a snake, it is helpful to your veterinarian if you have been able to identify the snake. The bites of non-poisonous snakes are usually U-shaped and look like scratches. While they do not produce signs of serious poisoning, a variety of bacteria are present in snakes' mouths, and your veterinarian will probably give systemic antibiotics and tetanus antitoxin.

In areas where pet animals are exposed to the bites of poisonous snakes, both owners and veterinarians are familiar with and alert for the typical signs — sudden and very painful swelling and tiny skin hemorrhages. Two fang marks can usually be found if the fur is trimmed away. Systemic signs that may develop quickly are unsteadiness or incoordination, convulsions, vomiting, bleeding from the nose and anus, blood in the urine, subnormal temperatures, and coma.

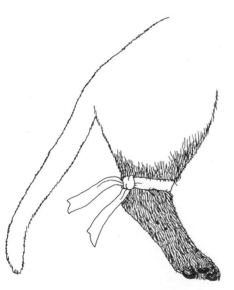

If you cannot get the cat to a veterinarian immediately and the snakebite was on the leg, tie a flat bandlike tourniquet, for example, a necktie, sock, or folded handkerchief, around the limb between the bitten area and the heart. There should be room for a finger to be slipped under the tourniquet, so that arterial circulation is not impeded but the flow of venous blood and lymph is prevented from spreading venom through the body.

The tourniquet may be left in place for two hours, by which time the cat should have reached a veterinarian for surgical treatment of the bite, injection of antivenin, and other symptomatic and supportive treatment to combat shock and the various effects of the poisoning.

Attempting to suck poison from the fang wound is not advised.

FOREIGN OBJECTS

IN THE EYE. A foreign body in the eye causes squinting, pawing at the eye, and inflammation of the conjunctiva. If it is one that the owner can see, it can perhaps be removed by flushing the eye with boric acid solution by means of a plastic medicine dropper, or by gentle manipulation of a moistened Q-tip.

Some foreign bodies such as wood splinters lodge in or penetrate the cornea, the glassy surface layer of the eyeball. Others may be present but are hidden by the lids. If flushing the eye with boric acid solution and then squeezing a small amount of White's A and D or boric acid eye ointment between the lids does not bring relief, take your cat to the veterinarian.

IN THE EAR. A foreign body in the ear makes a cat shake its head and paw at the ear. If you see what you believe to be a foreign object, possibly a tick or plant awn, try to remove it with a pair of small tweezers. If it is lodged deep in the ear canal, your veterinarian may need to give a local or general anesthetic to do the job.

IN THE MOUTH. Foreign bodies in the mouth cause a cat to paw at its mouth, work its jaws, and salivate. If an object is lodged in the tissues for any length of time the cat will drool a foul-smelling, blood-tinged slime. Small slivers of chicken bone, fish bone (especially small vertebrae), wads of fur twisted around the teeth, needles, and fishhooks are common.

Most dangerous and most often undetected is string or heavy thread that becomes looped around the underside of the tongue, the two ends then being swallowed. This can be seen only if the mouth is opened wide and the tongue is pushed well aside with the eraser end of a pencil. If the string does not easily pull out from under the tongue, the reason may be that a needle or knot on one end is lodged firmly somewhere in the digestive tract; persistent pulling could do great harm.

Unless your cat is cooperative and the foreign object is easily seen and removed, your veterinarian will have to do the job. Fishhooks, for instance, cannot be pulled back out but must be pushed on through the cheek or tongue. Often foreign bodies have disappeared into the soft tissues and may have to be searched for with a probe or radiograph. General anesthesia is frequently required.

IN THE THROAT. A foreign body in the throat can constitute an immediate life-and-death emergency, for if it lodges at the larynx, it impedes or cuts off the flow of air in and out of the windpipe. Usually the choking cat is in such distress that you have little chance for a good look down the throat, let alone grasping and removing the object. If the flow of air is completely cut off, the cat will struggle violently and asphyxiate. If this should occur before you can get to the nearest veterinarian, there is one final chance of a rescue: when the cat stops struggling and goes limp, apparently dead, quickly poke your index finger down into the throat to try to dislodge and remove the object, which is most often a small chunk of bone. If you are lucky enough to do so, chances are the heart is still beating, and artificial respiration may well get the cat breathing again (see page 82). Quick-acting veterinarians have succeeded in this maneuver, and there is no reason why a deft and desperate layman should not try.

A final caution: when feeling the outside of a cat's throat, do not mistake its rather large Adam's apple (larynx) for a foreign body!

ON THE SKIN. For removal of materials that may contaminate the skin or fur, see Poisoning (below). If a cat is sprayed by a skunk, soak the fur thoroughly with tomato juice for about ten minutes, then bathe with soap and water.

POISONING BY CHEMICALS, DRUGS, AND PLANTS

Poisons may be swallowed, inhaled, or absorbed through the skin. Poisoning occurs most often in cats that go out-of-doors and come in contact with a variety of substances that may not be known to the owner — plants, pesticides, herbicides, paint, and many other industrial chemicals. (See the chart for dogs, page 40.) Certain poisons that were once in common use as pesticides — strychnine and thallium, to mention only two — are now outlawed for general use, but many of the new pesticides and weed-killers, although labeled safe for pets, may under certain conditions prove poisonous. Perhaps the two poisonings most often recognized in dogs and cats at present are from lead and antifreeze, both of which may cause sudden and violent nervous signs as well as other manifestations of a less acute character. If your cat has swallowed antifreeze, see Automobile-Related Injuries, page 85.

Lead poisoning is acquired over a considerable period of time, most often from swallowing chips of old lead paint. There are no home antidotes or treatment.

A cat can sometimes be made to vomit up a poisonous substance if you administer a tablespoonful of a mixture of equal parts of hydrogen peroxide and water. If the poison is corrosive, do *not* try to stimulate vomiting — try to give the cat milk with a dropper, to help protect against the poison. It is far better to take the cat at once to a veterinarian, with all the information you have, including if possible the suspected poisonous material, and let the veterinarian give appropriate treatment.

If your cat swallows or comes in contact with some material that you suspect but do not know for certain to be poisonous, telephone your veterinarian or the nearest poison control center listed in your telephone directory, and follow the advice that you are given.

Nibbling on plants is a common activity with cats — housebound cats often substitute house plants. Unfortunately, many plants, both indoor and outdoor, are harmful, causing a variety of signs of illness. Salivation, vomiting, and diarrhea are typical effects of plants that irritate the digestive tract. Others may cause incoordination, blindness, convulsions, or coma. Common toxic plants include philodendron, dumbcane, elephant ear, Jerusalem cherry, poinsettia, ivy, mistletoe, hydrangea, laurel, rhododendron, boxwood, and oleander. (See also the table of plants poisonous to dogs, page 40.) If your cat proves to be a plant eater, you may have to limit yourself to such safe standbys as inch plant, spider plant, and Swedish ivy. Arboretums, botanical gardens, and university botany departments can furnish you with pamphlets on poisonous plants, their effects, and treatment.

Cats are more sensitive than many other species to the toxic effects of a variety of remedies and chemicals that are in common household and industrial use. The most important of these is aspirin, a very small amount of which can quickly kill a cat. There are virtually no indications for aspirin in cats; never use it except under a veterinarian's supervision. A number of other pain-killing drugs (for instance Anacin, Empirin, Tylenol) are chemically similar to aspirin and should not be used either.

Morphine and its derivatives may excite rather than calm a cat. Paregoric, a home remedy often used by humans for digestive upsets, is a morphine derivative and should never be given to a cat. Iodine and mercury-containing drugs also affect cats unfavorably and must be used with caution.

Phenol and related coal-tar derivatives are in common use as antiseptics, disinfectants, and preservatives. Among these are Lysol, naphthol, sylphonaphthol, hexachlorophene, hexylresorcinol, creosote, creolin, and tannic acid. Cats are unusually sensitive to these chemicals. They are most often poisoned when one is applied to the skin in treatment or by accidental contamination. The skin and fur should be flushed with warm water for at least fifteen minutes. If the material has been taken internally, milk and castor oil

(1 teaspoonful) should be given by mouth to inhibit absorption of the poison.

Many of the toxic contaminants that cats get into (paint, varnish, tar, creosote, oil, asphalt, kerosene) are sticky, oily, or have dried (paint). Chemicals such as gasoline, turpentine, and paint thinner are themselves poisonous and should never be used for removal. Sometimes contaminated fur can be cut off. Otherwise, massage mineral oil thoroughly into the contaminated skin and fur to loosen the material, then bathe well once or twice with a mild soap and warm water, and finally rinse several times. Since the material may well have been licked by the cat or absorbed by the skin, advice should be sought from a veterinarian or poison information center as to whether oral or other treatment is needed.

If you think your cat has been poisoned by any of these substances, in addition to first aid you can administer, be sure to call your veterinarian.

OTHER ENVIRONMENTAL HAZARDS

Innumerable common small household objects can be fascinating toys but dangerous if swallowed: threaded needles, elastic bands, buttons, nursing bottle nipples, marbles, paper clips, safety pins, wads of cellophane or foil, bits of crayon, Christmas tree ornaments.

Because of their curiosity cats can precipitate their households into panic by vanishing, getting shut into closets, attics, cellars, cupboards, and bureau drawers. Kitchens, cars, and laundries are often disaster areas. Sniffing something tempting on a stove, a cat may jump up and get its feet badly burned. Cats get shut in refrigerators, dishwashers, clothes washers, or clothes driers. They even find their way into crawl spaces, chimneys, furnaces, and elevator shafts.

Apartment cats are subject to what city veterinarians call the "high-rise syndrome," falling from unscreened windows or balconies. Outdoor cats scale trees from which they have not yet acquired the know-how to back down, and get built into buildings and embedded in freshly poured asphalt or concrete.

Occasionally cats suffer from a compulsion to chew on broom straw. Once in a while the stomach becomes so crammed that the straw must be removed surgically. Often fragments of straw perforate the intestinal wall and cause fatal peritonitis. In addition, eating broom straw may cause convulsions, possibly due to poisoning by material used in processing the straw. When not in use, brooms and brushes should be kept in tightly closed closets; as added precautions, the broom should be stood upside down, and brushes hung from a high hook.

parasites

The conscientious owner should be on the alert for signs of parasitism and follow a veterinarian's recommendations for routine examinations. In general, the problem will be far less if a cat lives strictly indoors.

The most frequently recognized internal parasites of cats are tapeworms, roundworms, and hookworms, all of which infest the small intestine and, if numerous, cause poor growth, weight loss, and often diarrhea and vomiting. Veterinarians can provide appropriate medication for all three.

TAPEWORMS

Tapeworms are acquired by swallowing fleas, or eating rodents or, less often, raw freshwater fish. They are flat, segmented worms many inches long. The sucking head is attached to the inner surface of the cat's intestine, but segments break off and appear in the cat's droppings or on the fur about the anus as tiny white moving segments about half an inch long. When exposed to the air the segments dry and contract till they resemble grains of rice. Microscopic examination of stool cannot be counted on to reveal the presence of tapeworm eggs.

The most important preventive measure is to keep cats and their environment free of fleas (see Fleas, page 97). Your veterinarian may advise that cats that regularly hunt and eat rodents should receive routine treatment whether or not segments are seen in their droppings.

ROUNDWORMS   Roundworms (ascarids) are slender, stringlike worms, yellowish white, from one to several inches long. They are sometimes seen curled up in vomitus or droppings, but are most often diagnosed by the presence of typical eggs in a sample of stool examined with a microscope. Heavy infestations, especially in kittens, cause potbellies, vomiting, diarrhea, and weight loss.

Ascarids may be acquired in several ways. Kittens swallow immature worms in an infected mother's milk. Older cats are infected by eating ripened eggs from other cats' droppings, or by preying on mice, which may be carriers. Medication may have to be given several times at suitable intervals before ascarids are entirely eliminated; repeated fecal examinations are advisable.

HOOKWORMS   Hookworms have a similar appearance to ascarids but are so small that they would be hard to see — in any case, they usually remain firmly attached to the wall of the intestine, where they may suck so much blood that the host becomes severely anemic and weak. They are most likely to cause serious trouble or death in very young animals and in the warmer areas that favor transmission. With proper warmth and moisture, tiny larval worms hatch from the eggs in stool and either penetrate the host's skin to reach the intestine eventually or are swallowed directly. Mice may perhaps serve as carriers.

Hookworm infestation is diagnosed by identification of typical eggs in feces obtained as fresh as possible, taken at once for veterinary examination, or refrigerated if delay is unavoidable.

Droppings should be removed and litter pans cleaned every day. Instances of human skin infection ("creeping eruption") have occurred when litter pans were left neglected in warm houses.

LESS COMMON PARASITES   LUNGWORMS (Aelurostrongylus). These parasitize the lung tissue itself and may cause coughing, wasting, severe pneumonia, and even death. They are acquired from eating carriers, among which are snails, slugs, and mice. The parasitism is diagnosed by microscopic finding of typical larval worms or rarely eggs in feces or sputum. Treatment is moderately successful.

Another type of worm, *Capillaria aerophila*, lives principally in the windpipe and larger airways of the lung. It usually causes no severe symptoms other than coughing, which is fortunate, because no effective treatment is known. Cats are infected by swallowing eggs from the stool of infected cats or foxes. Since the eggs of this parasite — coughed up, swallowed, and then eliminated in the stool — closely resemble those of the whipworm of dogs, frequent erroneous diagnoses have been made of whipworm in cats, although there is as yet no solid scientific evidence that the canine parasite infests cats.

TRICHINOSIS. Cats foraging in garbage and eating uncooked pork scraps, or preying on rodents that have done so, from time to time become infected with trichina larvae, but the parasitism, characterized initially by severe bloody diarrhea, adult parasites in stool, and migrating larvae, is rarely recognized except with special diagnostic procedures. Treatment depends on the severity of symptoms.

HEARTWORM. This is still almost entirely a disease of dogs, but is reported in cats (as well as man) with increasing frequency. Most infections in cats are recognized only at autopsy, after sudden unexpected death, but in a few cases the telltale larvae have been found in the blood of living cats, and treatment was given with apparent success. Exposure to mosquitoes, which carry this parasite, can be minimized by keeping cats indoors after dusk.

EYEWORM. *Thelazia californiensis*, the eyeworm, appears in wooded areas of certain western states. How it is acquired is uncertain. The worm, which is slender and may be from ½- to ¾-inch long, is found under the nictitating membrane ("third eyelid"). Its presence is irritating, and the cat's pawing at its eye inflames the conjunctiva and lacerates the cornea. After topical anesthesia, your veterinarian will remove the worm with a cotton-tipped applicator stick or forceps.

FLUKES (trematodes). These are tiny, flat, leaf-shaped worms. Infestation is acquired when an animal eats intermediate hosts such as snails, shellfish, and fish. The flukes most often reported to cause disease are those infesting the lung, liver, or pancreas. Characteristic fluke eggs may be found in sputum or feces. There has been little experience with treatment.

PROTOZOANS   Protozoans are one-celled organisms, visible only microscopically. The most important disease producers in cats are coccidia and toxoplasma.

COCCIDIA. Kittens or young cats kept in large groups in catteries or pet shops are the most likely to be parasitized. The infection arises from contamination of the environment by cat or dog feces containing infective eggs (oocysts). When swallowed, these undergo further development in the lining cells of the intestine, which then rupture, the stool containing blood as well as characteristic oocysts. Lack of appetite, diarrhea, and weight loss may lead to severe illness and occasionally death.

This parasitism can be diagnosed only by microscopic examination of stool. Although the infection is spontaneously eliminated with time, several drugs are used in treatment — and for a seriously ill cat, antidiarrheal medication and injectable fluids to correct dehydration and chemical imbalances. Reinfection can be prevented, if stringent sanitation is practiced — daily changing of litter, and cleaning of litter pans, cages, and floors.

TOXOPLASMA. This protozoan belongs to the same general group of parasites as the coccidia but differs in many ways. It infects a high proportion of warm-blooded animals and man worldwide but rarely causes illness. When illness does occur, it is usually so mild that it is not diagnosed, only severe and fatal cases being identified.

Although so many creatures can be infected, domestic and some wild cats seem to be the only species that complete the parasite's life cycle by transmitting infectious organisms (oocysts) in their stool. Cats, and other animals as well, are infected by swallowing oocysts from cat feces, by preying on birds and rodents infected the same way, and by eating uncooked or undercooked infected meat (mutton, pork, beef, fowl) and eggs. Roaches, flies, and other insects contaminated by contact with cat feces are also a possible source of infection.

Although 40 to 60 percent of cats (especially strays) become infected at some time, few ever become ill but simply shed oocysts in their stool. Shedding begins between three and forty days after infection, depending on how the infection was acquired, and continues for about ten to fourteen days. The oocysts are not infectious when shed, but become so within one to four days, depending on environment, temperature, and moisture. Under certain conditions oocysts may remain infective in contaminated soil for over a year.

Diagnosis. Diagnosis of infection is by (1) microscopic examination of feces, (2) inoculation of feces or other suspect tissue or body fluid into mice, (3) blood testing for antibody, and (4) microscopic demonstration of toxoplasma forms other than oocysts in body fluids and tissues obtained at biopsy or autopsy.

Because cats rarely become ill and discharge oocysts so briefly, veterinarians rarely find them in feces. Correct identification is crucial. Toxoplasma oocysts are much smaller than the two common coccidia of cats but must be distinguished carefully from similar small oocysts of different protozoans (Sarcocystis, Besnoitia, and Hammondia). If identification is uncertain, a stool sample may be sent to an expert for identification or mouse inoculation.

Blood (serologic) testing requires well-informed interpretation. Every infected creature develops antibodies as a defense against the infection. Most cats do so only after the shedding of oocysts in the feces. In cats ill with toxoplasmosis, the range in test results may be tremendous: the cat may not even have had time to develop a positive test, while at the other extreme, a single highly elevated test result is generally accepted as evidence of active disease. If, however, the test is negative or in the low or medium range, tests repeated at intervals of several days will show a rising level of antibody if the cat indeed has toxoplasmosis.

In the relatively few cats that become ill, the signs are myriad and vary in severity. A fever that stubbornly resists antibiotics is typical, and the white cell count is often below normal, sometimes causing confusion with panleukopenia. Acute, rapidly progressive toxoplasmal pneumonia presents a strongly suggestive appearance in radiographs and at autopsy. Acute illness may also affect the liver and pancreas, sometimes with jaundice. Inflammation of the intestine and associated lymph nodes may cause diarrhea in which oocysts may be shed. The inner eye may become inflamed in both acute and chronic toxoplasmosis. Infections of the heart and brain tend to be chronic, the latter producing varied signs including convulsions, incoordination, and personality change.

Toxoplasmosis can be strongly suggested by any of these signs, but active infection can be positively diagnosed only by one or more laboratory tests.

Treatment. If a cat sheds oocysts unquestionably identified as those of toxoplasma, it should be temporarily isolated and its feces carefully disposed of for two or three weeks, after which the stool should be reexamined to determine if shedding has stopped. Oocyst shedding can be suppressed by mixing sulfadiazine alone or together with pyrimethamine in the food for one to two weeks. The feces, however, should still be destroyed.

The same drugs are used, together with supportive measures, for active disease, but early diagnosis and treatment are essential. Pneumonia, characterized by rapid labored breathing, is almost always rapidly fatal. Infection of the heart, eyes, and nervous system is often so stubborn and deep-seated that adequate and prolonged drug treatment has fatal side effects.

Immunity. Many kittens have a low and short-lived supply of antibodies from their mothers. Cats once infected have considerable immunity to reinfection and if reinfected shed few if any oocysts; however, under certain circumstances impairing this immunity, the original infection may be reactivated and oocysts may again be shed.

Prevention. Control of food is the only practical way to prevent infection of cats. Risk to an indoor cat is virtually eliminated if it eats only dried or canned food, or meat and eggs cooked to 150°F. Freezing cannot be counted on to inactivate toxoplasma organisms.

An indoor cat that catches and eats mice or roaches must be considered in the same category as an outdoor cat.

Public health. In no single case of human toxoplasmosis has a cat ever been *proven* the cause. Still, all evidence indicates that cats' feces, as well as raw or undercooked meat and eggs, can be sources of infection for man.

Although humans once in a while become ill with much the same types of toxoplasmosis as cats, toxoplasma infection is of greatest concern to women who are or may become pregnant. Infection during pregnancy might pass to the child, who might at birth or later suffer from brain or eye disease. If a healthy woman tests positive, as many do, she should feel reassured: she has immunity that will most likely protect her from reinfection during pregnancy and from passing the infection to an unborn child.

Precautions for pregnant women. Few researchers advocate mass testing of women of child-bearing age, but emphasize the same precautions that should be observed by all humans:

1. Cook meat and eggs both for humans and cats to 150°F.
2. Dispose of cat litter daily by flushing in the toilet or burning, and disinfect the pan with boiling water. (If pregnant, wear plastic gloves for the task or delegate it to someone else.)
3. After handling a cat or raw meat or eggs, do not eat or touch your eyes or mouth until you have washed your hands thoroughly.
4. Eliminate from the home rodents and also roaches, flies, and other insects that may have had contact with cat droppings.
5. Use work gloves when working in soil that may be contaminated with cat droppings.
6. Cover children's sandboxes when not in use. Replace sand that has been contaminated by cat droppings.

FLEAS
Fleas are common external parasites of cats, especially in warm weather or in warm climates. They are small (about one-eighth inch long) but easily visible, hard, dark brown, rapidly moving and jumping insects, and live in the host's fur — sucking blood from the skin for nourishment (see illustration, page 45). Flea droppings, actually dried blood, appear as loose black grit. If this grit is evident in a cat's fur or on a light surface where it has been sitting or sleeping, it is good evidence that the cat needs treatment. When moistened the grit gives the red-brown color of dried blood. Minute white eggs may also be present.

Use only an insecticide preparation that is specifically labeled safe for cats, and exactly according to directions. Repeated powdering or spraying, with brushing to remove the flea grit, usually suffices. Almost never will you need to shampoo the cat.

Flea collars made specifically for cats are usually effective in eliminating and preventing flea infestations. They have, however, certain disadvantages. They do not stretch, so they can be a hazard to outdoor cats. They may wear down the fur, and, especially if they are not aired two or three days before use, get wet, or are too tight, they may cause a severe, occasionally fatal dermatitis underneath. Occasional systemic disturbances such as nausea and incoordination occur. Some owners remove a flea collar before allowing a cat out alone, and some remove them at regular intervals for indoor cats as well. If you bear all these facts in mind and check your cat's collar daily, it can probably wear one without risk. If a cat does not tolerate a flea collar, a flea tag attached to an ordinary collar may sometimes be safely substituted. Your veterinarian will be sure that a cat is not wearing a flea collar before he dispenses additional powder or spray — nor will he give certain internal parasite medications to a cat wearing a collar.

If tiny kittens have fleas, try to remove them by picking them off and crushing them between your fingernails. If the kittens are heavily infested, they may become severely anemic, and you should ask your veterinarian how they may be safely de-fleaed.

In getting rid of fleas, it is important to treat not only all cats and dogs in a household but also the animals' surroundings — their beds and floors and furniture where they lie. Fleas lay tiny white eggs which drop off the cat or dog, ripen for a variable period, and then hatch larvae that grow into adult fleas which will get back onto the animals. If an area is badly infested, the fleas may bite humans, too. Vacuuming is an effective way of removing flea eggs and larvae from floors, rugs, and furniture. This should be combined with spraying of any other haunts of your pets — garage, cellar, under the porch — with a household insecticide. The pets should be excluded for a time from the area sprayed so they do not inhale or come in contact with the moist spray.

Contrary to popular belief, cat and dog fleas ultimately can come only from other cats and dogs, or rarely from other animals or man.

LICE   Lice are exceedingly rare in cats and do not spread to humans or other animals. Resembling minute flakes of dandruff that cling to the skin or hairs without moving, they easily escape notice. Preparations effective against fleas are usually effective against lice.

TICKS   Ticks are far less apt to parasitize cats than dogs, but in areas and at seasons when ticks are unusually numerous in woods and shrubbery, some may be found on cats. Larger than fleas and easily felt by running the fingers carefully through a cat's coat, they are hard, flat, eight-legged arachnids, which burrow with their head into the skin, the female sucking blood till she is enlarged many times over.

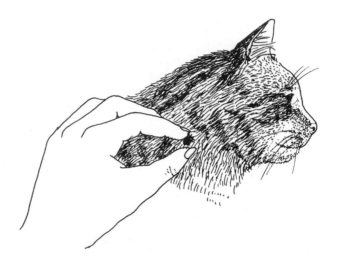

You can usually remove a tick, together with the head and mouth parts, by grasping it close to the skin and firmly pulling it away. Do not use lighted cigarettes or matches, kerosene, or gasoline! Flea collars and insecticide sprays and powders have some effectiveness in preventing or eliminating moderate infestations. Cats rarely need dipping. A rare complication of this parasitism is tick paralysis, caused by a neurotoxin. Removal of the ticks usually brings about recovery.

MANGE MITES   Mites can be distinguished only with a magnifying glass or microscope.

Ear mange, caused by the mite *Otodectes cynotis,* is discussed in detail in the earlier section on care of the ears (pages 73ff.).

Head mange, an itchy inflammation in which the skin becomes red, scratched, and thickened, and hair is lost, is a rarity. When it does occur it is usually in an adult tomcat, in which it may easily be confused with the thickening and scarring resulting from fights. When it reaches the advanced stage of heavy crusting of the face, eyelids, and ears, it presents a startling appearance that cannot be mistaken for anything else. Even at this stage your veterinarian can prescribe successful treatment. Rarely, it is encountered in litters of tiny kittens; in them, the entire body is involved, and any treatment that would be effective against the parasites is likely to be fatal to the kittens. *Notoedres cati* does not affect dogs and causes only a transient skin irritation in the rare cases in which it gets onto a human.

Demodectic (red) mange, a rarity in cats, causes a patchy loss of fur. It will respond readily to treatment your veterinarian can provide.

The larger Cheyletiella mite, most often found in the fur of rabbits, once in a while parasitizes cats. The irritation is mild and the evidence principally dandruff. The mites are eliminated by a flea preparation.

Trombiculid (harvest or chigger) mites are free-living as adults, but immature specklike orange, yellow, or red forms may infest the ears or other body parts of outdoor cats. Treatment is the same as for ear mites and fleas.

MAGGOTS Two less common but very disagreeable superficial parasitisms are caused by flies. A weak animal that cannot clean its body discharges, or one that lies injured and helpless outdoors in warm weather, attracts flies. These flies, which relish dried blood and serum or fecal matter, lay eggs on the animal. The eggs shortly hatch into small maggots, which eat into and undermine the skin, then work their way into deeper tissues. The sight and odor of such an infestation can turn the strongest stomach. The situation will eventually prove fatal unless *every last* maggot is promptly removed by your veterinarian and suitable treatment given.

Large flies of the genus Cuterebra ("bot flies") lay eggs in the soil, from which hatch larvae that continue their growth by burrowing under the skin of rodents such as rabbits and squirrels and occasionally kittens. Some time later a large swelling, an inch or more across, develops in and under the skin, usually about the head or neck of the kitten. At its center is a tiny opening in which the tip of a fat, inch-long larva can be seen moving. Do not try to squeeze the larva out. Take the kitten to your veterinarian, who will enlarge or incise the opening, remove the larva intact, and give appropriate treatment for the abscess.

disease Nonspecific signs that should alert you that all is not well with your cat are changes in its usual behavior and routine — hiding, lethargy, lack of appetite, absence of bowel movements, failure to urinate, thirst, vomiting, diarrhea, or decreased elasticity of the skin (dehydration).

Take your cat's temperature and then telephone your veterinarian with an orderly and accurate description of your cat's condition. The veterinarian may prescribe home treatment or advise a hospital examination.

PANLEUKOPENIA Panleukopenia, called in the past by many names — cat plague, cat distemper, cat typhoid, infectious enteritis — has been known for centuries as the great killer of cats and it still remains a disease that is easier to prevent than to cure.

Kittens and young cats are most often affected, although older cats that have led a sheltered life may also be susceptible. The typical course is short, characterized by severe depression, refusal of food, then vomiting of yellow fluid, dehydration, and often diarrhea. The cat may crouch with its head on the edge of its water dish but does not drink. At onset of symptoms there is high fever.

Because of the sudden onset and severe signs, and because other cats in the neighborhood may have been dying with similar symptoms, owners often suspect poisoning. Without immediate veterinary attention many cats die, usually within several days of the first signs of illness. If the cat survives the crisis, the temperature falls as recovery gets under way. If the disease is to prove fatal, the temperature may fall rapidly below normal.

The virus of panleukopenia (Greek for "lack of all white cells") destroys white cell–forming tissue, so a rapid white cell count is an important diagnostic test.

Intravenous and subcutaneous fluids, sometimes blood transfusions, vitamins, and antibiotics for secondary bacterial invaders are among your veterinarian's emergency measures. Early in the disease antiserum may also be of some benefit. Some veterinarians will hospitalize your cat, others will ask you to bring it once or twice a day for treatment.

As the cat recovers, the white cell count rebounds spectacularly. Feeding must be resumed with caution, as the cells in the intestinal lining have been damaged and have to heal before it can assimilate food.

Remember that your home has become thoroughly contaminated with the virus, which is present in all body discharges. It is a tough virus, highly resistant to light, heat, cold, and disinfectants and easily carried about on your person. Warn the owners of any cats that may have been exposed to have their cats given a protective inoculation at once. And do not bring any susceptible cats onto the premises, where the virus may linger for over a year, unless they have been vaccinated.

Considering that highly effective protective inoculations are available, this disease should never be allowed to happen (see page 74).

COLDS OR CORYZA   Upper respiratory infections (URI), often referred to simply as colds or coryza, are exceedingly common, especially wherever cats are kept in groups as on farms or in catteries, shelters, pet shops, and even in veterinary hospitals. These diseases may be passed through the air by sneezing cats and by direct and indirect contact.

Specific terms (pneumonitis, rhinotracheitis, "calici" infection) should be avoided, however, in favor of the general term "upper respiratory infection," since the different infections may produce symptoms that are much the same and may not be distinguishable except by laboratory procedures, some of them so elaborate that they are available only at research institutions. Happily the feline viruses are not transmissible to or shared with dogs or humans.

Symptoms of URI are sneezing, drooling, watery or purulent discharge from the nose and eyes, and frequently fever. Because the sense of smell may be lost, and tongue or mouth ulcers are frequent, cats stop eating, lose weight, and become dehydrated.

In no other condition is nursing care so important: frequent gentle cleansing of the eyes and nose with moistened cotton, patient hand-feeding, and demonstrations of TLC! Your veterinarian may also prescribe ointment for the eyes, a decongestant for the nose, vaporizing, and broad-spectrum antibiotics believed effective against pneumonitis (Chlamydia) and valuable in combating the secondary bacterial invaders that are responsible for as much damage as the viruses. A cat's sore mouth or throat often requires giving antibiotics, vitamins, and fluids by injection.

Except for the very young, ill, or elderly, the majority of cats do not become seriously ill with URI. Unfortunately, however, they may remain for indefinite periods carriers and shedders of the germs, infecting other cats even when they themselves have recovered and appear well. Under stress they may also break down again with infection themselves. Females carrying infection may be infertile or produce dead or sickly kittens.

Chronic bacterial infections of the nasal cavity, frontal sinuses, and middle ears are also occasional sequels to upper respiratory infections. If antibiotics fail, surgical drainage may be required.

The vaccines available have already been discussed (see page 74). For household pets, the best prevention is to avoid contact with other cats and to keep hospitalization and boarding to a minimum. Breeding stock should not be shipped about for mating.

RABIES   Rabies, caused by a virus which may affect the brain of all warm-blooded animals, is transmitted when virus-laden saliva enters a bite wound inflicted by a rabid animal. It is now established among many wild animals throughout the United States as well as much of the rest of the world. Because an outdoor cat roams and hunts at large, it may, unknown to the owner, be bitten by a rabid animal. In particular, bats that act odd and appear to be sick, floundering about in the daytime, if picked up and carried home by cats, sometimes prove to be rabid.

A striking change in disposition is the earliest sign of rabies in a cat. First it may become overly affectionate, then aggressive, then furious, tearing about and attacking and biting. The disease ends in a dumb stage with coma and death.

For their own protection and that of their human contacts, all outdoor cats should be protected with vaccines specifically designated as appropriate for cats (see page 75).

FELINE INFECTIOUS PERITONITIS

Known only for the past twenty years, infectious peritonitis has increased explosively in incidence until it has become one of the most serious diseases of cats, especially in multicat households and catteries, where it may become endemic and cause tragic and costly losses. The disease has an insidious chronic course, and the early signs are so varied and often nonspecific that weeks have often passed before a definite diagnosis was possible. The infection is most prevalent in cats between one and five years of age but occasionally affects kittens less than a month old or cats as old as fifteen years.

The earliest signs are lethargy, intermittent lack of appetite, and intermittent or persistent fever that fails to respond to antibiotics. In the most easily recognized form of the disease, inflammatory fluid accumulates in the abdominal or chest cavity or both, so that the cat's abdomen may gradually enlarge or the cat may experience increasing difficulty in breathing.

In some cases the characteristic fluid fails to develop and there are instead inflammatory changes in the eyeball, or nervous disorders involving the brain or spinal column — convulsions, personality changes, incoordination, and abnormalities of gait. Sometimes lumpy inflammatory lesions may be felt on the kidneys, liver, or abdominal lymph nodes.

If you or your veterinarian have reason to suspect the disease, confirmatory laboratory tests and sometimes exploratory surgery are essential to establish a diagnosis. A recently developed, specific blood test now makes earlier diagnosis possible.

If one animal in a group is found to have the disease, others may also be incubating it, even though, at the time, seemingly healthy.

Serological testing indicates that many apparently healthy cats have had exposure to the disease and suggests that such cats may also serve as carriers and shedders of the virus. Under natural conditions the incubation period of the disease is highly variable and may even be weeks or months.

Recent research suggests that there may be some very mild cases in which recovery occurs spontaneously, but practically all cats with serious forms of the disease die or are destroyed because of their steady deterioration. In a very few carefully selected cases, treatment with antibiotics, anticancer drugs, and heavy dosages of corticosteroids, in addition to drainage of fluid from the body cavities, has brought about a cure or greatly slowed the course of the disease.

Before attempting treatment, which is bound to be long and costly, an owner should take into consideration that the disease appears to be infectious among cats, and that an ill animal may be a hazard to others in its vicinity.

Since there is no specific or generally effective treatment, the greatest hope lies in development of a vaccine.

INFECTIOUS ANEMIA

Hemobartonellosis (feline infectious anemia, FIA) is caused by a rickettsial agent that parasitizes and destroys the red blood cells. It is apparently harbored in latent form by many cats and is activated by a variety of stresses or illnesses to produce acute or chronic disease. Young males with bite wounds are especially prone to develop the infection.

Lethargy, poor appetite, and weight loss may be the first vague signs. The temperature is usually found to be elevated, and the mucous membranes are noticeably pale. Since any anemia is a serious sign, take the cat to your veterinarian at once.

The spleen will likely be enlarged, and in most instances, the first blood film taken will reveal the characteristic rod- or ringlike bodies of Haemobartonella on the red cells. It is essential to demonstrate them in order to make a positive diagnosis.

The cat's most immediate need may be a blood transfusion. Broad-spectrum antibiotics and arsenical drugs are used in an effort to eliminate the infection but with varying results. Some cats, in which the disease is apparently uncomplicated by any other disorder, recover permanently. In others there may be recurrences, or if progress is poor, the Haemobartonella infection may prove secondary to a more serious condition.

SKIN The skin should be smooth, pliable, and free of blemishes. Except in areas of pigmentation, it should be pale pink. Yellow discoloration of skin or mucous membranes (jaundice, icterus) is a serious abnormality caused either by destruction of red blood cells (if the cat is anemic) or by liver disease.

DERMATITIS. After wound infections and bite abscesses (see Emergencies and First Aid, pages 82ff.), dermatitis is the disorder most often affecting the skin of cats. Most frequently it appears as tiny red eruptions which at first ooze serum and then scab over. It is apparently itchy, and the cat's licking, biting, and scratching aggravate the inflammation and may cause considerable loss of hair. The trouble often appears first at the base of the spine and may eventually involve the head and back of the neck and body. Increased eosinophil white blood cells often suggest allergy or parasitism as the cause.

Often the condition seems to be associated with flea infestation, but sometimes a certain food, for example, fish, horse meat, or milk, seems to be responsible. Fleas should of course be eliminated, and experimentation with diet sometimes provides a solution. In occasional cases, prompt remission follows emptying of distended, oozing, or infected anal sacs.

Fortunately, even when the cause remains uncertain, a regime of cortisone, given orally or by injection, will usually bring about long-term remission if not permanent cure. Bathing with a shampoo or soap with a moderate sulfur content hastens healing of the sores and is beneficial to the fur. The soap or shampoo must be prescribed by your veterinarian since many contain other ingredients that are poisonous for cats.

At certain times of year and in certain areas, the location of lesions of dermatitis (for example, face, belly, ears) suggests contact dermatitis. One cat may "break out" when it walks through the tomato patch, another from roosting on a television set, hot air register, or insulated heating pipe.

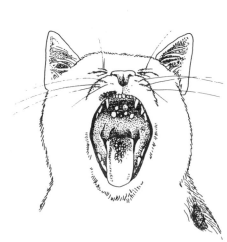

EOSINOPHILIC GRANULOMA. A chronic, sharply delineated, thickened inflammation of the skin, in which eosinophil white blood cells are numerous, is peculiar to cats. The irritant effect of their spiny tongue is believed to be a factor in the skin's reaction.

Eosinophilic granuloma may appear anywhere on the body where the cat licks, as thick, red, raised, sharply demarcated lesions. It may also appear on the upper lips above the fangs, as thick, leathery ulcers (so-called rodent ulcers), and in the mouth and throat as ugly red cauliflowerlike sores.

Like allergic dermatitis, most eosinophilic granulomas respond, at least temporarily, to systemic administration of cortisone. If a lesion can be bandaged to protect it from the cat's tongue, healing is hastened. Cauterization may also be helpful for lip and mouth lesions.

RINGWORM (dermatomycosis). This is a highly contagious skin infection caused by a fungus. Infectious for dogs and humans as well as for cats, it appears as itchy patches, often round, of dry, scaly, partially hairless skin. Lesions are most likely on the face, ears, and paws, although in very young kittens the whole body may be involved. The infection is especially prevalent and insidious in longhaired cats and is endemic in most catteries where longhairs are bred. Cats acquired from catteries and pet shops often infect both pets and people in their new homes.

A round, red, itchy spot on a human's neck or arm is often the first clue to inspect the cat. If any suspicious spots are seen, the cat should be taken at once to a veterinarian for positive diagnosis by fluorescence under an ultraviolet lamp, or microscopic examination or culture of particles of skin scales and fur.

Oral medication, ointment, and shampoo obtained from your veterinarian will eliminate ringworm in a month or two. The veterinarian will also recommend rigorous measures for treating and cleaning up the cat's environment.

Follow-up visits are essential to make certain your cat does not remain a carrier. An infected human should consult a physician.

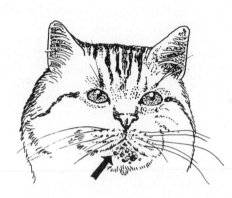

ACNE. Feline acne is an infection of large skin glands of the chin. The material produced by these glands often hardens into granules resembling the whiteheads and blackheads that occur in large pores in humans. These granules act as irritating foreign bodies in the skin, from which they often protrude and can be pressed out. This procedure, however, aggravates the secondary infection that is usually present. Severe bacterial infections, with pus breaking out from tracts under the skin, are not uncommon and are sometimes difficult to clear up.

If the condition is mild, your veterinarian will give you a suitable preparation with which to scrub the chin. Serious infection may require surgical drainage and infiltration with an antibiotic. Prompt attention when the condition is first noticed is most important.

STUD TAIL. Large oil-producing glands are present in the skin on the back of the base of the tail in all cats but usually make trouble only in unneutered males. Greasiness of the fur is conspicuous and attracts dust, making a dirty gray patch in light-colored fur. Secondary infection of the glands may result in discharging tracts similar to those described above on the chin. Treatment is similar.

For merely greasy fur, shampoo preparations for oily human hair are often effective.

MAMMARY HYPERPLASIA. A benign engorgement of some or all the mammary glands once in a while follows heat in a young cat. The breasts become swollen, warm, and tender. If cold applications are not helpful, medication may be required. Once the engorgement has subsided, the cat should be spayed to prevent recurrence after subsequent heats.

MASTITIS. This inflammation of one or more breasts is most often an acute complication of lactation and is described on page 119. Chronic nodular or cystic mastitis is usually asymptomatic and may or may not require surgical removal.

MAMMARY TUMORS. Beginning with a precancerous stage of glandular overgrowth, mammary tumors are frequent in older unspayed cats and are almost always highly malignant. Because of the cat's thick fur they often escape detection until well advanced. Starting as flat, hard, nodular areas in and under the skin and extending outward from the nipples, their surface ultimately breaks down into ugly, red, pus-covered ulcers. They also invade underlying muscle and spread by the circulation to other parts of the body, most often the lungs.

The tiniest lump in the vicinity of a nipple should prompt an immediate trip to the veterinarian. Early surgery has saved some cats, but unfortunately, radiographs may show that the tumor has already spread to the lungs and surgery is useless.

OTHER SKIN TUMORS. Although several highly malignant types may occur in young cats, most, whether benign or malignant, occur as the animal gets older. It is a good general rule that every lump should have immediate attention and, with few exceptions, be promptly removed.

UMBILICAL HERNIA. A soft fluctuating lump hidden under fur at the navel is not, strictly speaking, a skin lesion at all. A congenital failure of muscle to close in at the abdominal midline around the umbilical cord permits fatty tissue or occasionally a section of intestine to bulge out under the skin. Sometimes the opening is so small that as the cat grows it becomes negligible. If it is large enough, however, so that a loop of intestine might become trapped and pinched in the opening, surgical repair, which is very simple, is indicated. In a female cat the hernia can be closed at the same time that the cat is spayed, and through the same skin incision.

NEUROGENIC OR PSYCHOGENIC DERMATOSES. Some cats for no apparent reason pull out vast amounts of fur, chewing at themselves constantly. The skin itself is usually free of parasites and appears normal. Some veterinarians believe this condition results from feelings of frustration or inferiority, especially if the cat is low on the totem pole in a group. Very small and carefully adjusted dosages of male hormone may bolster the ego in cats of either sex, cause them to be normally assertive, and end the fur-pulling.

A peculiarity most frequent in Siamese but occurring occasionally in other pure breeds is an apparently itchy or painful sensation in the skin over the backbone and tail. The cat suddenly whirls around and looks back at the area, often biting at it. In the tail particularly, the sensation is apparently so acute that the cat cries out and chews in a frenzy at the flesh, practically to the bone.

Amputations of the damaged end of the tail are useless; the cat merely attacks what is left.

There is poor or transient response, if any, to antihistamines, cortisone, tranquilizers, Dilantin, or barbiturates. Very small doses of primidone, an anticonvulsant drug, carefully adjusted to the individual cat's response, are almost always quickly effective in controlling or eliminating the problem. Owners become very perceptive at recognizing when an attack, often triggered by some unpleasant event, is imminent, and prevent it by prompt medication.

A badly damaged tail may have to be firmly bandaged until it is healed.

In several instances acquiring a playmate for the affected cat has lessened or eliminated the attacks.

EYES   Kittens are born with their eyes closed. They open at between one and two weeks of age. All kittens have blueberry-colored eyes (irises); only after about three months does the permanent color become evident. Solid white cats with one or two blue eyes are often deaf. In darkness, with excitement, shock, blindness, certain drugs, or deep anesthesia, the narrow pupillary slit dilates to the maximum. Some researchers believe the cat is color-blind, others that it can distinguish red, but in any case it is very alert to any movement. It may fail to notice prey that remains still, but pounces quickly when the victim moves.

PROLAPSED THIRD EYELID. At the inner angle of the upper and lower eye-

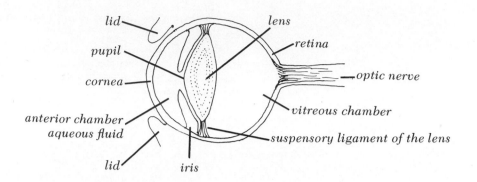

lid *lens*
pupil *retina*
cornea *optic nerve*
anterior chamber *vitreous chamber*
aqueous fluid *suspensory ligament of the lens*
lid *iris*

lids is the "third eyelid" ("haw," nictitating membrane). These membranes extend at times over a large part of the eyeball, giving rise to unnecessary fear that something is seriously wrong. Almost always they return to normal within several weeks without treatment. Prolapse is sometimes associated with severe parasitism, digestive upsets, or infectious disease — but in many cases the cat seems healthy and your veterinarian will not discover a cause.

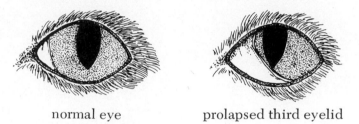

normal eye   prolapsed third eyelid

EPIPHORA. Epiphora ("tearing," lacrimation) involves one or both eyes, depending on cause. Possibilities are irritation, injury, allergy, presence of foreign material, or the early stage of upper respiratory infection. If tearing persists after flushing a few times with boric acid solution, your veterinarian should examine the eye for a possible scratch or foreign material.

In many Persians tearing is a congenital and permanent condition because the extreme flattening of the face kinks or blocks the duct which carries tears from the inner angle of the eye to an opening in the nose. Consequently, tears are constantly flowing over the lower lid margin and down the face, the fur of which may become sticky and stained. The skin may eventually become irritated and denuded of fur.

CONJUNCTIVITIS. This is an inflammation of the thin transparent membrane lining the eyelids and covering the eyeball. One or both eyes may be involved. Any of the causes listed above for epiphora may cause conjunctivitis, but the characteristic discharge is mucoid or purulent. If you cannot see an injury or foreign material, flush the eye with boric acid or salt solution (1 teaspoonful to a glass of water), and then squeeze a little boric acid ointment onto the eyeball. If two or three such treatments do not bring improvement, your veterinarian should examine the eye.

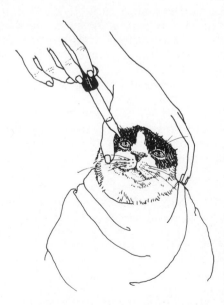

MEDICATION. Medicating of the eye is best accomplished with your cat rolled up in a bath towel and held upright in your own or someone else's lap. The towel immobilizes the cat and protects you both from soiling by the medication. A gentle preliminary cleaning of the eye is often needed. This can be done with a sterile cotton ball or swab moistened with warm water, boric acid solution, or salt solution. To medicate with a liquid, tilt the head back till the surface of the eye is approximately horizontal and with a plastic eyedropper drop the prescribed amount between the lids. Hold the cat's head in the same position for a few seconds so that the liquid will be well distributed over all the conjunctiva. Wipe away any excess that runs down the face.

Ointment is applied by parting the lids gently with the thumb and forefinger of one hand and with the other squeezing a thin line of ointment between the lids. The cat's subsequent opening and closing of the lids distributes the ointment.

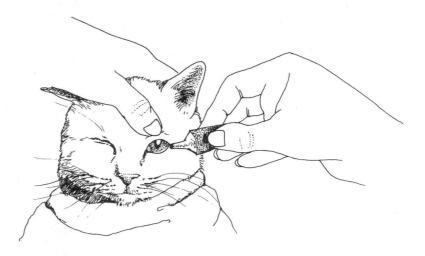

EARS   The pinna, or ear flap, consists of a thin sheet of cartilage covered inside and out with skin. The skin on the outer surface is covered with very short fur. Certain wounds or constant violent scratching at the ear because of mites in the ear canal may rupture a blood vessel between the cartilage and the inner skin of the ear flap. The result is an enormous blood blister, or hematoma, that gives the impression of a swelling involving the whole ear flap.

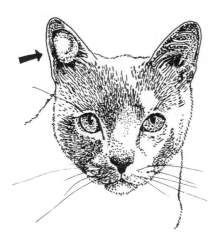

Surgical drainage and usually suturing are necessary if anything resembling the original shape of the ear is to be preserved. If the ear is untreated, contracting scar tissue produces a cauliflower ear.

CANCER.   Cancer of the ear occurs mostly in climates where white-eared cats have excessive exposure to intense sunlight. The tip and edges of the ear flap become inflamed and scaly, then scabby with dried exudate. At this stage, termination of exposure to the sun and protective ointment usually bring about a cure. Without these measures, an ugly, firm, red, ulcerated thickening gradually progresses downward, slowly eating the ear away. Generous surgical removal of the diseased edge usually brings complete cure.

INFLAMMATION.   Inflammation of the external ear canal is most often bilateral and due to the presence of ear mites. Treatment has already been described under Ears, page 73.

DISCHARGE FROM ONE EAR.   A discharge from only one ear may be a sign of a foreign body or growth deep in the ear canal where the owner cannot see or reach it. A veterinarian's aid is required for correct diagnosis and treatment.

MIDDLE AND INNER EAR.   Neglected disorders can have serious consequences if the barrier of the eardrum is broken: infection of the middle and inner ear and possibly fatal meningitis. When a cat circles or tilts its head down to one side, this is often a sign that the middle ear has become involved.

NOSE AND THROAT   See Respiratory (page 108) and Digestive ailments (page 109.)

MOUTH AND TEETH   The handsome whiskers on either side of the cat's upper lip serve as organs of sensation. Whiskers of poorly nourished cats sometimes fall out or crinkle. Occasionally a mother chews off her kittens' whiskers.

A cat's mouth, except where darkly pigmented, should be a healthy deep pink. In orange- or cream-colored cats, brown-black "freckles" may appear with age in the mouth and on the lips as well as the tip of the nose and the skin of the eyelids and ears. They are no cause for concern.

Eosinophilic granuloma (rodent ulcer) of the lips was discussed with eosinophilic granuloma of the skin (see page 102).

TEETHING. The twenty-six temporary kitten teeth first appear at two or three weeks and are all in at two months. By six months they have fallen out and been replaced by thirty permanent teeth. A visit to the veterinarian is needed only if the baby fangs refuse to fall out when the permanent fangs come in. Teething causes temporary soreness and redness of the gums.

The fangs (canines) are for grasping and tearing prey. The tiny front teeth (incisors) have little function except in grooming. The side teeth (premolars and molars) do not grind, as the Latin root of their name suggests, but mesh together so as to cut. Cats do not really chew their food but tear and crush it, swallowing much of it whole. The food is then broken down by digestive juices in the stomach and intestine.

Inheritance, food, and the bacterial flora in a cat's mouth are all factors in determining the health of teeth and gums. An owner should inspect a cat's mouth regularly.

CLEANING. Gnawing on dry, pellet-type food or on a bone that is big and strong enough so fragments cannot be broken off and swallowed helps to keep a cat's teeth clean and provides massage for the gums. A few cats permit their owners to brush their teeth or rub them with a rough cloth to remove the soft, slimy deposit that often accumulates near the gums.

Tartar is a gray-tan hard material that forms a shell at the base of the teeth next to the gum. It is often limited to the upper molars but may appear to some degree on the fangs and side teeth of both jaws. Sometimes an owner's fingernail is all that is needed to loosen tartar; otherwise the teeth should be "scaled" as often as necessary by a veterinarian. Neglected tartar provides ideal crevices for decaying food and infectious organisms that predispose to infection of the gum and tooth socket.

Infection of the roots of the molars, premolars, or fangs may betray itself as a discharging tract on the face or under the lower jaw. This is a condition that needs a veterinarian's treatment.

GINGIVITIS. Inflammation of the gums, gingivitis, is a common and often stubborn problem in cats. The gums, where they touch the teeth, are red and bleed easily. Sometimes thin sheets of red tissue grow over the base of the tooth. Under these sheets, the veterinarian is likely to find deep erosions of the surface of the tooth. Sometimes these erosions or cavities extend so deeply into a tooth that the tooth breaks off at the gum line, leaving a barely visible root as a permanent focus of gum and jaw disease.

Thorough cleaning of the teeth, perhaps under anesthesia, is required to remove all tartar, and eroded teeth and tooth roots should be extracted. The gums may be painted at the time with a strong antiseptic and the owner instructed to flush with an antiseptic mouthwash if the cat will tolerate it. A systemic antibiotic should be given to prevent dissemination of infection by the dentistry.

Occasionally a severely proliferate red, "meaty" type of gingivitis or stomatitis develops that is practically incurable, responding only temporarily to combined treatment with an antibiotic and cortisone. Many stubborn cases of gingivitis improve only when all the molar teeth and sometimes the fangs as well have been removed.

PERIODONTITIS. This refers to inflammation of the inner surface of the tooth socket. Predisposing causes are gingivitis and tartar. Many of the teeth prove to be rather loose in their sockets and should be removed.

TRENCH MOUTH. This is a virulent stomatitis caused by spiral organisms that normally live in the mouth but under certain conditions become aggressive pathogens. A malodorous drooling is the first sign. The infection progresses very rapidly, the cat becoming apathetic, feverish, and losing appetite. At first inspection of the mouth, one may note only the unusually foul odor. Rapidly, however, the edges of the gum and the angles of the lips become inflamed and slimy, then pale and devitalized. Unless prompt and vigorous treatment with antibiotics is started, the gums may become involved and rot away, leaving exposed areas of jawbone. Blood poisoning and death may follow.

TONGUE. The tongue may be injured by burns or foreign bodies or torn in fights. Ulcers in which the tip of the tongue may even slough away occur in severe cases of upper respiratory infection. Feeding with a stomach tube may be required.

Cancer developing under the tongue of an elderly cat may cause a foul odor and discharge and prevent eating. It is almost always too advanced for treatment when discovered.

RESPIRATORY

Upper respiratory infection, caused by several different agents, and giving rise to colds of varying severity, is by far the most frequent respiratory affliction of cats. It is discussed, together with chronic infection of the nasal passages and sinuses, under Colds or Coryza (see page 100).

Difficulty in breathing and abnormal sounds coming from the respiratory passages should prompt an owner to watch and listen carefully. Is the trouble in the nose, the throat, or farther down (lungs or chest cavity)? Snuffling and snorting or a unilateral nasal discharge of pus or blood may be a clue to a foreign body or an inflammatory or tumorous mass in the nose. Gagging and snorting suggest trouble in the nasopharynx.

A cat's purring is believed by most authorities to be due to vibration of the "false vocal cords," a pair of folds situated to either side of the true vocal cords. A change in the sound of the purr or inability to purr may be a sign of laryngitis or of a tumor involving the vocal cords.

LARYNGITIS. Laryngitis may be due to too much loud yowling, a chemical irritant such as smoke, or infection. It often accompanies upper respiratory infection and is an occasional complication of panleukopenia.

Tumors of the larynx (lymphoma, cancer) are, fortunately, rare. They cause increasing difficulty in breathing, and may end agonizingly in suffocation unless recognized in time.

CHRONIC BRONCHITIS, ASTHMA. Chronic allergic bronchitis (asthma) is rather frequent. Occasional cats are subject to sudden, frightening attacks of extreme respiratory difficulty, gasping for breath, and with mucous membranes turning blue, so that they appear to be on the verge of asphyxiation. Emergency handling of such cats has been described (page 83).

The majority of asthmatic cats simply have a chronic cough or wheeze, the depth of their breathing indicating varying degrees of respiratory difficulty — from scarcely noticeable to considerable. Cigarette smoke, aerosol sprays, and changes in weather or environment may aggravate the trouble. The dust from cat litter appears to be responsible in some instances. The cats are usually in good flesh, eating well, and without fever. Rarely is more than one in a household affected.

Radiographs, white blood cell counts, and fecal examinations are important in diagnosis. Your veterinarian will advise you to eliminate any possible irritant from the cat's environment — in particular, a change may be recommended from clay-type litter to paper or other material.

Initial treatment combines cortisone and an antibiotic. The dose of cortisone is gradually lowered. Periodic X-raying is advisable. The damage to the lungs can almost always be prevented from progressing, although the lungs may never again be quite normal. Many cats have recurrences unless kept indefinitely on a low dose of cortisone.

PNEUMONIA. Pneumonia may be acute or chronic and have many causes: inhalation of medication or foreign material, parasitism, and bacterial, viral, protozoan, or fungus infections. Signs are increased rate and depth of respirations, bluish color of the mucous membranes, depression, lack of appetite, and usually fever. Generally a cat is so obviously ill that an owner realizes it must be taken to a veterinarian without delay.

DISORDERS OF THE CHEST CAVITY. These are especially frequent in cats. Injury may cause the chest to fill with blood or air, or may tear the diaphragm, allowing abdominal organs to enter the chest and crowd the lungs. Most frequent in cats are infections of the pleura and leukemic tumors, which cause the chest to fill with pus or fluid and severely limit lung function. Whatever the cause, the compression of the lungs results in slow, labored breathing, in which the cat has great difficulty in expanding the chest.

The cat is in such danger of asphyxiation that any handling or attempt at medication may prove fatal. Get it to a veterinarian at once.

SKELETAL OSTEOPOROSIS. Osteoporosis (juvenile osteodystrophy, nutritional secondary hyperparathyroidism, paper-bone disease) has been shown to be a simple calcium deficiency caused by a diet too high in meat (phosphorus) and low in calcium. Kittens are the most frequent victims, but nursing mothers also develop the deficiency.

Signs are generalized soreness and reluctance to move or be handled. A jump from a chair to the floor or a tumble down the stairs may break several bones. The shoulder blades, rib cage, sternum, and spinal column may become severely deformed. If the pelvis narrows inward, bowel movements become impossible. Radiographs show thin-walled bones lacking the density of normal calcification. Unsuspected "greenstick" or "folding" fractures may be found. So soft are the bones that splinting and pinning are out of the question for fracture treatment.

Intravenous calcium brings prompt relief from soreness, and confinement to a cage and change to a balanced diet, supplemented for a time with oral calcium carbonate or calcium lactate prescribed by your veterinarian, will cure all but the hopelessly deformed animals.

EXCESS OF VITAMIN A OR D. This may produce abnormal, crippling deposition of bone. Hypervitaminosis D is rare, but overfeeding with liver, which is high in vitamin A, from time to time results in fusion of cervical vertebrae — which prevents a cat from bending its neck — and in abnormal thickening of the long bones of the limbs.

DIGESTIVE VOMITING. Many cats vomit occasionally if they eat food that disagrees with them personally, cold food straight from the refrigerator, or too much food at one time. Fur balls or parasites in the digestive tract also cause occasional vomiting and are sometimes brought up by the cat.

If a cat seems otherwise normal, there is no cause for immediate alarm. Fur balls may be helped to pass through the digestive tract by a dab of Vaseline or similar fur-ball remedy for the cat to lick off the nose or paw two or three times a week. Parasites require identification and specific treatment by a veterinarian.

Repeated vomiting associated with lack of appetite, depression, and developing dehydration may indicate severe infectious disease such as panleukopenia, poisoning, or obstruction by a foreign body, telescoping (intussusception) of the intestine, or possibly a tumor. Liver or pancreatic diseases are other possibilities.

Take your cat's temperature and note carefully the frequency of vomiting, and the color and content of the vomitus. Do not attempt to treat the cat yourself — telephone your veterinarian for advice.

DIARRHEA. Diarrhea may be caused by intestinal parasites (pages 93ff.), spoiled food, food that disagrees with certain cats (for example, liver, milk, horse meat), irritation from swallowed fur, a variety of poisonous substances, inflammation, infection, or tumor — and, finally, disease of the liver or pancreas, which may result in inadequate digestion or absorption of food and abnormal appearance of the stool. An occasional brief spell of diarrhea should be of no great concern, provided a cat seems otherwise well. For a day or two change the diet to small feedings of bland food, such as strained baby-food beef or chicken with rice. Many antidiarrheal preparations intended for humans have flavors abhorrent to cats, but ½ to 1 teaspoon of milk of bismuth several times a day orally by dropper or in the food may be accepted. A half teaspoon of bone meal obtained from your veterinarian or a health food store and mixed with each feeding also controls many diarrheas.

If the diarrhea persists, or other signs of illness develop, telephone your veterinarian for advice.

Violent exhausting diarrhea leading to dehydration and prostration is an emergency condition demanding immediate attention.

Whatever the type of diarrhea, be able to describe the frequency of movements and the character of the stool to your veterinarian. Better yet, take a sample with you.

FLATULENCE. Uncommon in cats, flatulence (gas) is usually due to the cat's food and if it persists, a change in diet should be tried. Feeding several small meals a day, rather than one or two large ones, which the cat may gulp, could also be helpful.

OBESITY. Most often obesity is due to overfeeding. If obesity is associated with thirst and excessive urination, a cat should be tested for diabetes. Obesity accompanied by sluggishness, constipation, a tendency to seek heat, and symmetrical loss of hair from the groin and thighs suggests hypothyroidism.

Because individual cats vary as much as humans in body structure and energy needs, hard-and-fast guidelines for ideal weight and amounts of food cannot be established.

CONSTIPATION. Constipation is often a problem in cats because most consume little liquid. Water, milk, or broth may be mixed with the food, and salt sprinkled on the food, as one would flavor food for humans, encourages intake of fluid. B-complex vitamins, believed to maintain intestinal tone and relished by many cats in the form of brewer's yeast tablets or powder sprinkled on the food, may be prescribed by your veterinarian.

A cat should move its bowels at least once every two days. Lubrication may be provided two or three times a week by dabbing on a cat's nose or paw some Vaseline or other petroleum jelly specially flavored for cats. If constipation is serious and persistent, a veterinarian may prescribe milk of magnesia or bulk-producing drugs, or advise the use of infant suppositories. Occasionally constipation advances to such a serious stage that it must be relieved under anesthesia.

Tiny kittens suffering from constipation due to congenital dilatation of the colon (megacolon) should be destroyed. Acquired megacolon in elderly cats, resulting from years of constipation and stretching of the intestine, is occasionally helped by surgery that takes a longitudinal tuck in the colon wall.

ANAL SACS. Under the tail on either side of the anus is a tiny sac corresponding to the scent gland of the skunk. These sacs produce a foul-smelling material. Normally they empty themselves, but if they do not they become uncomfortable and sore so that the cat licks at them constantly. In this case a veterinarian must empty them and, if there is evidence of infection, instill an antibiotic ointment. Occasionally they become painfully abscessed and must be incised, drained, and cauterized. If infections recur, complete removal of the sac provides a permanent solution.

Your veterinarian will check your cat's anal sacs as part of a routine examination. This is especially necessary in older cats, in which the secretion becomes so dry and hard that defecation may be impeded.

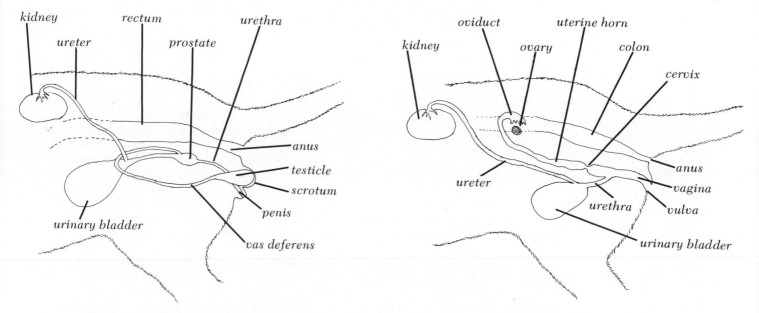

MALE GENITOURINARY SYSTEM

FEMALE GENITOURINARY SYSTEM

URINARY The urinary system begins with a right and a left kidney, which collect fluid and other materials from the blood to form urine. A ureter, a tiny, flexible, cordlike tube, carries the urine from each kidney to the urinary bladder. This is a very elastic, balloonlike sac, which contracts to about walnut size when emptied but can stretch to hold so much urine that a cat, if necessary, can go many hours without voiding. When a cat empties the bladder, the urine passes through the pelvis by way of the urethra. In the female it is discharged to the outside through the vulva, a slitlike opening just below the anus; in the male the urethra must pass all the way through to the end of the penis, being greatly constricted for about the last inch by the tiny caliber of the penis. Nature may justly be criticized for the small size of the cat's penis, for it is at this point that urinary blockages in the male cat originate.

Blockages occur in both intact and neutered males. In the female cat, they are extremely rare, because the urethra is of ample diameter throughout its short course.

UROLITHIASIS. Formation of "sand" or stone in the urinary tract is one of the most frequent and serious disorders in cats, especially adult males. Perhaps in part because they consume relatively little fluid, many apparently normal cats have tiny mineral crystals (phosphate salts) in their urine. For reasons not entirely clear, these sometimes clump to form sandlike particles or even small stones that may cause irritation in the bladder or urethra. Obstruction is tragically frequent, and often lethal, when accumulated crystals plug the fine-caliber terminal urethra of the male cat. Restlessness, discomfort, unhappy mewing, licking at the protruded penis, and frequent trips to the sanitary pan with straining and passage of only a few drops of urine, often bloody — these are danger signs for which the owner of a male cat must be ever on the alert.

A fatal mistake is often made when an inexperienced or uninformed owner misinterprets the condition as constipation and delays getting necessary treatment, perhaps even plying the unfortunate cat with laxatives. A urinary obstruction is one of the gravest feline emergencies — one about which an owner can do absolutely nothing; unless the blockage is relieved immediately by a veterinarian, the cat may die in a day or two from uremic poisoning.

If your veterinarian cannot relieve the obstruction by gentle manipulation of the penis or pressure on the bladder, he will try to catheterize the cat, usually with the aid of a tranquilizer, sedative, or light anesthesia. If that fails, urine must be drawn from the overdistended bladder by "tapping" — passing a needle directly through the abdominal and bladder walls, so that the urine can be drawn off by suction.

If the blockage is very solid and does not yield to repeated attempts at flushing, or if there are repeated episodes of obstruction, the last resort is surgery to provide a new urinary opening which bypasses the constricted end of the penis (perineal or antepubic urethrostomy). Although some urethrostomies fail because of recurrent bladder infection or poor function of the artificial opening, the operation enables many cats that would have died or been destroyed to live in complete or reasonable comfort.

CYSTITIS. The same tiny crystals that cause obstruction in males cause bladder irritation, inflammation, and secondary bacterial infection in both male and female cats. A cat with cystitis usually urinates so frequently that the bladder is practically empty all the time. It is therefore often impossible to obtain urine for analysis or bacterial culture, and treatment has to be given on a "shotgun" or trail-and-error basis. Luckily, this is very likely to be successful.

Your veterinarian will probably prescribe some combination of the following measures: (1) a broad-spectrum antibacterial or antibiotic drug for infection, (2) an acidifier to keep the urine acid (fewer crystals form in acid than alkaline urine), (3) cat foods with as low ash (mineral) content as possible, (4) a pinch of salt in each feeding to encourage greater water consumption, (5) avoidance of dry cat foods, since they lead to a more concentrated urine, and (6) availability of *fresh water* at all times. Recent research suggests strongly that one or more viruses may also be implicated, so that daily changing of litter and cleaning of the pan are advised.

If a case of cystitis stubbornly refuses to improve with these measures, your veterinarian may catheterize the cat to get a urine sample for bacterial culture and antibiotic-sensitivity testing. Radiographs are also indicated to make sure that the persistent irritation (and perhaps bloodiness of the urine) is not due to the presence of a bladder stone that will have to be removed surgically.

KIDNEYS. Chronic kidney disease due to inflammation and progressive scarring and shrinking of the organ is the other very important urinary disorder of cats. Occasionally, young adult cats are affected, but it is much oftener a gradually developing disease of middle-aged and older cats. Its first sign is increasing thirst and urine output, which may for some time escape the owner's attention. For variable lengths of time — months or years — a cat may compensate, by drinking and urinating more and more, for the kidneys' steadily decreasing ability to remove waste products from the blood. Laboratory tests are necessary to differentiate between kidney disease and other disorders characterized by thirst.

Although chronic kidney disease ends in fatal uremia, the compensated stage can often be prolonged by a low-protein, higher-starch diet, either canned commercially or improvised by you and your veterinarian.

URINE SPRAYING. True spraying must be distinguished from signs of cystitis (see above).

UREMIA. An accumulation of waste products in the blood, uremia may develop gradually or be precipitated suddenly by some stress such as injury, illness, surgery, traveling, hospitalization, or boarding. Signs of uremia are lethargy, lack of appetite, weight loss, and vomiting. Owners often ask about a kidney transplant or dialysis. Unfortunately, no kidney transplant technique has been developed for cats, and dialysis could only prolong life temporarily.

URINE SPRAYING. True spraying must be distinguished from signs of cystitis (see above).

When spraying, a cat backs up to a wall, doorframe, or other vertical object and lets go with a more or less horizontal jet of urine. Spraying is said to be the cat's way of asserting territorial rights. It is a natural development when a male kitten becomes a mature tomcat and is one of the chief reasons for neutering. It sometimes occurs in a female cat in heat, particularly if she is being frustrated in her natural desire to seek a mate.

Spraying in neutered males and females is a far more complex matter and can be difficult or impossible to deal with. Essentially, it is a cat's most effective way of expressing displeasure. The following long list of causes comes from real-life histories but is far from complete: inattention by loved ones, unappealing food, a dirty litter box, not being allowed out, not being allowed in, a new home, a new piece of furniture, a new pet, a new member of the family, or loss of a familiar object, animal, or person.

If it is impossible to satisfy the cat's desires, another solution rather recently reported has proven of benefit in many cats of both sexes — injections of female progestational hormone. Sometimes just one treatment will break the obnoxious habit, sometimes medication must be repeated after considerable intervals. This hormonal treatment is not recommended for *unspayed* females.

REPRODUCTIVE

FALSE PREGNANCY. This occurs when progesterone is released from the ovary although ova have not been fertilized. Because cats, unlike most animals, must mate in order to ovulate and release progesterone, false pregnancy can result only from some artificial stimulus to ovulation and is therefore rare. It lasts only five or six weeks, and the signs — mammary development and nesting behavior — are rarely pronounced enough to need treatment (with estrogen or male hormone).

UTERINE INFECTIONS. Acute infection of the uterus (metritis) may follow normal heat or mating, but most often results from a difficult birth, retained fetuses or placentas, or delivery in dirty surroundings. If a cat is nursing a litter, the first sign may be neglect of the kittens. Depression, fever, and failure to eat are accompanied by straining and foul vaginal discharge.

Both mother and kittens may be lost unless prompt and vigorous antibiotic and supportive measures are taken. Spaying is the wisest course to avoid the possible aftereffects of the infection.

CHRONIC METRITIS AND PYOMETRA. Chronic metritis and pyometra (pus-filled uterus) are occasional sequels of acute metritis (see above), but far oftener develop gradually and less spectacularly. Both may occur in breeding females, but are perhaps more frequent in unspayed females whose owners fail or refuse for a variety of reasons to have them spayed. Pyometra not infrequently follows the first heat in very young females.

Both chronic metritis and pyometra are often the result of constant ovarian stimulation, which causes abnormal development of the uterine lining and renders it susceptible to bacterial infection. In elderly unspayed females, breast cancer, ovarian cysts and tumors, and uterine tumors may all be associated with pyometra.

As long as the cervix is open and pus can drain, the cat may constantly lick herself clean and exhibit no serious signs of illness. If the cervix is closed, however, pus will eventually accumulate in the uterus. Increased abdominal distention may be the only sign, or there may be depression, poor appetite, and fever. With prompt and skillful veterinary attention even the oldest, sickest cats may often be brought through the necessary surgery.

CARDIOVASCULAR

CONGENITAL DISEASE. The heart and blood vessels of cats are subject to the same developmental errors that result in congenital defects in human babies — patent ductus, constricted valves, holes in the walls of the various chambers of the heart, fibrosis of the heart lining, and mix-ups in the large arteries and veins. In some lines of purebred cats the defect is clearly inherited, and conscientious breeders do their best to eliminate it from their stock.

Kittens and young cats with heart defects tire easily and are stunted in growth. Often the mucous membranes of their mouths are grayish or bluish instead of a normal pink. Occasionally an owner notices an unusually loud or extensive heartbeat, sometimes with a constant hum or vibration. Eventually, because the heart is incompetent to do its job, the chest or abdomen or both fill with watery fluid, and breathing becomes acutely difficult.

A veterinarian should be consulted as soon as any problem is suspected. An unobservant owner may just suddenly find a dead or dying kitten. If it is a valuable purebred, it should be autopsied by a veterinary pathologist to determine if the breeding stock carries an inherited defect.

ACQUIRED HEART DISEASE. Once considered infrequent in cats, acquired heart disease is recognized increasingly, thanks to modern diagnostic techniques.

Endocardial and valvular disease fairly often result from blood-borne infection that involves the lining of the heart and the covering of the valves. Signs are weakness, stubborn fever, and sometimes heart murmurs associated with or following a variety of infectious ailments.

Cardiomyopathy, inflammatory or degenerative disease of the heart muscle, is, however, the most notable form of heart disease in cats. As yet the causes are unclear, although in some cases it seems to develop after virus infections. Tiredness, weakness, labored breathing, and grayish or bluish color of the mucous membranes are among the signs. Your veterinarian will find abnormalities in the rate and rhythm of the heartbeat and in the size and shape of the heart.

Changes in diet and treatment with a variety of drugs are helpful to many of these cats. There is, however, the constant threat that the poor functioning of the heart will favor development of a clot (thrombus) which will break loose from the heart and pass rapidly to lodge as an embolus in large arteries of the lungs, digestive tract, kidneys, or at the end of the aorta, blocking the circulation to the hind legs.

The very sudden and catastrophic effect and signs of this condition have been discussed among Circulatory Emergencies (page 83).

BLOOD

The red cells of the blood are formed in the marrow cavities of the bones; the hemoglobin they contain transports oxygen to all parts of the body. Several kinds of white blood cells — essential for the body's defenses against injury and infection — also originate in the bone marrow, as well as the platelets, tiny particles essential to the clotting process. Other white cells, the lymphocytes, which are involved in the production of immunity to disease, are manufactured in lymph glands (nodes) throughout the body and also in the spleen, an abdominal organ. The marrow, the lymph nodes, and the spleen are crucially involved in anemia and leukemia, which are among the most frequent and serious diseases of cats.

ANEMIA. More than any other animal, the cat seems to react to the stress of disease and to exposure to a variety of chemicals and drugs by developing anemia. In a minority of cases, the anemia is due simply to blood loss (hemorrhage, parasitism), or is of a type in which the red cells are destroyed (for example, by hemobartonellosis [see page 101] or by certain chemicals, as in some urinary antiseptic drugs). In these anemias, if the cause is eliminated, a healthy marrow quickly produces new red cells.

The majority of feline anemias, however, are marked by depression of red cell (and sometimes also white cell) production that often persists and proves fatal in spite of all-out efforts at diagnosis and treatment. Among known causes are infections of many kinds, poisonings, chronic diseases, and malignancies. Cats that carry the feline leukemia virus may develop unresponsive depression anemia without ever becoming leukemic, and have lowered resistance to many disease conditions.

Anemia may develop so gradually that only when it becomes severe does the cat show signs of illness: weakness, lack of appetite, unwillingness to move, and respiratory difficulty accompanying the slightest activity. By this time the mucous membranes are chalky white, and any stress, strenuous activity, or struggle may prove fatal (see page 83).

LEUKEMIA. Leukemia, which may involve any one of the cell types mentioned above, is the most important cause of fatal anemia in cats and is caused by a virus. Malignant proliferation of red cells also occurs.

A simple test performed on a drop of blood from a cat demonstrates virus in about 90 percent of cats that have or may ultimately develop leukemia, but happily no more than 0.1 percent of the general cat population appears to carry the virus. A few very lucky cats develop protective antibodies that enable them either to harbor the virus without becoming ill or even eventually to eliminate it altogether.

It must be emphasized that a positive test merely indicates that a cat is carrying the virus of feline leukemia (FeLV). It confirms a diagnosis of leukemia or lymphosarcoma only if symptoms and other laboratory findings are characteristic.

Leukemia is a truly contagious disease. The virus may be passed from cat to cat in saliva or urine, so it is most dangerous in multicat households and catteries. Any sick cats or carrier cats — even though clinically healthy — should be eliminated or isolated from virus-negative cats.

Another reason for eliminating carriers is that while they may not actually have or ever develop leukemia, the presence of the virus in their system seems to lower resistance to other disorders and infections such as anemia, colds, hemobartonellosis, and mouth and wound infections. There is also reason to believe that the carrier state causes infertility and reproductive problems in mothers and unsturdiness and mortality among their kittens.

As yet there is no evidence that humans or other species can contract leukemia from cats that are ill with, or carriers of, the virus.

The average age of cats with lymphocytic malignancies is about five years, but more than 50 percent of cats are under three years of age when they become ill. Even young kittens develop the disease.

Depression, poor appetite, weight loss, fever, and anemia are typical. Nonhealing wound infections and infections of the mouth and upper respiratory tract are common. Tumors in the chest may cause respiratory difficulty, while growths in the intestine may give rise to vomiting or diarrhea. Occasionally owners notice enlargement of the lymph glands of the neck or of the kidneys, which may bulge visibly behind the ribs. Sometimes the malignancy chiefly involves the bone marrow and blood and is diagnosed by blood and marrow examination.

If a cat is seriously ill, many owners decide at once to have it destroyed.

Less seriously affected cats pose a problem. Several drugs offer the possibility of a prolonged remission, even once in a while of an apparent cure. Yet such a cat, even if seemingly restored to health, may continue indefinitely to shed virus, thus constituting a hazard for other cats. For this reason, treatment should probably be limited to "only" cats.

Once one cat in a household or cattery has been found to have leukemia, all should be tested for the virus.

mothers and kittens
PUBERTY AND HEAT CYCLE

The female cat is usually described as seasonally polyestrous — that means that in each of two or three seasons every year, she may have a number of heats. In much of the United States, the principal mating season for the female begins after the New Year, another is likely in late spring or early summer, and there is sometimes a third in late summer. If the cat has no opportunity to mate and conceive at the first heat, she will continue in heat for as long as two or three weeks or come back into heat at intervals, each heat lasting for several days. Typical signs of heat are restlessness, rolling, treading with the hind feet, and "calling." Inexperienced owners often telephone their veterinarian to report that the cat seems to be in pain! Season, breed, and environment are important determining factors: some cats may be as young as four months, but most cats come into heat between five and nine months of age.

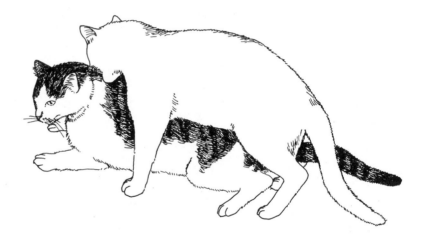

If a female mates with more than one male in a single heat, her kittens may have more than one father. They will be likely then to vary greatly in build, color, and temperament.

Before breeding, a female should be checked by a veterinarian and treated if necessary for both external and internal parasites, so that there will be no danger that these will be transmitted to the kittens. Breeders of purebreds are also testing increasingly for the leukemia virus.

Wise breeders of purebreds maintain suitable animals of both sexes in their own households or catteries and never ship or receive an animal for breeding. This avoids the stress of travel and exposure to infectious disease.

Moving a female to a strange environment for breeding may cause her to go out of heat, and she may have to remain with the stud's owner till she comes back into heat. If a male is taken to the female, he must usually be given time to feel at home in the new surroundings.

Because the abundant coat of Persians sometimes interferes with mating, breeders may do some trimming of the fur about the genital areas.

Unless one of the cats is inexperienced, the mating preliminaries, mostly antics of the female, usually take less than an hour. The mating itself, with the male mounting the female and grasping the back of her neck in his mouth, lasts only about ten seconds, but may be repeated soon after. Further characteristic antics by the female follow.

Domestic cats seem to have little trouble becoming pregnant. In breeding queens, however, varying degrees of infertility, resorption and abortion of fetuses, and loss of kittens are serious problems. Most likely endemic disease in the cattery is responsible — panleukopenia, upper respiratory infection, toxoplasmosis, and the virus of feline leukemia.

PREGNANCY AND DELIVERY

The duration of pregnancy for the cat is usually said to be sixty-three to sixty-five days, but it may vary within a range of fifty-eight to seventy. Siamese and Abyssinians are likely to have prolonged pregnancies. Pregnancies tend to be shorter, the more kittens are being carried. Occasional cats act slightly out of sorts in early pregnancy.

About two weeks after mating, the nipples gradually become darker and more prominent. At about five weeks developing kitten skeletons are first detectable by a radiograph; before that time X-raying could harm the fetuses, and only a veterinarian's manual examination can detect the enlargements in the uterus.

Abdominal enlargement is first noticeable at about five or six weeks. After seven weeks, the kittens' heads may be felt, or even seen moving, within the distended abdominal wall.

Now and then a cat comes into heat and mates during pregnancy. Additional kittens may even result from the mating and be born some days after the earlier ones.

As pregnancy advances, the cat should be given all she will eat of a nutritious and balanced diet, because her developing kittens need an abundant supply of protein and calcium.

As the time for delivery approaches, the cat becomes slower and more deliberate in her activity. This is all to the good, because sudden violent movements such as a jump to or from a high place, or a fall, have been known to cause a twist in the uterus that was followed by shock and death within a few hours. Fortunately, such bizarre disasters are rare.

In the last week of pregnancy, the nipples swell so that drops of milk may ooze from their tips. The cat may wander about restlessly, either because of uncomfortable distention or because she is looking for a secluded place to have her kittens. This is the owner's cue to choose a suitable spot and provide a roomy box lined with a towel — a box big enough so that the cat can stretch out comfortably at full length, and with sides high enough so that the kittens will be unable to climb out for several weeks. Do not be surprised, though, if in the end your cat decides on another place — a dark closet, a basket of clean laundry, your bed, or under a dining room chair at mealtime!

The day before giving birth some cats stop eating. Some, but not all, have a drop in body temperature.

When labor begins the cat may move around restlessly, mew, lie first on one side, then the other, and occasionally squat and strain in her litter box. When abdominal contractions begin, the cat will pant, strain, and groan, sometimes lying on her side, sometimes squatting.

When the water sac of the first kitten breaks, the cat is likely to lick energetically under her tail. At this time the kitten's head may be seen emerging.

If the sac remains intact, it will protrude like a fluid-filled balloon which the cat easily breaks by licking, freeing the kitten and stimulating it to breathe.

Kittens may be born either head or rear first. A good mother chews promptly through the umbilical cord and cleans the kitten thoroughly, causing it to breathe regularly, move, and mew. A cat having a first litter may need some supervision and prompting from her owner. Once in a while the inexperienced mother, chewing on the umbilical cord, may go too far and injure or even devour a kitten. Some believe that a mother sometimes intentionally destroys a kitten that she senses is abnormal.

If a mother shows a tendency to lie on kittens already born as labor continues, they should be temporarily removed to a safe warm box of their own. Once in a while a mother neglects or perhaps does not have time to sever the umbilical cords of kittens born in rapid succession. The result is a confused tangle of kittens in which kittens may be strangled or legs cut off by tightly twisted umbilical cords. In such a situation the owner must sever the cords.

The duration of labor and the intervals between kittens may vary enormously. Once in a while an apparently normal labor may be interrupted for as long as two days and then be resumed satisfactorily, the cat meantime taking food and nursing the kitten or kittens already born. Most often, however, delivery is completed within several hours. Nursing by the kittens may start immediately after birth, or the mother may not encourage it until all the kittens have arrived.

Indications that should prompt concern during delivery are: passage of a red discharge without onset of labor; labor characterized by weak diminishing contractions, or four hours of strong contractions resulting in no births; no further effort following partial birth of a kitten; continued strong labor several hours after birth of the first kitten or kittens.

If all goes normally the afterbirth (placenta) accompanies or follows shortly after each kitten. Many cats eat the placentas, sometimes developing diarrhea as a consequence. Retained afterbirths can cause serious illness.

POSTDELIVERY CARE OF THE MOTHER

Within a day after the birth, the mother should be eating, and actively and contentedly nursing and washing her kittens. Neglect of the kittens, vomiting, listlessness, a foul discharge, or fever call for prompt veterinary attention.

For the first six weeks after delivery, the mother will need as much or even more food as during pregnancy. Litters of four are the average. With larger litters, some supplemental bottle-feeding with a commercial kitten formula will take some of the stress from the mother and assure steady growth of the kittens.

At first the mother will spend most of her time with the kittens, but should soon be encouraged to leave them for exercise and, if she is an outdoor cat, for short stays outdoors.

Occasional cats come into heat, mate, and conceive within a few days of delivery, even though they are nursing kittens. Most, however, do not come into heat until after the kittens are weaned. If all the kittens die or are destroyed within a day of birth, recurrence of heat is accelerated.

MILK FEVER. Hypocalcemia (eclampsia, puerperal tetany, milk fever), rather frequent in bitches nursing large litters of puppies, is a rarity in cats, even those that have not had as much extra food and calcium as is generally considered desirable. Although it has been reported to occur before and during delivery, it is most likely at two to four weeks after, when the kittens' demand for milk is at its maximum. Signs are restlessness, lack of appetite, and progressively unsteady gait. Later the cat pants, trembles, twitches, and finally goes into convulsions that can cause the temperature to soar. If emergency treatment is not given, shock ensues, with dilatation of the pupils and subnormal temperature.

Calcium gluconate, given intravenously by your veterinarian, will almost always bring about miraculously rapid recovery. The cat should not be separated from her kittens, but should receive calcium tablets as a supplement, and weaning or bottle-feeding of the kittens should rapidly reduce their need for the mother's milk.

LACK OF MILK. Lack of milk (agalactia) occurs occasionally, usually in new mothers. Pituitary hormone (oxytocin) provided by your veterinarian as either an injection or nasal spray will cause the milk to flow within minutes.

CAKING. "Caking" of the breasts once in a while results from insufficient nursing, especially if the nipples are inverted, so that the kittens cannot suckle. Warm moist packs and gentle massaging are helpful in releasing the milk, and kittens should be guided to make use of the affected nipples.

Inversion of nipples is best dealt with during pregnancy, the owner drawing them gently outward and massaging them.

ENGORGEMENT. Engorgement of the mammary glands occurs if an entire litter dies or is suddenly taken from the mother. Massaging or milking out the glands is contraindicated because it stimulates additional milk production. If the cat is intensely uncomfortable, treatment with estrogen or with male hormone slows the production of milk. If kittens are still nursing when it is time to start selling or giving them away, they should not go all at once, both to prevent the engorgement with milk and also because the sudden loss of all the kittens is seriously distressing to the mother.

MASTITIS. Inflammation and infection of the breasts, mastitis most often occurs during nursing and involves only one or two glands. The owner's first clue may be that the kittens are doing poorly, perhaps even dying, as a result of changes and bacteria in the milk. The infected gland is inflamed, swollen, and painful, and may abscess. Your veterinarian will treat the cat with a systemic antibiotic and if an abscess is present, drain it surgically. Any surviving kittens must also receive antibiotic treatment and be bottle-fed with kitten formula to protect them from further exposure to the toxins in the mother's milk.

CARE OF THE NEWBORN KITTENS

Healthy kittens, as soon as they have been cleaned and stimulated by their mother's licking, instinctively start nosing their way to her nipples. It is most important for the kittens' future health that they suckle the mother's first milk (colostrum), for it contains antibodies that will give them protection for several weeks against panleukopenia and perhaps some of the upper respiratory infections as well.

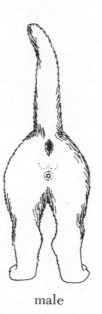
male

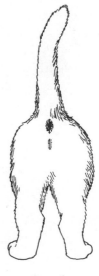
female

Weak, inactive kittens should be rubbed gently by the owner. Any fetal fluids that are blocking their throats should be swabbed out with tissue or a Q-tip. Some breeders warm weak kittens in a water bath at about 100°F., until they breathe regularly, mew, and move actively.

It is said that each kitten in the beginning chooses its favorite nipple. If the kittens seem dissatisfied and mew hungrily, the owner should check to see that the nipples are indeed producing milk.

A kitten's sex may be determined by looking beneath its tail. The male has two small dots like a colon; the female has an upside-down exclamation point (see sketch on previous page).

Soon after the birth, fresh bedding may be put in the box. Until the kittens learn to use a litter box at three to four weeks, the mother will be responsible for keeping them and the box clean. For the first two weeks the kittens should be handled very little, lest the mother become alarmed and decide to move or hide them, but they should become accustomed to the sound of voices and gradually they may be stroked and fondled more and more.

As they grow, the more their contacts with people and other pets in the home, the better their start toward a well-adjusted life.

Flourishing kittens should be nursing vigorously at frequent intervals and mewing little. If they cry loudly and often, are not nursing, or feel cool to the touch, your veterinarian should be consulted at once. Diarrhea and failure to suckle, both serious symptoms, cause kittens to dehydrate and fail rapidly.

If one kitten dies, it is sometimes the prelude to further deaths or loss of an entire litter. If you wish to safeguard the rest of the litter, the dead member should be carefully autopsied to determine, if possible, the cause of death and to prevent further losses.

FEEDING AND WEANING ORPHANS

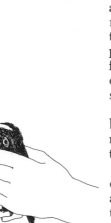

If it is necessary to bottle-feed very young kittens, because they are orphaned or the mother is unwilling to care for them, commercial kitten formula (such as Borden's KMR) is available from many veterinarians. If not, a good substitute may be devised with nonfat dried milk (⅓ cup), cottage cheese (¼ cup), and corn oil (⅛ cup). Add water to make up to 2 cups, blend, and refrigerate, making the mixture fresh every two days. (Cow's milk does not have enough protein — and also may cause diarrhea.) Before feeding, heat to body temperature; and feed in a doll's bottle. Two teaspoonfuls of formula per ounce of kitten will meet its daily needs. Vitamins may be supplied by a fifth of the daily dose of an infant vitamin preparation added to the formula or placed on the back of the tongue. At first the kittens should be fed five or six times a day, but after two weeks, three or four times should suffice.

Kittens too weak to suckle may be fed with a plastic dropper; they should be held upright during feeding so that they do not choke. Bubbles at the nostril are a sign that your technique is faulty. Give only a few drops at a time, lest the kitten drown or inhale the fluid and develop pneumonia.

Baby kittens, at four or five weeks of age, may be offered cow's milk (if it does not cause diarrhea), commercial kitten formula, strained baby meats, and moistened commercial kitten pellets. After weaning (at about six weeks to two months) they should receive moderate amounts of food several times a day. The number of meals is gradually cut till a grown cat receives one to three.

Because orphaned kittens have no mother to keep them warm, they are sometimes kept in a box heated by an electric light bulb. After each feeding the perineum should be rubbed gently to stimulate bowel movements and urination, until the habits are established.

Kittens that have been orphaned or taken too young from their mothers form the strongest attachments to their humans. They are also prone throughout their lives to infantile habits such as suckling on fingers, woolly garments, and their own or other animals' toes or tail.

BIRTH DEFECTS AND INFECTIONS

Birth defects are too numerous to be listed in full and vary from the trivial to the fatal. Extra toes (polydactyly) are considered an attractive feature by many owners. A variety of serious deformities of the limbs and of the spine (for example, spina bifida), however, are inconsistent with a healthy life. The most spectacular deformities are seen in the double-headed, double-trunk, or Siamese-twin "monsters." Not infrequently, kittens have a huge head that is partly double but with a single "cyclops" eye. Cleft palate and harelip prevent normal nursing and eating. Deformities of the breast bone are often associated with a congenital hernia of the diaphragm that is life threatening. Abnormalities of the tail and shallow hip sockets, on the other hand, handicap a cat little or not at all.

Eyes may be absent, or too small, or crossed. Blue-eyed white cats are very often deaf. Defects that soon prove fatal in young kittens are imperforate anus and multiple cyst formation in the kidneys or liver ducts. Abnormalities in the structure of the heart are frequent causes of early death in kittens and a number of these defects are believed to be inherited.

What causes many of the defects is unknown. Some are inherited, some are due to faulty fetal development, some may be associated with the mother's illness during pregnancy or her treatment with certain drugs, for example, griseofulvin, which is the remedy of choice for ringworm.

Cerebellar hypoplasia, an underdevelopment of the part of the brain concerned with balance, is an effect of the virus of panleukopenia on certain of the brain cells, occurring if a pregnant mother contracts the disease or if her kittens become infected in the first month of life. The staggering gait and bobbing head become apparent when the kittens first crawl out of the nest and try to get about and eat from a food dish. Most kittens are so severely afflicted that they cannot function well enough for life's daily activities and have to be destroyed.

Feline viral rhinotracheitis contracted by a mother during pregnancy may be the cause of congenital infection in her kittens or may be transmitted to them while they are still young.

Mothers may also be inapparent carriers of other respiratory infections and pass them on to their young. The respiratory infections are perhaps the most tragic of all, for they may pass from generation to generation in a cattery for years, apparently subsiding, then flaring up, and presenting a constant disease problem.

old age

Cats in general age more gracefully and with less obvious signs of wear and tear than dogs or humans. Gray hairs are few, stiffness, deafness, and blindness are uncommon. Wasted temporal muscles, a pearliness of the lenses of the eyes (sclerosis), and thickening of the bones of the jaws are the few signs by which one can sometimes recognize a very old cat. Well-fed, well-cared-for neutered cats that lead a life without stress frequently live into the late teens and even twenties with virtually no signs of aging, some even playing at times like kittens.

PREVENTIVE CARE

Dental care, scaling of tartar and removal of diseased teeth, should be routine, if a cat is to continue to eat well and maintain healthy gums. Many very old cats have excellent teeth, but do not be apprehensive if eventually your cat loses most or all. Cats don't chew their food, and the stomach and intestine will take care of digestion.

Claws that do not get enough wear should be clipped.

Regular brushing is important to prevent swallowing of fur and formation of mats in the coat.

The anal sacs may need to be emptied several times a year. In older cats the contents can become so firmly inspissated that defecation may be interfered with.

The owner should be very observant about any changes in the cat's condition or habits. Many oldsters suffer a moderate weight loss unassociated with any disease process, but sudden or severe wasting must be investigated.

Increased intake of fluid is frequent. Most often it is a sign of chronic progressive kidney disease. A urinalysis and blood urea nitrogen and creatinine determinations will distinguish whether the cat is for the time being compensating for the disease, or is already uremic. A cat with compensated kidney disease should be shifted if possible to a diet with a greater proportion of carbohydrate, in order to lessen the amount of protein waste products to be processed by the kidneys. Low-protein prescription diets are available for cats, but in case they prove not to an animal's taste, possible substitutes are New England clam chowder, tuna-noodle casserole, spaghetti with meat sauce, and macaroni and cheese.

Once significant uremia develops and a cat stops eating, vomits occasionally, and becomes anemic, it should be humanely destroyed.

Diabetes mellitus is another important cause of extreme thirst. Usually the cat is eating ravenously. Early in the disease it may be obese but eventually loses weight. Urinalysis and a blood sugar test are necessary for diagnosis. It is often rather easy to find the suitable dose of insulin for a diabetic cat that leads a quiet indoor life, and if an owner is interested enough to check urine for sugar occasionally and to give daily injections of insulin, a cat's life may be prolonged for some years.

Urinary incontinence is often a consequence of the greatly increased urine excretion associated with either chronic kidney disease or diabetes mellitus. A few extra sanitary pans put around the house often solve the problem.

Aged spayed females occasionally develop involuntary urinary incontinence. Small doses of estrogen are effective.

Constipation is one of the most frequent problems in old cats, and a variety of remedies may be tried. Increasing the moisture content of food comes first. Vaseline or a yeast-flavored petroleum jelly laxative marketed especially for cats may be placed on a cat's nose or paw two or three times a week to be licked down and act as a lubricant. Other cats take well to bulk-producing laxatives. With still others, an infant suppository two or three times a week is effective.

As general tonics for old cats, brewer's yeast as powder sprinkled on the food or several tablets a day often seems beneficial. Even more so, in many cases, are anabolic yeast-flavored tablets which contain a number of vitamins, minerals, and small amounts of thyroid extract and male and female hormones.

Osteoarthritis and calcified intervertebral disks are frequently seen in radiographs of old cats but do not often cause serious trouble. For severe stiffness or pain, a veterinarian may try small doses of cortisone or phenylbutazone (Butazolidin). Aspirin, which would be the preferred drug for humans, is so toxic for cats that it is very rarely used.

Malignant tumors spell the end for many old cats. Most likely to be noticed by an owner is the breast cancer that occurs chiefly in unspayed females. Most frequent are the leukemias and leukemic tumors. Other fairly common tumors are those of the mouth (under the tongue), liver, pancreas, and skeleton.

Take your veterinarian's word if he advises you that your old friend has come to the end of the road; do not insist on heroic and most likely useless measures that will mean procedures and hospitalization to which your cat would undoubtedly prefer a peaceful death.

EUTHANASIA

As long as your cat is not actually suffering or in pain, you may wish to let it have some last peaceful days at home, but it will be cruel to you both to let the illness go on to a long drawn-out end.

You yourself will know when the time has come to put your cat away. If it is fearful or hard to handle, your veterinarian may give you a sedative to administer at home to quiet the cat before the veterinarian comes or before you take it to the veterinarian.

Euthanasia is most easily and gently performed by an intravenous or intraperitoneal injection of an overdose of the same kind of anesthetic that would be used for surgery. If you stay with your cat and stroke and speak to it during the procedure, it will fall asleep quickly and without apprehension.

further readings

CATCOTT, E. J., ed. *Feline Medicine and Surgery.* Santa Barbara, California, American Veterinary Publications, Drawer KK, 1975.

CROUCH, J. E. *Text-Atlas of Cat Anatomy.* Philadelphia, Lea and Febiger, 1969.

Encyclopedia Britannica. Chicago, William Benton, 1971.

Feline Practice: The Journal of Feline Medicine and Surgery for the Practitioner. P.O. Box 4457, Santa Barbara, California.

FOX, M. W. *Understanding Your Cat.* New York, Coward, McCann and Geohegan, 1974.

GERSHOFF, S. N. *Nutrient Requirements of Laboratory Animals,* 2nd ed. Washington, D.C., National Academy of Sciences, 1972.

————.*Nutritional Problems of Household Cats.* J. Amer. Veterinary Medical Association, 166, 1975, 455–458.

HABEL, R. E. *Applied Antomy.* Ithaca, New York, 1963.

JOSHUA, J. O. *The Clinical Aspects of Some Diseases of Cats.* Philadelphia, Lippincott, 1965.

KIRK, R. W., ed. *Current Veterinary Therapy,* vol. 6. Philadelphia, W. B. Saunders, 1977.

KIRK, R. W., AND BISTNER, S. I. *Handbook of Veterinary Procedures and Emergency Treatment,* 2nd ed. Philadelphia, W. B. Saunders, 1975.

McGINNIS, T. *The Well Cat Book.* New York and Berkeley, California, Random House–Bookworks, 1975.

ROBINSON, R. *Genetics for Cat Breeders.* Oxford, Pergamon Press, 1971.

SCOTT, F. W. "Feline Panleukopenia Vaccinations," *Feline Practice,* II, 2, March–April 1972, 10–13.

WOLSTENHOLME, G. E. W., AND O'CONNOR, M. *The Lifespan of Animals.* Boston, Little, Brown, 1959.

Skunks

LESTER E. FISHER, D.V.M.

An animal wisely shunned in the wild for more than one reason, the skunk has come into increasing vogue as a household pet in the past decade. While possibly not so demonstrative as dogs or cats — though individuals have marked differences in personality — these animals can make handsome, interesting pets. Skunks, because of their highly effective natural defense, are far less excitable than most wild animals and, if secured as pets from domestic stock, are ready to give a considerate owner their trust. Do not bring home a wild skunk.

Over recent years, growing epidemics of rabies among wild skunks have made it far too dangerous to attempt to capture a kitten for yourself. The high percentage of rabies in the skunk population is undoubtedly a result of the animal's fearlessness. It relies on a weapon that is useless against a maddened, rabid animal, however, and is therefore a prime prospect to get bitten and infected. Furthermore, skunks are highly sociable with their own kind.

There are four skunks native to the United States:

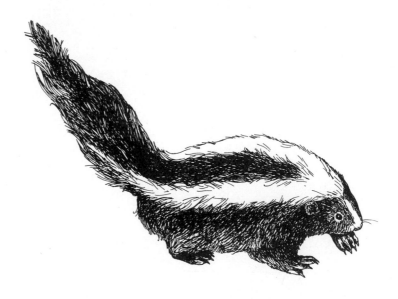

STRIPED SKUNK The striped skunk is found in southern Canada and throughout the United States, with the exception of southern Florida and the Coastal Plain. This heavy-bodied animal reaches a length of 30 inches, including 7½ inches of bushy tail. Its glistening black coat is marked by two white stripes that go from the base of the tail to the nape of the neck, where they meet. There is a narrow, white stripe on the head, from the tip of the nose to the nape. Striped skunks weigh up to 10 pounds.

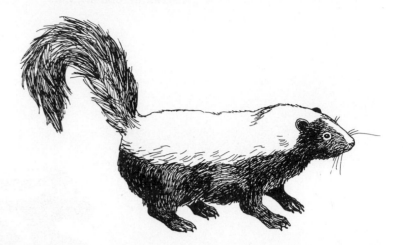

HOODED SKUNK   The hooded skunk is confined to southwest New Mexico and southeastern Arizona. It is similar in appearance to the striped skunk, except there is a single white stripe beginning at the nape of the neck. The narrow stripe on the head is the same. Both the striped and the hooded skunk belong to the genus Mephitis.

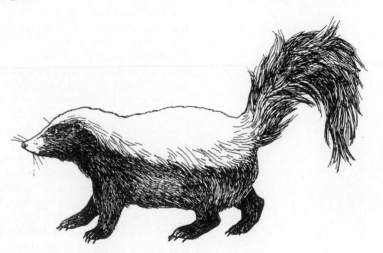

HOG-NOSED SKUNK   The hog-nosed skunk of southwestern Arizona, Colorado, and Texas, while generally similar to its Mephitis kin, belongs to a separate genus, Conepatus. The otherwise handsome appearance of this animal is aesthetically marred by its bare hoglike snout — which is an excellent attribute in a life spent largely in rooting for food.

SPOTTED SKUNK OR CIVET   The remaining genus is Spilogale, also represented by a single species, the spotted skunk, or civet. These animals are found west of the Mississippi — with the exceptions of Montana and most of Wyoming — as well as along the Gulf Coast and up into the southern Appalachians. The spotted skunks reach 22½ inches, but the tail on such a specimen takes up 9 inches of that length. The animal gets its name from the fact that the stripes along its sides and down the tail appear to be broken; actually, they look more like dashes than dots.

Of these different species, only one has earned popularity as a pet, the striped skunk — not only because of its wider distribution, but because an increasing number of breeders are raising these animals for the pet market. The less luxuriant coat of the striped skunk undoubtedly robs it of some of its commercial appeal.

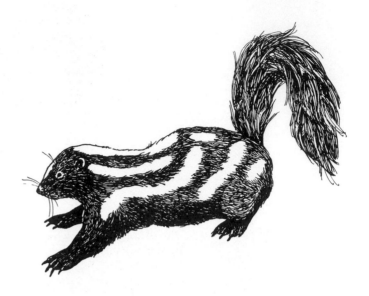

Only the entry of these breeders into the market makes skunks suitable as pets. In addition to the danger of rabies, in many areas conservation regulations forbid the capture of skunks, for these ecologically valuable animals kill large numbers of vermin and destructive insects. Because of the threat of rabies, there are also regulations in many communities completely forbidding skunks as pets, whether bred in captivity or not. Before making a purchase, you should check with both state and county health authorities.

While skunks are naturally nocturnal animals, they can be trained, as will be discussed, to change their habits. Also, skunks in the wild go into a state of semihibernation in wintertime. (They never reach the deep state of sleep some bears do, though, and will arouse themselves whenever there is a short spell of milder weather.) This habit, too, can be changed.

To live a completely healthy life as a pet, a skunk should be given a fair degree of freedom. They can be housebroken easily, and by nature they are clean animals. Around the home they are no more of a problem than a cat. They can be taken out for walks as well, though skunks should always be kept on a leash at such times. The urge for an excursion into the wild could be dangerous, on two counts: first, if the skunk has been de-scented, it would be defenseless; second, there would be the danger of its contracting rabies. While rabies inoculations are effective in dogs and cats, there is some question whether they produce solid immunization in skunks.

De-scenting is not strictly necessary, by the way. Skunks raised from kittens show no inclination to use their weapon on those they consider friends, and many have lived a full life, up to ten years, without giving the slightest cause for offense. They are calm animals, slow to assume danger because in their natural state they have the universal respect of their neighbors. They are not likely to go off half-cocked. It is only good sense, though, to recognize that life is full of surprises. There is no way to guarantee your kitten (the operation should be performed at six to eight weeks) will never encounter a situation that in its judgment constitutes an emergency calling for extraordinary action.

The consequences are not something that can be shrugged off lightly. The respect given the skunk is well deserved, for its weapon is impressively effective. The secret lies in two musk glands — a characteristic of its family,

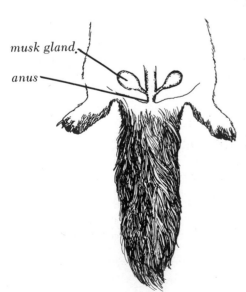

musk gland

anus

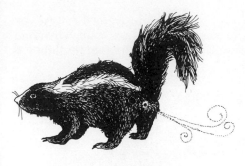

Mustelidae, which includes the minks, weasels, and polecats — that lie just under the skin beneath the tail. These protrude from the anus, and the angry skunk can project a spray of noxious fluid for 10 feet or more without getting a drop on its own lovely coat. This is strong enough to burn the skin and, if it gets in the eyes, to cause temporary but painful blindness. There is nothing temporary about the smell. It can be removed from clothing, but on household furniture the memory of an accident lingers on.

Should you decide to leave your skunk in a state of combat readiness, an essential part of your household equipment should be a generous stock of tomato juice. This is the secret to deodorizing. Clothes or, more likely, the family dog that went too far in asserting its rights should first be thoroughly soaked in the juice and then washed or shampooed to remove the odor.

preventive medicine
GENERAL CARE

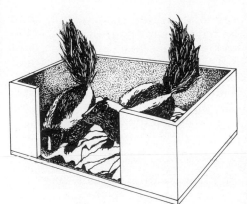

While the comparison to a cat as a house pet is valid in most instances, the skunk does have habits that are different enough to require special consideration. In the wild, for instance, skunks live in dens — which they either burrow in the ground or take over from previous tenants. As household residents, they need some form of substitute for the den in order to gain a sense of security when they sleep.

Fortunately, these quarters can be quite simple and are easily provided. Virtually any small box or even a barrel with a door cut into the end or the side will serve. For a kitten, this should be partially filled with clean, dry cloths to provide a warm bed. It will be necessary to introduce the kitten to its sleeping box but the little skunk will quickly grasp the box's purpose. The box should always be left in the same place. As the skunk grows to maturity, soft hay can be substituted for the cloth bedding. This should be changed weekly for cleanliness.

If you get more than one skunk, it is not necessary to keep adding beds. Skunks lack the territorial instincts of some animals and in the wild, several females often share their dens without the slightest sign of friction. This same friendliness may carry over to their relations with other pets in the household, incidentally. If they are introduced to the family as kittens, they will become amiable companions to cats, dogs, or any other animals that do not become aggressive toward them.

HOUSEBREAKING. Skunks are easily housebroken. The kitten will instinctively pick a corner of its cage or of one of the rooms in your house for use as its toilet. Do not attempt, at first, to change this — rather, put it to use. You can put either a newspaper or a litter box in the chosen corner. Because skunks are burrowing animals, the newspaper would probably be best. If you do use a litter box, remember that there is bound to be spillage, and it will be necessary to put something under the box to catch this; thus the box may end up merely as a supplement to the newspaper in any case.

When you clean the box or replace the papers, leave some of the kitten's wastes there at first, until it has thoroughly learned that this is indeed the right place. Once it has the idea firmly in mind and is well housebroken, you can try moving the box or papers to a place of your own choosing. When the move is made, leave some of the wastes in. Then show the kitten the new location. Watch it and, should it try to return to the original place, carry it to the proper one.

DISCIPLINE. Do not attempt to spank the skunk should it make an error. Discipline of this type is totally unsuited to a skunk. No matter how well adapted these animals might seem to life with humans, always remember that they are still wild by nature. Dogs and cats have been selectively bred over many centuries not merely for their appearance but for temperament. The skunk has not. Spanking could totally destroy your pet's trust. Once this happens, there is no means of correcting the error.

Otherwise, handling your skunk is in no way different from the way you would handle a puppy or a kitten. While some skunks are more shy than others, in general they love fondling and petting and often become devoted lap-sitters, actively seeking affection.

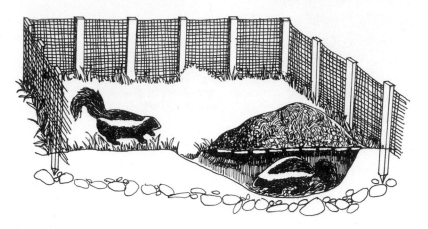

If you intend to give your pet an enclosed outdoor run, again bear in mind that it is a burrowing animal. A pen must have a wire floor to prevent the skunk from digging out. If the pen is to be kept in one place, the floor could be sunk into the earth if the wire is galvanized so that it will not rust and weaken. Another approach would be to bury a layer of heavy rocks beneath the cage. An outdoor den can be easily made by digging a trench and covering it with boards, over which earth can be spread. It must be underlaid by either wire or rocks to prevent escape, and be where there is no possibility of the den becoming flooded.

FEEDING
In its natural state, the skunk is a true omnivore, eating virtually anything that is available — insects, small rodents such as mice or even rats, as well as fruits and vegetables. There is no point whatsoever in attempting to duplicate this diet for your pet skunk, however, since an adult skunk can thrive on anything man, dog, or cat will eat.

Processed dog and cat foods available in your local supermarket are a perfectly acceptable diet. Table scraps are excellent. These basic meals can be supplemented occasionally with a raw egg, a chicken head or neck, and fresh fruits and vegetables in season. To keep its teeth in good condition, occasionally give the skunk dog biscuits or a fresh bone with the fat and most of the meat trimmed off. While skunks are extremely fond of milk, they should be given a saucer only rarely; too much milk gives them diarrhea.

Once a week, add ½ teaspoon of cod-liver oil to the skunk's meal to keep its coat in condition. If it still seems to lack luster, this can be stepped up to additional meals.

WEIGHT-WATCHING. By the time they are six months old, skunks can be fed only once a day, preferably in the late afternoon or early evening. Skunks are gluttons and their diets should be carefully controlled. A normal meal will consist of roughly one cup of food. While it is not necessary to measure this out, any leftover food should be removed as soon as the skunk has finished eating to prevent its returning for snacks later.

Regulating the skunk's diet is especially important in the fall. Instinctively, the pet will prepare itself for hibernation at this time, an adaptation designed to get it through the winter when food is scarce and hard to find in the wild. This is, of course, not necessary for a pet that has a consistent food supply.

To counteract this natural tendency, the skunk's food should be cut in half during September and October. This can be done either by halving its daily ration or by feeding it only every other day. If it is not allowed to accumulate fat, the skunk will remain an active and amusing pet throughout the winter.

WATER. Fresh water should always be available. If you are keeping your skunk in a cage or run, a watering bottle (available in pet stores) will provide a good, unspillable supply that cannot be contaminated. Otherwise, both the water and food dishes should be flat-bottomed and broad enough to make them difficult to turn over.

GROOMING Brushing will help assure that your skunk's coat will remain healthy and beautiful. This need not be a daily routine but should take place at least once a week. It will be regarded by your pet as a treat, as it sits in your lap receiving welcome attention.

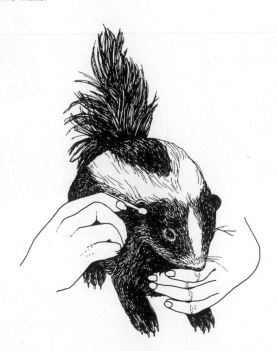

DEODORANTS, SHAMPOOS, AND HAIR DRYERS. The slight smell of a skunk's coat has nothing to do with the musk glands and is easily removed by using the deodorants for dogs that are available in pet shops. Bathing is not necessary, but should you decide to do so, your pet must be introduced to it while still a kitten. Use a baby shampoo that will not irritate the skin. Rinse and dry the animal thoroughly. Your kitten can become accustomed to a hair dryer if you do not expose it to air that is uncomfortably hot.

CLAWS. Your skunk's claws should be regularly checked to see if trimming is needed. They should be kept about ¼ inch beyond the quick. The quick can be located by holding the claws near a light, which will show pinkness within the nail.

EARS. To minimize the possibility of bacterial infection, check the interior of the skunk's ears occasionally to see if there is an accumulation of dirt or wax. Any accumulation should be cleaned out, using a cotton swab dipped in a mixture of equal proportions of water and hydrogen peroxide.

TRAINING While they are naturally playful animals, skunks show little inclination to learn tricks — which is not to say that they don't have their own. It is more a matter of the owner's learning to appreciate what is happening than teaching the pet. Foot-stamping, for example, is something many owners report their skunks do in play. In a wild animal, this is a warning to get out of range as quickly as possible, for it is the skunk's equivalent of the rattlesnake's buzzing alarm. There is no danger from a pet skunk that is playing, though, even if the skunk has not been de-scented. The human parallel that comes to mind is bluffing.

The only real training possible is alteration of the skunk's nocturnal habits, so that it will become a daytime pet. This is quite simple and takes only a few days. After your pet has slept for about an hour in the morning, take it out of its den and offer it a favorite food. When it has accepted it and eaten, take the skunk on your lap and pet it for a while. By this time the contented pet will have waked up and will be happy to stay up for a few hours. Continue this on a daily basis and within a short time, the animal will have completely changed its sleeping habits.

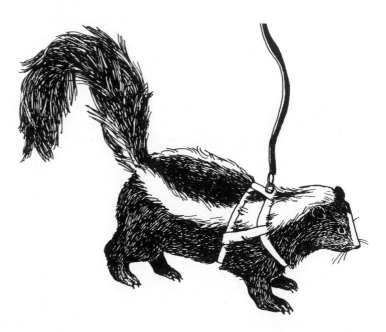

It is not necessary to train skunks to walk on leashes; they are quite willing and able, simply waiting for the opportunity. Dogs are a far more difficult problem, because the owner has to overcome the energetic puppy's inclination to strain and jerk in its efforts to run and investigate strange smells and sights, or simply to race around. The more lethargic skunk is quite willing to amble along peaceably at your side. Don't expect the skunk to learn to heel, though, or to sit on command.

Because the skunk's head is relatively narrow in comparison with its neck, dog and cat collars are not practical. A harness or halter that loops under the chest and attaches behind the forelegs will solve the problem. Only the lightest of nylon leashes is needed, because the skunk will have no tendency to resist or to strain against you.

optional operations
DE-SCENTING

Between its sixth and eighth week, de-scenting, the operation to remove the skunk's musk glands, is simple, quite safe, and relatively inexpensive. It should not be performed if the animal is younger, and it becomes progressively more dangerous as it grows older. Any veterinarian is capable of performing this operation, and the animal may be taken home afterward.

It should then be allowed several days' rest in its den. Let it set its own pace for becoming active again — don't try to force it to play until it is ready.

SPAYING AND CASTRATION

The sex of your skunk can be determined by examining the external sex organs in a manner similar to checking a kitten (page 119). In a very young animal it may be difficult. While it is possible to spay females and castrate males, the circumstances pet skunks live under make such operations questionable. When would they have the opportunity to mate haphazardly? If an animal were to escape during the spring mating season, when the females are in heat, the danger of its contracting rabies would far outweigh that of its having unwanted offspring. In such circumstances the skunk should be taken to a veterinarian and kept under observation until it has been determined whether the pet might have become infected, even if it had been immunized. (See Disease, pages 133ff.)

the home clinic

Since skunks are similar to cats, the same principles for stocking a medicine cabinet and taking their temperature and heartbeat (page 77), giving pills and liquid medicine (page 79), giving artificial respiration (page 82), making bandages and dressings (page 86), and protective restraints (page 80) apply.

first aid

Except for the following addition — rectal prolapse — you can apply the same principles of first aid to skunks as to cats. (See pages 82ff. for discussions of internal bleeding, shock, unconsciousness, paralysis, convulsions, fractures, dislocations, burns, extreme heat and cold, bites, and poisons.)

RECTAL PROLAPSE

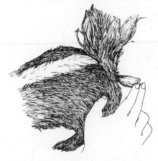

For reasons which may be connected with its means of self-defense, skunks are occasionally subject to an accident in which the anus protrudes as much as four inches, literally turning inside out. The animal seems unable to correct this condition and needs human help, for these delicate mucous membranes could become infected if left exposed. Bring the animal to your veterinarian. If you can't do this, then wash your hands and carefully bathe the area around the rectum with warm, soapy water. Rinse the area off and apply mineral oil liberally. Then gently try to push the protruding anus back into its normal position. You may have to use one or more fingers or even both hands, for as you push some of the tissue back into the animal, other tissue will attempt to come out.

parasites and fungus

Studies of the wild skunk population have shown that these hardy animals are remarkably resistant to parasitic infestations. A pet skunk living in a home or a pen in the yard is protected even further by its isolation. If it is in frequent contact, though, with pet dogs and cats, which are allowed greater freedom, the possibility of its picking up parasites does exist.

ROUNDWORMS

The likeliest pests are various roundworms, or nematodes. While they are not usually a major problem for a healthy, well-fed adult skunk, they must be taken more seriously in kittens. Furthermore, humans, particularly young children, could pick up the parasites from the animal. The best means of prevention is sanitation, preventing accumulation of the pets' feces in either boxes or yards, for it is through contact with these that the parasite is spread from one animal to another.

There are a number of symptoms, depending on the particular parasite, but signs you should watch for include emaciation, slow growth, loss of energy despite a normal appetite, dull coat, and potbelly. Consult your veterinarian whenever possible for all parasite examinations and treatments.

If the pet coughs and vomits, the vomit should be examined for worms, which look like very small or large earthworms. These may also be visible in the feces at times.

Piperazine tablets, available from pet shops and veterinarians, are effective in treating skunks for worms if you follow the manufacturer's directions for use with cats of the same weight. If any one pet shows signs of worms, all should receive treatment.

TAPEWORMS
Tapeworms are far less likely to be a problem and can be avoided by keeping your pet free of fleas (see below), which spread the parasite's eggs. Loss of appetite, nervousness, dull coat, swollen belly, and diarrhea are all symptoms. Rectangular segments of the worm or a string of segments, which looks like a flattened strand of tissue, may be visible in the animal's feces and in the hair surrounding the anus.

Commercial preparations containing dichlophen are effective and may be obtained from pet shops or veterinarians. Again, follow the instructions for their use with cats. Two treatments, one week apart, will usually be sufficient. Again, all pets should be treated if any one shows symptoms of having tapeworms.

TICKS
Since it should not have the freedom given dogs and cats, a pet skunk is not so likely to be exposed to ticks — certainly not to the point of infestation. On the off possibility that somehow a single parasite or two might be picked up, removal is a simple process. Precautions must be taken, though, to make sure the tick's head does not break off where it has penetrated the skin — this can cause infections that are far more difficult to treat. Therefore something more is involved than grabbing and pulling. To remove the tick safely, the first step is to get the tick to withdraw its head. One of the best means is to coat it with petroleum jelly. After half a minute, it can be picked off with tweezers. Another technique is to place a piece of cotton soaked in ether or lighter fluid over the parasite, taking it off in the cotton when a half minute has passed. Should the head break off, clean the area around it with soap and water and remove it in the same way you would a splinter. Then disinfect the wound.

FLEAS
The presence of fleas is easily discovered — their bites will result in furious scratching to relieve the itch. The tiny, dark brown insects can be spotted as they run or leap for cover when you part the animal's hair (see illustration, page 45). Their favorite lurking places are around the ears, the neck, and the base of the tail.

A shampoo containing selenium sulfide, available at drugstores, or other effective medications your veterinarian can prescribe will be helpful in removing them. Bathe the skunk every three days for two weeks. Be sure to rinse out all the shampoo. Flea powder containing rotenone — rotenone will be listed on the label — should be used on the other days. Dispose of the bedding that has been used and dust the pet's den with flea powder. Check other pets to see if they need defleaing as well.

LICE
Lice, while similar to fleas and also detectable by scratching, are gray and move slowly. They tend to be found around the base of hairs. A selenium sulfide shampoo twice a week for two weeks will usually be sufficient to remove them. If not, you can obtain other effective products from your veterinarian.

MANGE AND RINGWORM
Mange, caused by tiny parasites closely related to spiders, is too easily confused with ringworm to be treated without professional diagnosis. The para-

sites are too small to be visible to the naked eye. The first obvious symptom, as with other skin parasites, is frenzied scratching. Parting the fur at the points of irritation will reveal breaks in the skin. Bald reddened patches will appear. With ringworm, which is caused by a fungus rather than a parasite, there will also be flakes of skin similar to dandruff caught in the animal's hair. If you suspect either mange or ringworm, wash your hands thoroughly after making an examination, for both conditions can be transmitted to humans. Do not attempt diagnosis or treatment with patent medicines on your own initiative. Because of the possibility of contagion, it is vital that these conditions be handled promptly and properly. A veterinarian should examine the animal at the earliest opportunity and will prescribe the correct medication.

disease

If it is properly cared for, the possibilities of your skunk's contracting a disease are extremely slim. The concentration must be, therefore, on prevention — once the damage is done there is little the owner (or, in some cases, even the veterinarian) can do to help the pet. Taken in order of importance, the diseases with which you should be most concerned are:

DISTEMPER

Skunks are vulnerable to both dog and cat distemper (pages 25 and 99–100). Once an animal has contracted it, death is a possibility, for there is no effective treatment. Fortunately, your pet can be protected effectively by immunization. At two months, a kitten should be inoculated against both forms.

RABIES

Skunks, as was said earlier, are extremely susceptible to rabies. Not only is rabies invariably fatal to the animal, in the course of the disease prior to its death the pet becomes a serious danger to humans. Since there is some doubt about the effectiveness of rabies vaccine in immunizing skunks, you must do everything possible to ensure that your pet cannot become infected. Have the skunk inoculated anyway, and keep it under control at all times, not allowing it to wander just as you protect a de-scented skunk from dangers against which it has no defense.

It bears repeating that if there is the slightest possibility your pet might have been exposed, this is a problem for the veterinarian. If it returns after temporarily escaping, it should be carefully examined by the veterinarian for any signs of bites and, if they are present, isolated until safely past the incubation period for the disease. Your veterinarian will decide how long this should be — rabies symptoms may show up within ten days but in some cases have been delayed for as long as seven months after exposure.

COLDS

Loss of appetite and a moist nose are classic symptoms of a cold. While this need be no more serious than it would in a human, there is the possibility of its developing into pneumonia. The pet should be taken to the veterinarian, who will determine whether antibiotics should be administered.

GENERAL SYMPTOMS OF DISEASE

The range of symptoms of disease in a skunk is relatively limited — and most are also possible indications of parasitic infestation, which is far more likely. The owner's first step should be to look for other symptoms, as outlined above. If there are no other indications that a parasite might be the cause, however, the animal should be taken to a veterinarian for a definitive diagnosis and treatment. Antibiotics are the prime weapon today in treating animal diseases, and these invariably require either administration by a veterinarian or a prescription to obtain. The symptoms for which you should watch include:

DIARRHEA. This could be a symptom of pampering rather than of disease. If you've been indulging your skunk's taste for milk, stop at once. Give the pet 1 teaspoon of regular Kaopectate or place it in its food (if you have Kaopectate for animals, follow directions for use with cats). If this is not effective within forty-eight hours, and there are no indications of internal parasites, the animal should be taken to the veterinarian.

DULL FUR. By itself this could be nothing more than an indication of a dietary deficiency, and if you find no other symptoms present, the animal should be given cod-liver oil to correct the condition (see Feeding, page 128).

LOSS OF APPETITE. In animals as fond of eating as are skunks, this is an immediate alarm bell. Check for signs of intestinal parasites (see Parasites and Fungus, pages 131ff.). If results are negative, the pet should be taken to a veterinarian.

Other signs that the pet should be seen by a veterinarian are:

Difficulty breathing or short breath
Lack of growth in kittens
Weakness
Signs of muscular stiffness or soreness
Weakness of the hind limbs
Abnormal thirst
Bleeding in stools

breeding and kittens

While skunks are bred in captivity commercially, this is definitely a job that should be left to experts and not attempted with animals reared as household pets. There are two sound reasons for this. First, experience has shown that there is very little chance of success. Pet skunks show little inclination to mate. Even when mating does take place, litters rarely result. One theory professional breeders offer is that their animals live outdoors, experiencing the year's full weather cycle, in large runs with adequate room for exercise. Conditions are therefore much closer to what the skunk lives under when wild than they can be in the average home.

Even though chances of producing a litter are slim, it might still be worth making the attempt but for the second problem: breeding skunks can be dangerous to the animals, especially when they are not inclined to cooperate. In the natural state, even though mating may have taken place, after two or three days the female shows increasing hostility toward the male. Finally, if he is slow to leave, she will actually attack him. If the male is bitten, unless he quickly receives antibiotics the wound almost invariably will become infected. In such cases, the rate of fatality is extremely high. Oddly, the skunk's bite, for a human, is no more serious than that of any other animal.

There is a theory to account for this. Some naturalists believe it may be a population-control mechanism unique to these animals. In the wild, the skunk has no natural enemies. Its ability to eat a broad range of food and the habit of hibernating during the lean winter give it a high survival potential. Some means of preventing overpopulation is therefore essential. The fact that it is the female who almost invariably attacks the male tends to confirm that the lethal effect of the bite is an overpopulation preventive. Skunks are polygamous. The females share dens, and during the mating season one male may move in to fertilize as many as five females. From a species-survival standpoint, there need be only a relatively small number of males.

WHEN AND WHERE TO GET KITTENS

Fortunately, there are adequate sources for skunks. They can be secured through licensed commercial breeders. It is important to get them before they are weaned in order to avoid taming problems. The best age is between five and six weeks after birth.

Since litters — usually four or five kittens in each — are born in early May, you should plan on getting your kitten around the middle of June. Because they haven't been weaned and require special care, orders must be made in advance and you should prepare yourself with all the things you need to take care of the little animal. If you plan on being a two-or-more-skunk family, obviously you would be best advised to get all females. In some states, if you own more than one skunk you will be required to get a breeder's license. Fees for these are nominal, however.

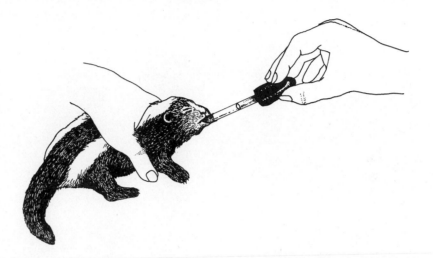

Kittens may be nursed with either a plastic doll's bottle or an eyedropper. If glass is used, a small piece of rubber tube should be placed around the tip of the glass tube in order to prevent the possibility of its being shattered by the kitten's teeth.

Fresh cow's milk should not be used in nursing kittens because of the danger of diarrhea. Instead use evaporated milk mixed with an equal portion of water and sweetened with Karo syrup rather than sugar. This should be given at body temperature, testing it against the inside of your wrist. Feed until the kitten rejects the nipple.

Very young kittens must be fed every four to five hours, again, to capacity. At four weeks, they can be spoon-fed Pablum or other cereals to begin the weaning process. As the kitten begins to feed itself, you can start reducing the bottle feedings and gradually convert to an adult diet (see Feeding, page 128). When it has been weaned, for the first two months it should be fed twice a day. This can then be cut to a single feeding.

Housing for the new kitten has been covered earlier (see page 127). The primary object in outfitting the kitten's den should be to assure that it will not become chilled at night.

further readings

COLBY, C. T. *A Skunk in the House.* Philadelphia, J. B. Lippincott, 1973.
HUME, C. *How to Raise and Train a Skunk.* Neptune, New Jersey, T. F. H. Publications, 1967.
SNEDIGAR, R. *Our Small Native Animals.* New York, Dover, 1963.

In tanks and terrariums

Fish

JAY D. HYMAN, D.V.M.

An aquarium makes it possible, without leaving your own home, to observe fish in their natural environment and study the ways in which different species move through the water, their mating, nesting, and feeding habits, and their attitudes toward territory. You don't need to travel to the Bahamas, South America, or the Philippines to enjoy the beauty of fish native to their waters, and you can do so without the risks of scuba diving or snorkeling. Often it is possible to bring together species from throughout the world that would normally never come in contact with one another, though you should watch them closely at first to make sure they can coexist peacefully.

The first step, before you get your fish, is to plan your aquarium with care. Naturally, the characteristics of the species you intend to buy will determine the kind of setting you should provide, but how you set up and maintain the tank are most important aspects in giving your fish the care upon which their lives depend. And it is essential, as will be discussed, to have the tank ready before you get the fish so that the water can age properly.

If you happen to live in the vicinity of the ocean or a bay, or even a lake or pond, you can do your own collecting and set up your aquarium with local fish. The popularity of tropical fish is due to the beauty and variety of colors of species living in warm water. Although most come from parts of the world we consider remote, native species can be obtained in Florida. The sunfish, which is found throughout the United States, is a handsome addition to any tank.

Your first decision will be whether to keep freshwater or marine (saltwater) species.

freshwater fish

Because they are so widely available and are the most common in home tanks, tropical species will be the focus of this chapter. Fortunately, temperate-water species such as sunnies, minnows, or bass will thrive in a home tank.

One of the most common fish raised in home aquariums is the goldfish — some of which are tropical. Much of what will be said about fish in general applies to them, too, though goldfish are both hardier and easier to raise.

Tropical, or temperate water, fish can be divided into two categories, depending on how they bear their young.

LIVE BEARERS

Species in which the mother drops the fry (young fish) alive are known as live-bearing, or viviparous. Live bearers are much more likely to breed than egg-laying species. Mating among these fish is haphazard, and most are quite promiscuous, the male fertilizing virtually any available female of breeding age. There is little attachment between the parents, and sex appears to be a mechanical function rather than a pleasurable act.

In many cases the female will store the sperm and produce a series of separate births from a single mating. Many animals, including even mammals such as seals, have this ability to store sperm. An octopus in the New York Aquarium laid eggs that hatched despite the fact that there had not been a male in her tank for almost a year. Gestation periods vary, with water temperature appearing to be an important factor. Females will give birth much sooner when the tank is kept between 75° and 80°F. than they would at lower temperatures. In most live bearers, a three- to five-week gestation is normal, though sometimes it may extend to six weeks. At temperatures below 65°F., it can be dragged out as much as three months. When the mother gives birth, the fry emerge folded in half and will usually float in this position for some time before they begin to swim.

For a first tank, there are four species that can be highly recommended. They are available in most tropical fish stores or from fish breeders, and they mix well in a community tank.

GUPPIES (*Lebistes reticulatus*). These fish come in a wide range of colors and forms. Because they have been bred to obtain varied characteristics, such as fan or veil tails, it is almost impossible in this country to find a guppy of the size, shape, and color of those in the South American streams and ponds from which their ancestors came. The males of this hardy species grow to a length of 1½ inches, while the less colorful females are from ½ to ⅔ inch larger. Guppies are quite resistant to disease, are lively swimmers, easily bred, and inexpensive.

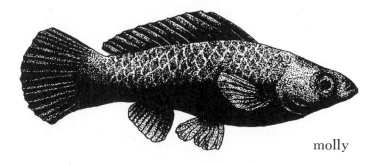

molly

MOLLIES (*Mollienisia*). These fish are usually around 2 to 3 inches long, though some grow to as much as 5 inches. They are handsome fish, most commonly black or green, usually peaceful, and inexpensive. If living plants or algae are not available in the tank, vegetable foods must be provided for mollies. This is an essential part of their diet. Plants are preferred.

platy

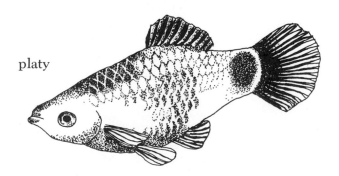

PLATYS (*Xiphophorus maculatus*). These fish are quite peaceful. Colors range from orange and red to silver and black, and mixtures are common. Like the guppies, these fish bear little resemblance to their South American forebears. Breeding has resulted in so many variations no two seem to be exactly the same color.

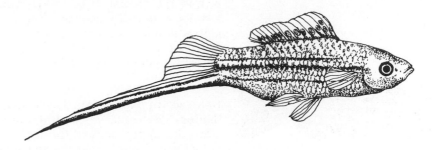

swordtail

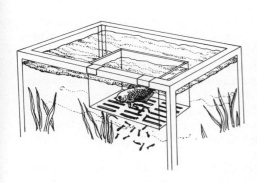

SWORDTAILS *(Xiphophorus helleri).* These fish closely resemble the platy, but are larger. The length of the male, not including the magnificent sword-shaped tail from which it gets its name, ranges between 3 and 3½ inches. Despite their militant name, swordtails are a docile fish. In common with the mollies, they like vegetables in their diet. For purposes of breeding and rearing, swordtails do best in a higher temperature range, near 80°F.

While mollies require a separate tank for raising the fry, young platys, guppies, and swordtails can be kept in the community tank if there is a rearing pen to isolate them for their protection. These are available in any fish hobbyist store and are easily installed. With most of these small fish, a life span of a year should be considered good.

EGG LAYERS The majority of fish kept in home aquariums are egg layers. In reproducing, the female deposits her eggs, which are then sprayed with sperm by the male. The eggs are protected by one of two means: in many species, they are sticky enough to attach themselves to a supportive surface, such as a plant or rock. In others, nests of bubbles are built — usually by the male — in which the eggs are placed. When the male is ready to breed, he takes air in his mouth and coats it with saliva to form a bubble. The bubbles are ejected and accumulate on the surface as a mound of foam.

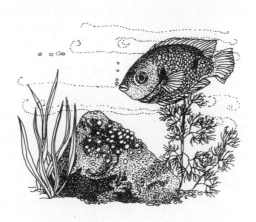
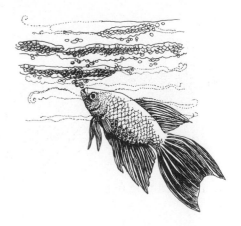

Unlike the live bearers, egg layers are quite selective in their pairing. Many of these fishes have courtship or mating rituals — they vary with the species, and they are always interesting to watch. Here are some of the most readily available egg layers, most of which make excellent choices for a first tank and are compatible with one another:

BARBS OR TIGERS *(Capoets tetrozon)*. These golden red fish have black stripes, a dramatic contrast that makes them an attraction in any tank. These active swimmers, which grow to a length of 2 to 3 inches, move in schools. Barbs do have a tendency to be aggressive if another fish in the tank lacks vigor. By pecking at the fins of a weakened fish, they will further debilitate it.

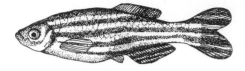

zebra fish

DANIOS *(Brachydanio)*. These fish are also known as zebra fish or striped danios. These natives of India are very fast swimmers and tend to stay toward the upper third of the tank, frequently breaking the surface with their dorsal fins. Their rapid darting movements and their handsome appearance — blue or gold stripes on a silver background — make them a popular addition to any tank. They grow to 2 to 3 inches. Danios are extremely hardy and can stand a temperature range that probably exceeds that of any other tropical fish — between 62° and 102°F.

HATCHETFISH *(Carnequilla strigat)*. Like the danios, these fish are surface swimmers. They lack the hardiness of the danios, however, and are better suited for the experienced aquarist than the novice. Furthermore, they have a tendency to leap out of the water; it is imperative that the tank have a glass cover to keep them from escaping and dying. The fish's shape, a deep chest tapering to a narrow tail area like the head of a hatchet, is the source of its name. The basic color of this South American species is silver, overlaid with broad black stripes.It grows to 2 or 3 inches.

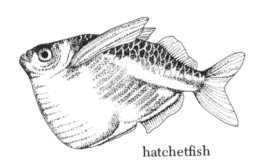

hatchetfish

TETRAS. These fish include a number of unaggressive, schooling fish, which add color and activity to any aquarium. They range in size from ½ to 2 inches. Among the more common varieties are the neon tetra, cardinal tetra, black tetra, lemon tetra, and glolite tetra.

BLIND CAVE FISH OR BLIND CHARACIN *(Anoptichthys jordani)*. These fish are, as their names imply, totally blind, though there is a barely visible eye spot. Yet this small whitish fish with its pink underbelly swims without bumping into things and feeds voraciously on anything that comes its way. Because they are bottom feeders, they make excellent scavengers for a tank. It is a good idea to provide a cave in the tank by putting several rocks together if you intend to keep these fish.

LABYRINTHS (Anabantidae). Unlike the egg layers above, these are bubble-nest builders. Not only does the male select one specific female for his mate, he will kill off all those that do not suit him. Therefore, a male should be removed to a separate tank as soon as he starts to build a bubble nest. Should you desire to breed bubble-nest builders, experience shows that a 20-gallon tank gets the best results.

Siamese fighting fish or bettas *(Betta splendens)* are the most popular of the labyrinths, and they are, of course, native to Thailand. These brightly colored fish — red, blue, green, white, and mixtures of the four — with their large flowing tails and fins, grow to around 3 inches in length. While the males will immediately attack another of their own species, they are quite compatible with other fish. Obviously, there can be only one king of Siam in a tank.

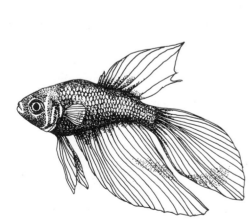

Siamese fighting fish

Gouramis *(Osphronemus goramy)* also rate highly among the labyrinths in popularity. There are several species, beautiful in both their coloring and their movements, all of which mix compatibly in a community tank. The largest are the kissing gouramis *(Helostima temmincki)*, named because of their habit of bringing their lips together in what appears to be a kiss. These range from 1 to 6 inches. The blue gourami *(Trichogaster trichopterus)* also reaches 6 inches. The smaller dwarf gourami (*Colisallia*) and the pearl gourami (*Trichogaster leeri*) are especially striking in their coloring. Gouramis are quite hardy and have been known to live for as long as five or six years in community tanks.

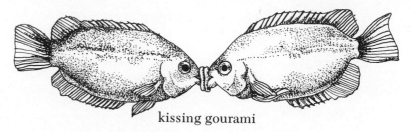

kissing gourami

Another labyrinth, the Egyptian mouth breeder (*Haplochromis multicolor*), has especially interesting mating habits. After the eggs are deposited and fertilized, the female picks them up in her large mouth and carries them — often 100 at a time — for as long as fifteen days after hatching! She does not eat during this period, but makes a peculiar chewing motion with her jaws which serves to change the water in her mouth and keep the young free from parasites. Her lips do not open wide enough to allow the fry to escape. Mouth breeders can be kept at temperatures between 70° and 80°F.

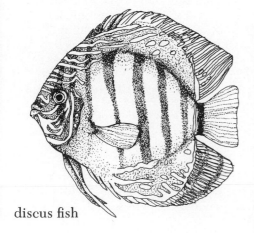

discus fish

DISCUS (*Synphysodon discus*). These are among the most beautiful fish kept in home aquariums. Extremely flat, around 6 to 8 inches in diameter, they resemble oversized silver dollars. The large blue stripes across the body are especially vivid in the male during the breeding season. These timid fish should not be kept with other species but should be by themselves, no more than four to six in a 40-gallon tank. They are quite difficult to keep and will eat only live food, such as brine shrimp.

ANGELFISH SCALARE (*Pterophyllum scalare*). This fish would resemble a discus but for the long dorsal and ventral fins. The basic color arrangement is black bands over silver blue, but selective breeding has produced varieties such as the black and black-veil angels and others with spectacularly long tails. Angelfish have been described as sailing through a tank like swans and their appearance justifies their popularity.

While they can be somewhat aggressive toward smaller fish in a tank, angels tend to be peaceful if kept in schools and are usually fairly easy to keep in a community tank. They prefer live food such as daphnia or brine shrimp.

If frightened, angels will often play possum, floating on the surface as though they were dead. In their native South America, they can be caught by slapping the water with the flat of a hand. After the loud noise, whole schools of angels will rise to the top, where they are gathered up.

The egg layers discussed up to this point have been, so far as other species are concerned at least, relatively peaceful fish. But there are some that can be classified as vicious. There must be those who find something admirable in the qualities that make these animals efficent predators, for they do have their "fans."

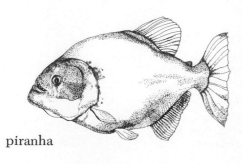

piranha

PIRANHAS (*Serrsalmus spilopleura*). These fish thoroughly deserve their bloodthirsty reputation. A school has been known to attack and devour a cow completely in a matter of minutes. They show the same viciousness toward other fish — therefore, they are not suited to a community tank. Characteristically, the piranha will first bite off its victim's tail fin, which serves as a rudder, destroying its maneuverability. Then it will gouge out great chunks until the fish is consumed.

Piranhas, which come from the Amazon and La Plata river basins of South

America, have never been known to breed in captivity, so all those sold have been caught in their home range. Despite their habits, these are handsome fish, silver or lemon yellow, often with a bright red or orange underside. They can be kept in water with temperatures between 72° and 78°F.

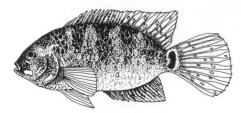

Jack Dempsey

JACK DEMPSEY *(Cichlasoma biocellatum)*. This is probably the most popular among the predator fish, and certainly it is beautiful with its strong head and the blue spots on its long body. Another South American, the Dempsey can nevertheless take a wide range of temperatures — between 65° and 85°F.

While Jack Dempseys can be kept together or in company with other aggressive fish, they should never share a community tank with smaller species such as guppies or bettas. Within a day, most of the small fish will have been eaten. Jack Dempseys are voracious. They will feed on large pieces of raw hamburger and dried as well as live fish. As hardy as they are pugnacious, Jack Dempseys have been known to live as long as ten years in tanks. They average about 6 inches in length.

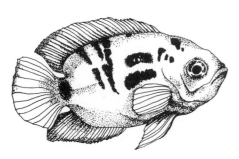

oscar

OSCARS *(Astronotus ocellatus)*. The oscar, from the same continent and particularly the Amazon basin, if kept in a 50- to 100-gallon tank, can reach over 18 inches in length and weigh over 1½ pounds. An oscar is capable of consuming a whole hamburger if it is dropped in the tank. Unlike most fish, the oscar does not have scales. Its velvety skin is often black, reddish, or gray-green in appearance, with a large spot at the base of the tail fin. Like the Jack Dempsey, oscars should be kept to themselves rather than in a community tank.

SCAVENGERS: CATFISH, LOACHES, AND SUCKER FISH. Scavengers are desirable additions to your aquarium and every tank — even tanks of predators — should have at least one (scavengers are well disguised and can take care of themselves). These gentle bottom-feeders act as living vacuum cleaners, eating the food that drops down to the floor of the tank. Catfish, generally of the family Corydoras, are the most common scavengers. These fish come in a variety of colors and sizes (1 to 3 inches) and are attractive as well as useful additions to a community.

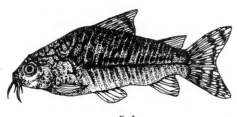

catfish

Loaches, particularly the clown loach *(Botiamacracanthus)*, which with its orange body and black bands resembles some marine fish, have an interesting swimming motion as well as being colorful. They are about 2 to 3 inches in size.

Sucker fish or suckers (family Otocinclus) not only clean up the bottom of the tank but keep the sides free from algae, which interferes with viewing. Suckers are rarely seen during the day — they prefer to hide behind any available rocks. They can grow quite large. A specimen only an inch long when put in the tank may reach 6 inches. While suckers are somewhat aggressive, they will not injure other fish, simply drive them off.

marine fish

Marine, or saltwater, fish, found in the ocean or seas, are generally more colorful than the freshwater species. The small fish you see in the pet shop, in its natural environment, might grow to a tremendous size. There are far too many species to be covered even in a large textbook, but the following are among those you would be most likely to find in your local fish store:

DAMSELS *(Dascylous)*. These fish are among the best for the aquarist making his first attempt at setting up a saltwater collection. They are hardy, beautiful, and small enough — 2 to 3 inches — to make them suitable for the average home tank. Damsels come from Africa, India, China, and the Pacific Ocean. Some favorites are *Dascylous aruanus*, silver with black bands; *Dascylous trimaculatus*, with three white spots on a brownish black background; and yellow damsels *(Ponacentrus melanociur)*, a bright iridescent

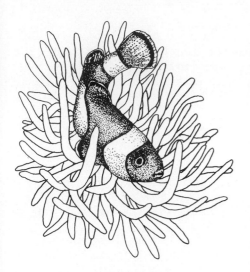

clown fish in anemone

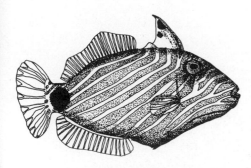

trigger fish

blue with yellow tail. Other commonly available varieties include blue and green. Damsels, while fairly peaceful, will not tolerate more than one or two of their own kind in a tank.

CLOWN FISH OR ANEMONE FISH (*Amphiprion*). These are possibly the most popular of the marine species. Not only are they generally available and vivid in appearance, their "life-style" is a subject of continuing interest. These handsome little (1 to 3 inches) fellows have three white stripes on an orange background. Clown fish live in a symbiotic relationship with the sea anemone, an invertebrate marine animal that resembles the flower after which it is named.

Anemones are carnivores that inject poison into their victims through petallike tentacles before eating them. Only the clown fish, which establishes a relationship with certain species of anemone, is immune to its venom. The anemone provides the clown fish with a refuge to which it can flee on being chased by a predator. It nestles in the cavity at the center of the tentacles, safe from attack. At the same time, the brilliantly colored clown fish acts as a lure, bringing other fish within striking distance of its voracious but immobile host. Several species are sold in fish hobbyist stores, among them the jumatum clown, the sebae clown, and two varieties of bandit clown fish.

TRIGGER FISH (*Balistes*). This is a brightly colored species characterized by a sharp, spiny fin just behind the usual soft dorsal fin. As is often the case, the fish's name is misleading. In reality, the stiffened fin is not used as a weapon in any sense, apparently serving only as a stabilizer for the softer dorsal. These fish can grow quite large (20 to 22 inches), though they are usually about 1 to 6 inches, and they come in a number of different colors and shapes. They are quite aggressive fish and are not recommended for a communal marine tank.

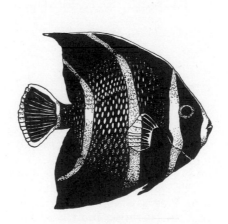

French angelfish

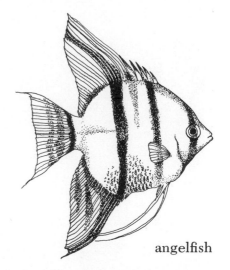

angelfish

butterfly fish

ANGELFISH (*Panacanthus*). These are, in the opinion of many aquarists, the most beautiful of the marine species. They too come in a variety of colors, sizes (2 to 18 inches), and shapes; they have in common the flat body found in the freshwater angels and discus fish. The species most frequently encountered in fish stores are the black, the blue, and the French angelfish.

BUTTERFLY FISH (*Chaetodon quriga*). This is a close cousin to the angels, sharing the same flattened form. They range from 4 to 8 inches in length and are noted both for their beautiful coloring and for their large dorsal and ventral fins.

preventive medicine

The novice aquarist's most common error is to buy both fish and tank at the same time. In order for the chlorine in the water to dissipate and for the filter system to start the bacteriological growth necessary for the removal of ammonia, the tank should be in operation for at least a week before fish are introduced.

The first decision is where to put the aquarium. It should be where the fish will not be disturbed constantly and where it will receive from three to six hours of natural light during the day (they need artificial light too — see Light, page 148). Too much sunlight will mean a constant battle against algae; too little will result in the fish losing their color. Drafty areas should be avoided and a tank should never be placed over a radiator. Extreme temperature changes are very bad for fish. They cause stress, which can weaken the fish, and could even put the fish into shock.

A tank can rest on a sturdy stand or desk top but the best approach, if feasible, is to build it into a wall. The important thing is to ensure that you have access to either the rear or top for ease of feeding and periodic cleaning, as well as for introducing new fish.

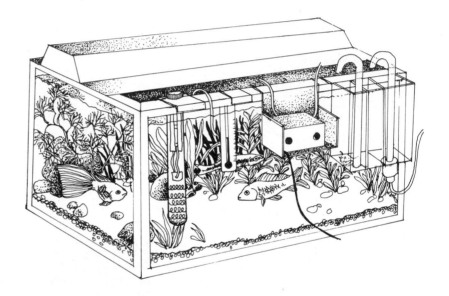

There are many sizes and shapes available. It is best to start with a tank holding at least 20 gallons of water, and then to advance to 50 or even 100 gallons. Smaller tanks are quickly abandoned when owners want to add more fish for a better showing.

The most common and easiest tanks to work with are rectangular. In addition to the familiar glass models with stainless steel trim, there are also all-glass or Plexiglas tanks (which are better for marine aquariums since salt water would corrode the trim). The basic accessories are a reflector, or light source, usually mounted on the top of the tank; a glass cover to limit evaporation and keep fish from jumping out; a filter and pump, plus the valves and plastic hose to connect them; a thermometer; and, if you live in an area where daytime or evening temperatures drop below 65°F., some form of heater.

On the bottom of the tank, there should be sand or gravel. While artificially colored products are available and may look nice in the pet shop, they do not give you the realistic setting possible if you use natural material. There should be between 1 and 2 pounds of gravel or sand per gallon of water — a 20-gallon tank, therefore, would need between 20 and 30 pounds.

While they are not essential, rocks make an interesting display and can be used as a hiding place if there are aggressive fish in the tank. You can use rocks found in your neighborhood or purchase them from the pet store.

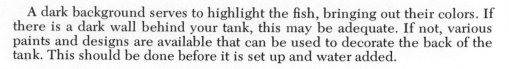

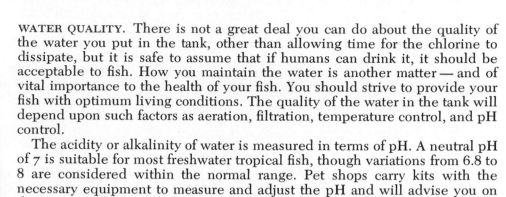

A dark background serves to highlight the fish, bringing out their colors. If there is a dark wall behind your tank, this may be adequate. If not, various paints and designs are available that can be used to decorate the back of the tank. This should be done before it is set up and water added.

WATER QUALITY. There is not a great deal you can do about the quality of the water you put in the tank, other than allowing time for the chlorine to dissipate, but it is safe to assume that if humans can drink it, it should be acceptable to fish. How you maintain the water is another matter — and of vital importance to the health of your fish. You should strive to provide your fish with optimum living conditions. The quality of the water in the tank will depend upon such factors as aeration, filtration, temperature control, and pH control.

The acidity or alkalinity of water is measured in terms of pH. A neutral pH of 7 is suitable for most freshwater tropical fish, though variations from 6.8 to 8 are considered within the normal range. Pet shops carry kits with the necessary equipment to measure and adjust the pH and will advise you on the range healthiest for the fish in your tank. Extreme changes in pH are to be avoided for they may lead to debilitation and, as a result, disease.

The filtration system, which removes metabolic wastes, odors, and coloration, is of prime importance in maintaining water quality. There are three types available.

The most efficient means of filtering is known as the open system. Water enters the tank over a spillway at one end and leaves it over another at the opposite end. There is a continuous flow and little chance for it to become contaminated, stagnant, or to accumulate toxic by-products of the fish metabolism. The problem is that such a system depends on the availability of a large supply of chlorine-free water, and for most home aquarists it simply is not practical.

The other filtration systems both depend upon bacteria to break down the ammonia, a normal metabolic waste product that the fish excretes. Living in the filter, the bacteria convert the ammonia first to nitrites and then to nitrates. While this removes the problem of the highly toxic ammonia, nitrites and nitrates themselves in sufficient concentration can be injurious to the fish's health, causing sluggishness, susceptibility to disease, and even death.

The outside bacterial filter system consists of a simple plastic box connected by hoses to the tank. As the water circulates through it, rock wool or spongy flocking not only acts as a strainer to catch debris but serves as a home for the bacteria that make the essential chemical conversions. Below the flocking is a layer of charcoal to remove odors and undesirable stains from the water, which is then returned to the tank.

The pump used for propulsion also oxygenates the water, improving the fish's environment. Some filters, such as the Aqua-Flow, have built-in pumps; others must be hooked up with plastic tubing.

When the flocking becomes strongly discolored by accumulated debris, the filter system should be disconnected and the flocking removed and washed. It should then be used again rather than replaced with new material that lacks the necessary bacteria. It takes from a week to ten days before bacteria will begin to grow on new flocking. If you do choose to replace it, bacteria growth can be speeded up by putting a thin layer of the old flocking under the new. The filter should be cleaned every six weeks — more often if there is a rapid accumulation of dirt.

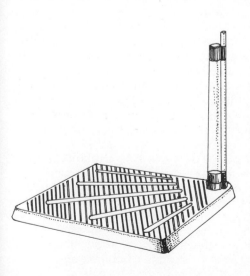

The underground filter system consists of a perforated plastic sheet covered with a gravel bed, which provides a home for the bacteria. Air pumped under the plastic sheet bubbles up, circulating the water through the gravel. The shortcoming of this system is that it is necessary to completely dismantle the tank before it can be cleaned, removing fish, rocks, and plants to another tank. To avoid any more disruption than is absolutely necessary, these filters should not be cleaned more often than twice a year, though also

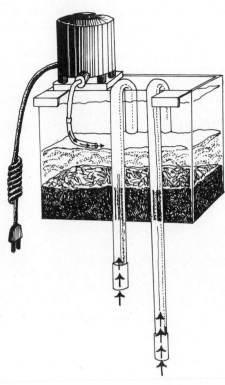

not less than once. Since many experts object to the buildup of metabolic wastes over so long an interval, it is probably wise to check the nitrate/nitrite level of your tank once a month with a kit that is available from an aquarium shop.

Whichever system you choose, make sure to get a strong, sturdy pump. This may prove to be one of the most expensive pieces of equipment you buy, but it will be well worth the cost. The inexpensive little vibrators or aerators are both noisy and subject to frequent breakdowns.

The pump can also be connected by valves and plastic hose to any of several accessories for the bottom of the tank to provide additional aeration. Depending on your tastes, there are figurines of divers, sunken ships, and the like, or simple air stones. The bubbles rising through the water create an interesting effect and attract the fish. Bear in mind, however, that your fish will be more highly visible in a naturalistic setting with a minimun of visual distractions that compete with their beauty.

LIGHT. Most tanks are equipped with a fluorescent fixture at the top to supplement the natural light. While these are excellent for display, remember that in nature fish are exposed to a cyclical pattern of light and darkness. It is best to try to simulate this, giving the tank only between eight and twelve hours of light — natural plus artificial — a day. The light should never be left on for the entire twenty-four hours.

If you are giving your tank too much light, the warning signal will be an accumulation of green algae on the glass sides of the tank or on the rocks on the bottom. While this rarely harms the fish, it is unsightly and obstructs the view of the tank's interior. If it continues to build up in large amounts, the algae could reach the point of competing with the fish for oxygen. While it would be most unlikely in a home tank, algae growth in ponds has been known to wipe out the fish population.

Algae can be removed without disturbing the fish by scraping the sides of the tank. While there are instruments for this purpose available in pet stores, a paper towel or cloth will do the job adequately if rubbed vigorously on the glass surfaces. Rocks and stones can be removed, washed in the sink, and replaced. In small amounts, however, algae can be beneficial to the fish, especially to the vegetable-eaters.

If the tank is receiving too little light, you will be alerted by the appearance of dark brown algae. This can be removed in the same way and the light exposure increased.

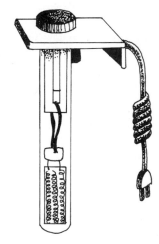

TEMPERATURE. In most of the United States, temperature fluctuations make a thermostatic heater an essential item of equipment. It is important to maintain as constant a temperature as possible — between 70° and 80°F. for most freshwater tropical fish. Variations of no more than 8° can set up a stress pattern that will lower the fish's resistance to disease. Excess heat can be even more critical: the danger signs are fish swimming near the surface that do not ordinarily do so; immobility; refusal of food; and ultimately death. Too cold fish usually just seem to move slowly.

The thermostatic heater is hung from the side of the tank and extends down into the water. It should not be placed near an aeration system — if bubbles get into the mechanism, they can cause a short, which can wreck the unit or, worse, cause it to overheat the water.

PLANTS. The next decision is whether to have live or artificial plants in your tank. Plastic plants are convenient because they can be moved around and arranged as you like, but live plants in your freshwater tank are more beneficial to the fish. And, if you have fish that need vegetables, the trouble plastic plants spare you is offset by the fact that you must add dietary supplements to the fish food. (There are no live plants suitable for saltwater tanks.)

Plants are necessary for purposes other than beauty or food. They give smaller fish a refuge if their larger neighbors in the tank become aggressive

— and surface plants are essential if the fry of live bearers are to survive to maturity.

Living plants also serve as an oxygen balance, supplying the tank with oxygen during the day and giving off carbon dioxide at night. A wide variety are available and you should have no difficulty selecting some that appeal to you. They should receive at least six hours of light a day. With plants, as with all the other elements that make up the environment of the tank, the important thing is to maintain stability rather than to make changes constantly.

SETTING UP THE TANK. Gravel is the first thing you will add to your tank, and it must be rinsed throughly (in water only) before you put it in. (Soaps not thoroughly removed might be toxic to the fish.) It should be given five or six washings, either with a garden hose or under the tap in your tub or sink. Stir it continually to loosen sediment while the water is running. The tank should be thoroughly washed out, too, and any equipment or rocks going into it must be cleaned in advance.

When you have poured the gravel in, either level it or create a slight hill, making sure the terrain is smooth. Cover it with newspaper or clean white paper and add the water slowly enough to minimize disturbance. When the tank is about half-filled, the paper can be removed and the rest of the water added. Start the pump and filter system, and then wait a week before introducing any fish.

At the same time, you should set up a second, smaller tank (about 5- to 10-gallon capacity) to hold replacement water and to serve as hospital or breeding tank when needed. If you lack either the space or money to do this, fill several gallon jugs with water, which can age until needed. Chlorine killers such as Chlor-out are not necessary with most municipally supplied water. Time and the aerator will efficiently eliminate chlorine before you introduce your fish to the tank.

The heater should be mounted at the back of the tank and the thermometer on the side where it will be easiest to read.

CHOOSING YOUR FISH

When your tank is ready to receive fish, visit several stores to see what species are available.

The important thing is to ensure that the fish you get are healthy. Your first basis for judgment is the store itself. If there are several dead or dying specimens in the tank, the fish are not receiving proper care. Healthy fish are sleek and bright-eyed, and move vigorously. If they are weak, they will lie on their sides, move slowly, and lack color. A fish that is picked on by others is a poor bet. After an hour or two observing in several shops, you will be able to judge for yourself.

The dealer is a middleman, buying fish from breeders or collectors and holding them until they are sold. If he has had them for some time, he should know whether they are healthy or not. Find out how long they have been in the shop — and avoid taking fish that are newly arrived. Furthermore, moving stresses a fish and increases the chances of its becoming ill or dying. It should have a chance to recover from the effects of an earlier move before you take it home.

The more carefully the fish is handled, the better. Watch how the fish handler removes them from the tank. They should be scooped up gently and the net should be large enough to accommodate them comfortably. If you are not able to get the fish home quickly, compressed air or oxygen should be added to the top of the plastic bag in which they will be carried.

Add all the fish you originally plan to keep at the same time. Then wait until natural attrition or disease has reduced the number by at least half before introducing more. Any new fish increases the possibility of diseases to which the inhabitants of the tank may not be immune, thus increasing the death rate.

PUTTING THE FISH
IN THE TANK

As soon as you arrive home, place the plastic bag containing the fish in the tank and allow it to float until the temperature of the water inside is about equal to that surrounding it. Then small holes should be poked in the bag to allow the water to mix. After these steps have been taken, the bag can be opened and the new fish allowed to enter the tank.

A fish that is too aggressive must be removed. It is particularly important at such times to have places where smaller or shyer fish may hide. Also, there should be a top on the tank for, in the excitement, fish will frequently jump out.

Newcomers are bound to cause a commotion. The older inhabitants may attack them or, if the new fish is aggressive and they are small, be attacked.

The size of the fish will determine how many can be kept in a 20-gallon tank. For fish up to 2 inches, a rule of thumb is that there should be no more than one per gallon, though even this might be excessive. With smaller fish such as neon tetras and cardinal tetras, on the other hand, twenty might be conservative. Overcrowding is a stress factor, however, and lowers the fish's chances of surviving and flourishing. With larger species, such as the mature angel or discus, it would be wise to limit the number to no more than four. Crowding will limit the growth of your fish; the more water per fish, the larger they will grow.

You can assume that fish purchased from a pet store have been fed recently, but if they have been shipped they may need food. The important thing is to avoid overfeeding. If the fish do not eat quickly, allow several hours before giving them more food. Once they are acclimatized to the new tank, you should feed them twice a day.

THE MARINE AQUARIUM

Setting up a marine (or saltwater) aquarium involves the same steps and precautions as preparing freshwater aquariums — with the following important differences.

First, no metal should be in contact with the water — use an all-glass or Plexiglas tank.

In a marine aquarium the ideal pH is between 8.2 and 8.5. Any gravel other than coral or beach sand will have a negative effect on the pH. If you live near the coast, you can collect this yourself, as well as sea fans, coral, or coral rock to decorate the tank. These are also available in pet shops and will help adjust the pH of the water, which is particularly important in marine tanks, as well as giving the fish hiding places. Anything to be put in the tank should first be carefully rinsed in water.

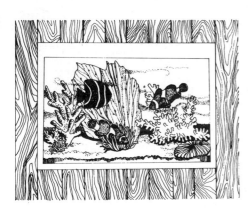

Either natural or artificial salt water can be used to fill the tank. In mixing the latter, be sure to follow the manufacturer's instructions.

The specific gravity of seawater is 1.026. While this is fine for most tanks, by reducing the specific gravity to around 1.020 you can do an even more effective job of protecting your fish's health. The protozoans, which cause many diseases, will not develop at this specific gravity, though the fish can tolerate it easily. An inexpensive hydrometer can be used to measure specific gravity. If it drops too low, artificial marine salts can be added to the tank to bring it up.

No more than four to six of the smaller marine fish, such as clowns or damsels, should be kept in a 20-gallon tank. With larger species, angels or butterflies, for example, three would be the maximum. Five gallons of water to each fish is considered the optimum ratio.

ACCLIMATING THE WATER. A marine tank should be kept at around 75°F. It is particularly important to acclimate the water in the plastic bag containing the fish before putting it in the tank. Place the bag on a chair or table by the tank. Then inject a plastic hose, puncturing the top of the bag. Put a clamp on the hose, to allow water from the tank to drip slowly — about six to eight drops per minute — into the bag. If the bag is too small, use a clean plastic bucket. Several hours should be allowed for the waters to equalize.

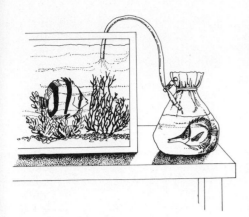

New water for replacement as evaporation takes place should be brought to the proper temperature — around 75°F. — before it is added; and let it sit forty-eight hours to eliminate the chlorine.

While it is a good idea to have a reservoir of salt water available, if you don't have a supply it is quite safe to add fresh water up to 10 percent of the tank's capacity. New salt must be added periodically — commonly, about once a year — to maintain the specific gravity. Too much salt can be harmful; the salinity should be checked with a hydrometer. You will be most successful if you make an effort to keep conditions in the tank — temperature, specific gravity, daily light exposure — constant.

Marine fish are considerably more expensive than most of the freshwater species, costing up to fifty dollars each. Most cannot be bred in captivity at present and must be collected either by hand or in nets. They are often shipped great distances, and mortality is high even before they reach your local pet shop. Obviously, good care is sound economy.

FEEDING The quality of the food you give your fish is important in determining their health, and you will find a wide variety on the shelves of your pet shop or fish store. Live food — such as brine shrimp, daphnia (water fleas), or tubifex worms — is best for freshwater fish. These may be available in pet stores.

In some areas, daphnia can be collected from local ponds during the summer using a very fine-meshed net. While it is not difficult to hatch brine shrimp from eggs in your home, it does require considerable time and an extra tank for the purpose. Ordinary earthworms, shredded or cut into small pieces, make an excellent and inexpensive food.

Beef or lamb liver, heart, and kidney are all good fresh foods for fish. For smaller fish, they should be finely ground. Tiny pieces are suitable for larger species. Any seafood, such as shrimp or clams, will be excellent if cut into small pieces.

All these foods can be kept frozen for convenience, but if you put them right into the tank from the freezer, the fish will eat them before they are defrosted. It is best to thaw them in a dish or glass of water before they are put into the tank so that they are closer to what the fish would get in nature.

The third and least desirable choice is commercially prepared dry food. Whichever of the commercial dry foods you use, be sure to remember that some fish, such as the mollies and others mentioned earlier, also require vegetation. Either crushed lettuce or spinach is an excellent diet supplement for these. Algae is also ideal for newly hatched fry. Local pet stores carry commercial fry preparations as well, usually in gelatine or liquid forms.

Although marine species will eat the same foods as freshwater fish, their basic diet should be live or frozen brine shrimp. Any marine crustacean, such as shrimp or crabs, and shellfish — clams, oysters, or mussels — will make a good food when chopped up. Variety is quite important in your fish's diet. Try to serve them at least two, and preferably three, different foods during the week.

Avoid overfeeding, particularly of live foods. As it deteriorates, uneaten food will make the water cloudy and may deplete the oxygen content. If the fish have not eaten all the food you put in the tank within ten to fifteen minutes, you should give them less. If they do consume the food within this time, you may try adding more or, if you are feeding them only once a day, go to a second feeding. It is always better, however, to err on the side of underfeeding initially.

first aid and the home clinic

What should you do when your fish appear sick or start dying? If it were your dog or cat, the normal thing would be to call your veterinarian. Unfortunately, because veterinary schools have neglected fish diseases in the past, you probably wouldn't get much help.

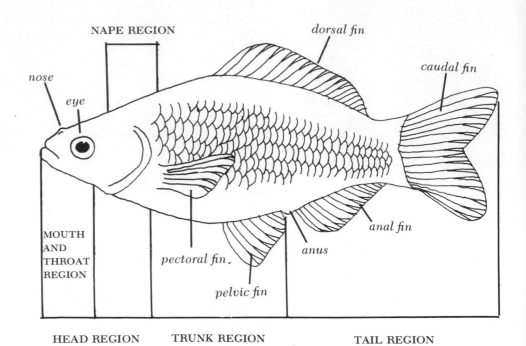

NAPE REGION

dorsal fin

caudal fin

nose

eye

MOUTH
AND
THROAT
REGION

pectoral fin

pelvic fin

anus

anal fin

HEAD REGION   TRUNK REGION   TAIL REGION

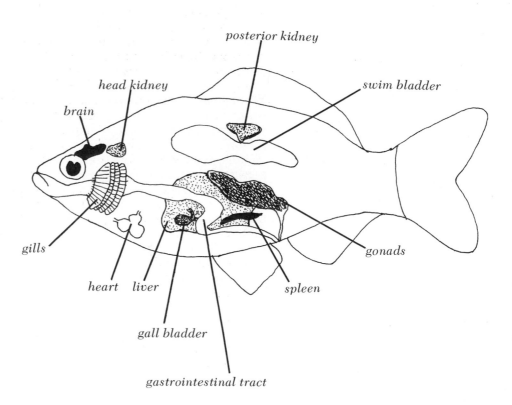

posterior kidney

head kidney

swim bladder

brain

gills

heart   *liver*

spleen

gonads

gall bladder

gastrointestinal tract

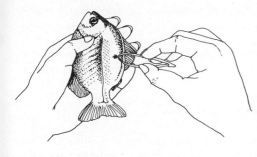

This situation is improving, though, and the home aquarist of the future can look forward to talking with a veterinarian who can give authoritative information and help.

If your fish has suffered external wounds or cuts or has visible parasites, you can treat these yourself. First gently remove the fish from the tank with a fine-meshed net. (The net should be washed thoroughly after each use, preferably in a disinfectant solution.) Remember that you have between thirty seconds and a minute to take action before the fish must be returned to the tank. Hold the fish firmly in your cupped hand, putting your thumb over its gill with enough pressure to restrain it gently. Remove the dead tissue or parasite with small scissors, tweezers, or thumb forceps. After removing tissue, apply an antiseptic solution—Mercurochrome, iodine, or an antibiotic spray—and quickly return the fish to the water. Common sense and speed are your best devices for treating an injured fish.

There is little you can do to prepare yourself in advance so far as equipment for first aid is concerned. You will either have what you need already on hand or will have time to obtain it from a drugstore or aquarium shop. The two medications you are most likely to use are:

> Mercurochrome, the same 1 to 2 percent solution you buy for yourself, which will either be applied directly to the fish or be added to the tank in a 1 to 10 ratio with the water
>
> copper sulfate, added to the water in a ratio of 1 part copper sulfate to 1,000 parts water

Broad-spectrum antibiotics, such as tetracycline, can be obtained only with a prescription from your veterinarian. Pet shops carry many fish remedies, most of which are useless. One exception, however, is Aqua-Cure,* which is very effective for protozoan diseases. Follow the instructions on the label.

As a last resort, if your fish are dying, you cannot diagnose the problem, and no veterinarian is available to help you, there is an old remedy that often works wonders in a freshwater tank, though no one knows why: ordinary table salt added to the tank in a ratio of 1 tablespoon to 12 gallons of water.

In many cases, your only course will be to destroy a diseased or injured fish. The best method is to place it in a 10 percent solution of formalin after removing it from the tank. Death is rapid and the fish will be preserved if you wish to seek a diagnosis of what caused the problem.

diseases

Preventive medicine—avoiding a disease rather than treating it—is the fish owner's best course. The starting point is good husbandry, doing what is necessary to keep your fish healthy and improve their resistance to disease.

You can also take precautions to avoid exposing them to disease by setting up a second tank in which new fish can be isolated or quarantined before they join the community in the tank. This tank can alternatively serve as a hospital for fish that appear to be ill, and you should not hesitate to transfer them to it.

Just as do other creatures, fish contract a wide range of diseases. There are viral, bacterial, and protozoan diseases, as well as parasites and tumors.

SYMPTOMS OF ILLNESS

By studying how your fish behave normally, you will soon learn to tell when something is wrong with a particular individual. Among the signs of disease are the following:

LOSS OF APPETITE. The fish stops eating, or picks listlessly at its food.

* Available from Marine Tropical Import, 9503 Fourth Avenue, Brooklyn, New York 11209.

IRREGULAR POSTURE. The fish loses its equilibrium and swims in an odd posture or without seeming to be able to maintain its balance.

SURFACING. The fish stays near the surface or seems to be frequently gasping for air. If more than one fish does this, however, this may indicate overheating. Some species customarily swim near the surface, some in the middle, and others toward the bottom of the tank. You will soon learn where each fish can normally be expected to be found. A deep swimmer near the top of the tank is clearly in trouble.

LOSS OF MOBILITY. A fish swimming more slowly than is normal.

VICTIMIZATION. The fish is singled out and picked on by the others. This should not be confused with the territorial defensiveness common to fish, however.

FADING. Loss of coloration is a definite sign of disease. When a brightly colored fish begins to look pale, it is usually a sign of trouble.

SPOTTING. The appearance of spots or new areas of coloration.

BREAKING FINS AND TAILS. Pieces break off the fins and tail.

BODY ABNORMALITIES. Bulges, swellings, bumps, or external wounds.

VIRUS Viruses are so small they will pass through filters that screen out bacteria. Only the most powerful electronic microscopes are capable of detecting them. Because it has become possible to observe them only within the past few years, viral diseases remain the least known, and veterinary medicine has not yet come up with a scientific means of attacking them.

Trial-and-error has produced one answer nonetheless, though why it succeeds is still an open question. An example is viral papillomatosis, a disease that produces growths on a fish's sides that resemble cauliflowers. If the fish is removed from the water and one or two of these papillomas, as they are called, are crushed, the others will often wither away. If not—and at this point it is purely a matter of chance—the fish may die.

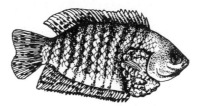
viral papillomatosis

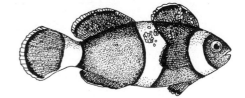
lymphocystis

Marine fish are subject to lymphocystis, which, fortunately, occurs more frequently in the ocean than in home tanks. Coral fish are particularly likely to contract this disease, which produces a raspberrylike growth or pearl-shaped nodules on the body. At present, there is no known cure for these infections.

BACTERIAL Even though there has been more opportunity to study bacteria, which can be trapped by filters and cultured out on media plates, the study of diseases in fish is still too new—they require the expertise of the fish pathologist for diagnosis. In many cases, cures have yet to be discovered. While it is known that bacterial hemorrhagic septicemia, an infectious disease which causes abdominal swelling, is caused by Aeronomas bacteria, it is still usually fatal for no antibiotic has been found to counteract it.

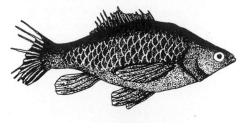

FIN OR TAIL ROT. Some strides are being made, however. Fin or tail rot is a common disease in tanks, and when pieces of these parts of the body begin to break off you have good reason to suspect that your fish have been infected. There may be a hereditary factor that makes one fish more likely to contract this disease than another, but the direct cause is known to be Pseudomonas. While introducing antibiotics into the tank has not proved really successful in combating this disease, more valuable fish have been saved by injections of kanamycin (prescribed by a veterinarian).

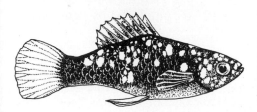

COTTON WOOL OR MOUTH "FUNGUS." Columnaris, caused by a myxobacterium called *Chondroccus columnaris*, is particularly widespread among freshwater fish. The characteristic symptoms are known as cotton wool of the mouth, or mouth fungus, though bacteria are responsible rather than fungus. Large white spots are found on the head, mouth, fins, gills, and sides of the fish. These become ulcerous in time. At present, sulfa drugs as well as antibiotics are being used in an attempt to control this disease.

FUNGUS

A gray or white fuzz on a fish's skin is often a sign of a disease caused by a fungus. This can usually be treated fairly easily, either by applying medicine to the single fish affected or by putting chemicals into the water of the tank if the problem affects many fish. To treat the individual fish, remove it from the tank and apply a solution of 1 to 2 percent Mercurochrome to the affected area. Potassium permanganate can be added to the tank to disinfect it. Your veterinarian will give you a prescription and advise you on the amount to use. Fungus diseases are not usually fatal.

PROTOZOAN

CORAL FISH DISEASE. Protozoans probably are the greatest cause of disease in fish tanks, and oodinium cause one of the most common protozoan infections, coral fish disease. The skin becomes cloudy and the gills will show hemorrhages or swelling. Frequently there will be patches of dead skin. This disease is usually introduced into the tank by a new fish carrying cysts.

The disease must be diagnosed by a veterinarian or marine biologist who can look at the cyst microscopically, and who will usually prescribe adding acriflavin to the water in a strength of 1 gram to every 100 liters. This is repeated every twelve hours until the cysts disappear. Antibiotics such as Achromycin are effective, as well as additives such as copper sulfate (1 part to 1,000 of water), which may help to reduce the salinity of the water and prevent cysts from hatching.

VELVET DISEASE. Fish with velvet disease, caused by another species of Oodinium, lose their color. When the disease becomes advanced their skin may have a dark grayish or yellowish velvety appearance. At times it may peel away. They will lose weight and tend to rub themselves against rough surfaces such as rocks. Again, definitive diagnosis and treatment should be left to a veterinarian.

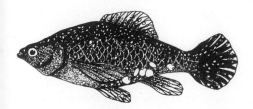

ICH OR WHITE SPOT. The most common protozoan disease in tanks is ichthyophthirius, usually referred to as ich or white spot. The whitish or gray spots which appear on the fish's skin or fins are actually areas where the protozoan's cyst has penetrated, which sets off intense irritation. In advanced cases, the spots will grow larger and appear on the gills.

Ich will usually appear when there is overcrowding or there has been a sharp temperature change in the tank. It can be treated by frequently changing the water and adding a 10 percent solution of malachite green—1 ounce for every gallon of water in the tank. Treatment must be repeated at intervals of five to seven days in order to destroy the encysted protozoans as they hatch. Two or possibly three treatments should be enough. It is helpful to also raise the temperature of the water, by stages, to 90°F. First, take it up to 80°F. If the fish seem to be doing all right, continue to raise it slowly. Adding a 1 percent solution of methylene blue to the water, a commonly sold remedy, has spectacular effects visually but the results are questionable.

The wisest course is to isolate new fish for around two months to make sure the infection is not introduced to the tank. Ich is as common as it is only because most aquarists lack the patience to take this precaution.

BLACK SPOT. Also a protozoan disease, this is caused by Diplostomiasis. Small brown or black spots, containing the larvae of the trematode worm, appear on the fish's fins and body. This should be diagnosed by your veterinarian, who will prescribe treatment.

PARASITIC   ARGULUS. One of the most common parasites in home tanks is a fish louse known as argulus, introduced when daphnia are a part of the diet. Because of this, many aquarists will not use this food. The parasite attaches itself to the fish's skin by two large suckers, and can be removed by small tweezers or a thumb forceps. Although it is visible to the naked eye, you should have a magnifying glass handy both to confirm your diagnosis and to help in removing the parasite. Another method is to apply a 1 percent solution of iodine or kerosene directly to the louse. Care should be taken not to damage the fish while handling it.

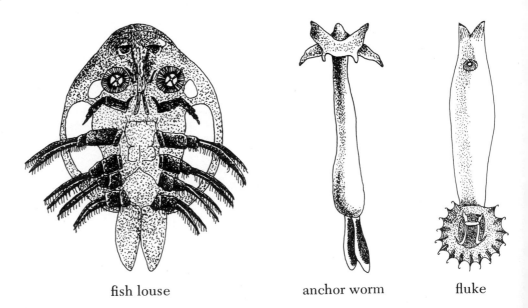

fish louse   anchor worm   fluke

ANCHOR WORMS. These larvae of *Lerngea cyprinagea* get their name from the anchorlike appendage on their heads. These parasites are common but are easily killed by a 1 percent solution of potassium permanganate applied directly or added to the tank in a ratio of ½ ounce to 1 gallon of water. One treatment should be enough.

SKIN FLUKES. While skin flukes (family Gyrodactylid) are not visible to the naked eye, they can be seen with a magnifying glass. The first symptom is fading color. Then the fish's fins will droop and become torn. The skin becomes slimy and there may be hemorrhages at the base of the fins. The greatest danger occurs when the gills are affected. The usual treatment today is to add formaldehyde to the tank in a 1 percent solution in a ratio of ½ ounce to 1 gallon of water. One or two treatments several days apart should be enough.

DIAGNOSIS   If you are a serious aquarist and cannot find local veterinary help, getting an accurate diagnosis of your problem can often require some time and trouble.

Your first step should be to put a fish which has died of mysterious causes in a 1 percent formalin solution. Find the nearest diagnostic laboratory and send it there for examination. The veterinary college, school of marine biology at your state university, or your state and local wildlife services may be able to help you. Find out if a fee is required for diagnostic services.

If you are scientifically inclined, you may wish to find what was wrong by dissecting the fish yourself. A simple schematic of the fish's internal organs appears on page 152. For the smaller fish, a magnifying glass is helpful and, if you have access to one and know how to use it, a small microscope will make it possible to examine the organs and other parts of the fish closely.

further readings

AMES, F. *The Fish You Care For: A Manual of Fish Care.* New York, New American Library, 1971.

AMLOCHER, I. *Textbook of Fish Diseases.* Neptune, New Jersey, TFH Publications, 1970.

AXELROD, DR. H., AND BURGESS, W. *Saltwater Aquarium Fish.* Neptune, N.J., TFH Publications, 1963.

INNES, DR. W. T. *Exotic Aquarium Fishes.* New York, Dutton, 1966.

REICHENBACH-KLINKE, H. H. *Fish Pathology.* Neptune, N.J., TFH Publications, 1973.

SINDERMANN, DR. C. J. *Principal Diseases of Marine Fish and Shellfish.* New York, Academic Press, 1970.

SPOTTE, S. *Keeping of Saltwater Fish: Marine Aquarium Keeping.* New York, Wiley Interscience, 1973.

Reptiles
snakes, lizards, turtles, tortoises, alligators, crocodiles, and others

FREDRIC L. FRYE, D.V.M.

Generations of amateurs have been fascinated by reptiles, and today there are numerous local, national, and international herpetological societies for anyone interested in making them a serious hobby. Reptiles have become increasingly popular as pets because little space and time are required to keep them healthy. Most have little or no odor, make little or no noise, are not allergenic, and do not demand regular excursions outdoors. Generally, reptiles may live longer in captivity than in their wild state because they are not subjected to their natural predators. Although data are scanty, most small reptiles live for about twenty years, some chelonians survive for a hundred years, and the tuatara is thought to live for over a century.

There are four living orders of reptile, in which there are approximately 5,500 individual species. They range from a few inches long to well over 8 yards for the larger pythons and crocodiles. Their most striking common feature is that they are cold-blooded — their body temperature rises and falls in response to the environment. Reptiles are categorized as:

ORDER CHELONIA   Tortoises, turtles, and terrapins. Generally, tortoises are land animals, which enter water only to drink or soak for brief periods. Turtles and terrapins — names that are basically synonymous — are far more aquatic. All members of this order tend to be short, wide creatures with modified flipperlike feet. The tortoises' legs and feet are better adapted to walking than to swimming; the limbs of the aquatic forms are adapted more for swimming than for walking, and often they have webbed toes.

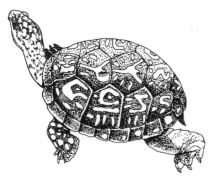

box turtle

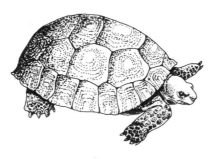

desert tortoise

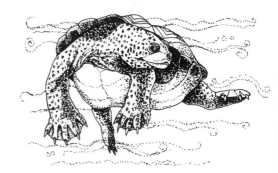

diamond back terrapin

Most chelonians have a bony shell covered with horny plates, which gives them good protection from predators. Some, however, have a soft, more leathery body covering, which, while it gives less protection, is streamlined and much lighter than the bonier armor plating.

Chelonians range in size from about 1½ inches and a few ounces to well over 2 yards and several hundred pounds. They may be carnivorous (meat-eating), herbivorous (plant-eating), or omnivorous (meat and plants).

All chelonians are oviparous, egg-laying.

ORDER RHYNCHOCEPHALIA

There is only one living species in this order, *Sphenodon punctatum*, the tuatara. This lizardlike animal, which can grow to 30 inches at maturity, is not really a lizard, but rather a "living fossil," more closely related to the crocodilians. The tuatara is interesting both for its unique anatomical features and because, unlike the majority of reptiles, it prefers low environmental temperatures.

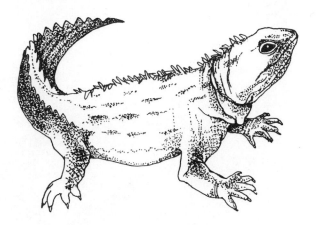

Tuataras live on a few isolated islands off the coast of New Zealand and are strictly protected by the government. Only a very few animals are granted to carefully selected institutions. There are a few captive breeding programs under way now in the United States, and it is hoped that attempts to get this rare, endangered species to reproduce will be successful.

The tuatara is oviparous; the eggs require about one year to hatch after they are laid.

ORDER SQUAMATA

This is divided into two suborders: Sauria, or lizards, and Serpentes, or snakes.

The lizards range in size from tiny geckos of 1½ inches to the giant Komodo "dragon" monitor lizards which can grow to 9 feet and 250 pounds. Most members of this suborder have four legs, though some have only two: the forelimbs. Others have no legs at all, and look superficially like snakes. All lizards have a dry, scaly, or tubercular skin — which may be plated like that of a small alligator, spiny as though studded with hobnails, soft and rubbery like plastic, or almost as smooth as glass. Most have movable eyelids and external eardrums or ear canals.

Lizards can be aquatic (freshwater), marine (seawater), terrestrial (land), or even arboreal (tree-dwelling) such as the "flying dragon" that can glide from treetops to the ground on an outstretched skin flap supported from its ribs. The Sauria are the most diversified order or suborder within the entire class of reptiles.

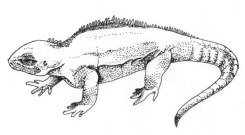

iguana

Most species are harmless — the two known venomous lizards are North Americans: the Gila monster of Arizona and northern Mexico and the Mexican beaded lizard.

Lizards can be strictly herbivorous, carnivorous, or omnivorous. Certain species, which are highly specialized, eat only specific insects, mollusks, or marine vegetation. Some lizards are oviparous (well-developed shells on the eggs), and others ovoviviparous (membranous shells on the eggs) — the fer-

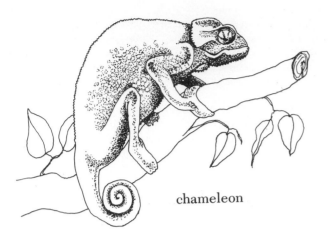

chameleon

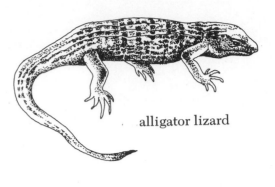

alligator lizard

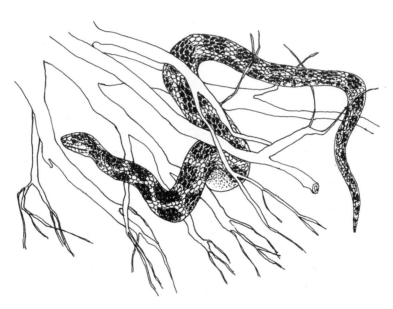

rat snake

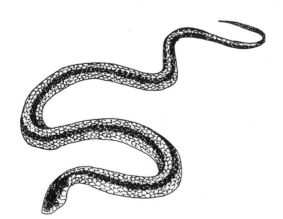

garter snake

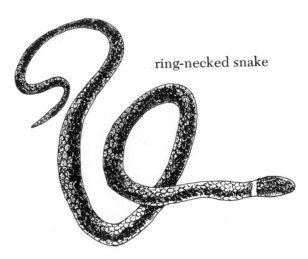

ring-necked snake

tilized eggs stay inside the female body until embryonic maturity; when the babies are born they are fully competent lizards.

Suborder Serpentes — the snakes — includes about 1,700 different species. Slender, elongated, legless creatures with dry, scale-covered skin, snakes may be only a few inches long or several yards. The skin may be very smooth to rough, depending upon the nature of the scales. Snakes do not have movable eyelids or external ears.

There are aquatic, marine, terrestrial, subterranean, and arboreal snakes. Many thrive near human habitations because they find rodents attractive, and they greatly reduce the destruction of agricultural products these animals cause.

Snakes are basically omnivorous, their diet including mammals, birds, other reptiles, amphibians, fish, or invertebrates. There are snakes with specialized dietary habits, though, and with highly specialized adaptations in anatomy and habitat. The smallest snakes dine upon small worms, slugs, and termites; the giants, such as the anaconda, boa constrictor, and the larger pythons, may eat creatures as large as pigs, deer, and other game animals. Some snakes that eat only whole eggs have jaws that can stretch wide to accommodate these large objects, and specialized toothlike ridges in their throats that break the eggshell neatly when the neck muscles contract. Once the egg is crushed, the snake swallows the fluid portions and disgorges the shell.

Poisonous snakes have several different venom-delivery systems — all variations of fangs (rigid or movable) connected by ducts to venom-producing organs, which are basically modified salivary glands. Some snakes merely strike at their prey and immediately begin to swallow it alive, not waiting for the venom to produce its lethal effect. Other snakes are constrictors, which throw one or more coils around the victim and rapidly squeeze until it is unable to breathe — causing swift death by asphyxiation. Contrary to popular opinion, they do not crush their food.

Snakes may be oviparous or ovoviviparous, and demonstrate a wide variety of reproductive habits.

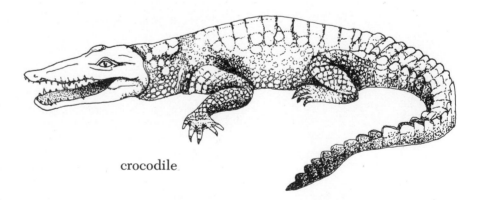

crocodile

ORDER LORICATA (CROCODILIA)

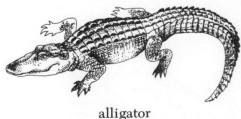

alligator

These are alligators, crocodiles, and the lesser-known caimans and gavials. These four-legged, semiaquatic animals have heavily armored skin complemented with bony armor plates, particularly upon the back. In size, some of these species may grow longer than 20 feet and weigh several hundred pounds.

All crocodilians have jaws studded with short, rootless, conical teeth that are shed periodically. One of the characteristics differentiating alligators from crocodiles is the way in which the fourth tooth on each side of the lower jaw is accommodated by the upper jaw: in the alligator, the tooth fits into a pit in the gum; in the crocodile, it merely fills a groove located between the corresponding upper teeth.

All members of the order are carnivorous — most have a varied diet of

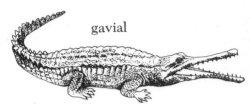
gavial

mammals, birds, fish, and other reptiles. The vegetable matter they consume is incidental or contained in the bodies of their prey. Some gavials and crocodiles are strict fish eaters.

All crocodilians are oviparous. The females prepare a nest in which the eggs are deposited and hatched into miniature replicas of the adults, emerging with hearty appetites and feisty tempers.

SELECTING A REPTILE AS A PET

Personal preference should play the main role in selecting a reptile, but there are other factors to consider: the initial cost of a specimen; the habitat and diet it needs; what is necessary to properly house and care for it (for some species, a great deal); whether it is potentially hazardous to humans (such as poisonous snakes and lizards, large alligators and crocodiles); and local health and safety regulations and codes. Turtles have been banned as pets in some areas because they carry a disease, salmonellosis, which can be communicated to humans. Ideally, a veterinarian should check over a turtle found in nature. Children should not be allowed to handle terrapins, and their water should not be poured down the kitchen sink or allowed to come in contact with any place where food is prepared.

It is — absolutely — not safe to allow children to have pet turtles that are commonly sold. There is too great a chance of salmonella, which is quite dangerous.

For the beginner, the wisest choice is to start with a species that lives naturally in your own area and has a diet that can be easily obtained throughout the year. Unfortunately, many people start their hobbies with reptiles whose diets are so specialized that a ready food supply is either not available for months at a time, or only at such great cost that the unfortunate animal may, of economic necessity, go hungry much of the time.

When reptiles native to tropical South America are brought several thousand miles north of their natural habitats, they often begin a long period of decline ending in eventual death. Whether the immediate cause of death is pneumonia, malnutrition, vitamin- or mineral-associated deficiency, the underlying cause is related to the tremendous difference between the "native" and the "foreign" habitat in captivity.

Strict attention must be paid to *all* the subtle conditions that make up the animal's natural ecosystem. Most mammals and birds, faced with such overwhelmingly negative environmental conditions, quickly sicken and die, but a reptile may survive for a prolonged period — perhaps for months — before it succumbs to respiratory infection or malnutrition. This is why the beginner is wisest to start a collection with species that live nearby.

Some of the best reptiles for the beginner are garter snakes, alligator lizards, box tortoises, and freshwater turtles. Each has a varied diet and is relatively easy to keep healthy while in captivity. A wide variety of color patterns or markings may exist within a single genus and species, and many collectors specialize in studying these.

Never gather more animals than you actually need, and disturb the collecting site as little as possible. Local game laws must be obeyed, and necessary permits obtained.

As you gain experience with captive reptiles, you may want to add some of the more exotic forms to your collection by trades with other amateurs or purchases from animal dealers throughout the country. New specimens must be quarantined properly so that diseases will not be transmitted to resident animals. Obviously, prey species are never housed with their natural predators unless you are looking for a diminishing return.

HANDLING CAPTIVE REPTILES

Ideally, reptiles should not be handled unless absolutely necessary. Most reptiles have teeth, and even the toothless chelonia have biting mouth parts that can inflict serious injury. Nevertheless, usually the safest way to handle reptiles is by hand. Gloves and nooses pose the risk of unintentional injury to the animal from failure to control the amount of pressure on their bodies. Venomous snakes and lizards pose another problem, but these animals are not recommended except for the most serious and experienced amateur herpetologist. When necessary, a snake hook can be used with aggressive or sharp-toothed snakes to gently lift the snake from one location to another or to pin down its head and neck if it is likely to harm the handler.

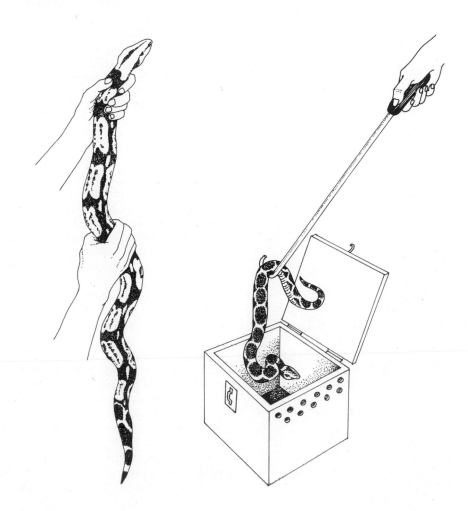

Since reptiles have only one bone that connects the skull to the spinal column, rough handling can dislocate or fracture the neck. Support the head and neck area gently in such a way that the rest of the body's weight is not suspended from it, especially when handling large, heavy-bodied boas and pythons.

preventive medicine

HOUSING

The natural habitat of a particular species dictates housing—but in all cases, avoid overcrowding. There must be adequate space to allow for freedom to move, gather food and water, and select living room without encroaching on the territories of cage mates.

Different orders, species, and sexes can be mixed. One must take care, however, not to house prey and predator together, tiny animals and big ones, freshwater and marine animals.

AQUATIC REPTILES. Pelagic sea snakes and some turtles are totally aquatic; the marine iguanas of the Galápagos Islands and some of the marine crocodiles are semiaquatic but leave the water at times to bask and reproduce. Most alligators, crocodiles, caimans, and gavials require "hauling-out" and basking sites.

For aquatic reptile management to succeed, particular attention must be paid to water quality. Uneaten food and feces soon provide a rich breeding medium for disease-causing organisms of many kinds. Scavengers such as snails, freshwater clams or mussels, crawfish, or bottom-feeding fish are useful cleaners and also serve as a ready source of food. If clams are used, they should not be large enough to be a danger to small turtles, which might be drowned if they got their toes caught between the shells of an especially vindictive bivalve. High-capacity filters usually will handle the waste load, if cleaned and checked regularly. The pH should be maintained near 7.0. Normal oxygen saturation of the water will promote the growth of plants and animals and impede the growth of deleterious bacteria and fungi. The oxygen may be supplied entirely by thriving living plants through their photosynthesis and/or may be supplemented by bubbling air through air stones and pump.

Marine reptiles should be maintained in salt water. Otherwise they may develop a sodium chloride deficiency or severe eye disease.

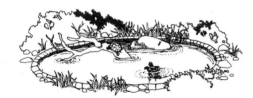

Permanent large aquarium tanks are often used, but are not necessary for the aquatic or semiaquatic species of turtles or crocodilians. A child's plastic wading pool can house these animals satisfactorily for quite some time. It may not particularly appeal to your aesthetic sense, but this type of pool is both inexpensive and practical.

(For more detailed information on aquarium water, filters, pumps, and the like, see "Fish," pages 146ff.)

More permanent outdoor ponds may be constructed from concrete, reinforced with steel, according to readily available plans. There must be adequate drainage and basking surfaces. The surface may be dressed with textured epoxy resin or latex-based swimming pool paint. Latex paint is more economical initially, but has poor resistance to abrasion from claws, carapaces, and everyday wear and tear; also, it must be reapplied more frequently. The textured epoxy surfaces last almost lifelong, and when coated with algae, which will grow by itself, look far more natural. Another advantage of epoxy is its resistance to cleaning abrasion and chemical disinfectants. Either type of surface may be cleaned with steam or high-pressure water streams.

Outdoor ponds are not too cold for reptiles in summer months, but whether they are in spring and autumn depends on the region of the country.

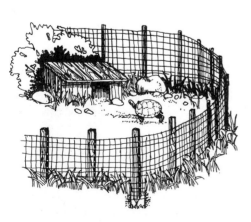

TERRESTRIAL REPTILES. Terrestrial chelonians can be kept outdoors in temperate weather if they are housed within a movable wire-fenced corral. The enclosure should be moved regularly to fresh "pasture" to provide clean forage and to prevent the accumulation of disease-producing organisms. Shade must be available to prevent overheating. Some species will attempt to burrow beneath the wire fencing. This can be prevented either by burying the fencing material an inch or two underground or by driving wire staples down around the fence perimeter. John Hoke's book, listed at the end of this chapter, gives a more detailed description of these techniques.

Standard aquariums and terrariums with a screen top can be used to house small turtles, lizards, and snakes. For larger species you can buy reptile cages from biological supply or pet stores or you can build one yourself. Commonly the front is made of glass, the bottom, back, and ends (or just the bottom and back) of wood — with a screen top hinged along the back and locked in front. To prevent the snake from rubbing its snout, plastic screen or small holes high up on the cage edges should be used for ventilation.

Whenever possible, outdoor enclosures tailored to the requirements of the species are preferable to these artificial, indoor quarters. Reptiles are more inclined to feed and reproduce under natural conditions.

ARBOREAL REPTILES. Clean, nonresinous, hardwood tree branches are an essential part of the environment for arboreal reptiles such as vine snakes, rat snakes, chameleons, iguanas, and the like, whose usual natural habitat is the forest, dwelling in bushes and trees.

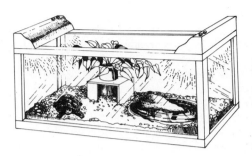

DESERT-DWELLING REPTILES. Some desert-dwelling species should be provided with natural sand litter in which to burrow and rocks on which to bask. These reptiles often regulate their own body temperature not only by basking but by changing the angles of their bodies in relation to the source of radiant energy — and pigment-containing chromatophores in the skin also play a major role in heat regulation. The source of radiant energy may be unfiltered natural sunlight or artificial light of the proper wavelength, such as ultraviolet fluorescent lamps (Grolux from Sylvania; Vita Lite from Durotest Corporation, North Bergen, New Jersey; Chroma Series from General Electric). Some shade must always be available. When overheated, many lizards cool themselves by panting, but their tolerance to heat is limited. See the section on Photoperiods, page 167.

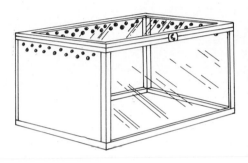

BURROWING REPTILES. A floor covering of forest litter, potting soil, leaf mold, and so forth, should be provided for burrowing species (some tortoises, for instance, desert snakes, and lizards are burrowers). Check frequently for decaying vegetation and remove it because the acids released as it decomposes can be harmful to the reptiles. Some of these animals appear satisfied merely with hiding boxes or crevices into which they may retreat, while others may require material they can actually burrow into in order to remain content and healthy.

DECORATION. While not ideal, some of the more realistic artificial plants can do much to enrich a cage's appearance and have the additional advantage of being able to withstand chemical sterilization. Rocks, sand, and gravel may be sterilized by dry heat in an oven, by steam from boiling water, by formaldehyde in 10 percent concentration (though this is irritating to the mucous membranes of both people and reptiles), or by household bleach at 5.25 percent sodium hypochlorite — the strength of all commercial bleaches. Household bleach is effective and inexpensive and, after thorough rinsing and drying, leaves no residue.

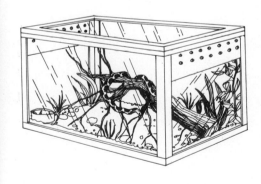

If you have more than one cage or tank in a room, a clean, orderly layout will make care and hygiene simpler. All handling utensils, implements, and so forth, should be thoroughly disinfected between use with different animals. Again, household bleach is good for this purpose, but should be rinsed off to prevent skin, respiratory, and eye irritation.

WATER SUPPLY. A water supply must be designed specifically to meet the needs of each animal. Tortoises get most of the moisture they need from the succulent content of their food. Generally, savanna, prairie, or desert reptiles drink readily from shallow containers; arboreal reptiles will lap only dewdrops from leaves, petals, or cacti; while most snakes, crocodilians, chelonians, and a few lizards enjoy soaking. Mist guns work well in producing dewdrops. Waterfalls and artificial streams are both useful and aesthetic in the more elaborate cage environments. If the water is to be recycled, you must take care to prevent cross-contamination and the accumulation of potentially hazardous bacteria, viruses, protozoans, and other parasites—and even the most elaborate systems have been known to fail, with disastrous effects.

LITTER AND WASTE MANAGEMENT. Cage litter undoubtedly poses a difficult problem. Depending on the environmental preferences of a particular species, forest litter, leaf mold, humus, moss, sand, gravel, pebbles, kitty litter, wood shavings, newspaper, ground corncobs have all been tried—and *all* have been shown to have disadvantages. There is no universally acceptable litter material. Some do not absorb well; some are easily eaten, causing obstructions and impactions of the gastrointestinal tract; and some are too readily converted into culture media for organisms that cause diseases.

Unless display is particularly important, clean newspaper or butcher's wrap — changed frequently as it becomes soiled—makes a very satisfactory cage litter. In cases where appearance is the primary object, synthetic, artificial turf (available from at least two manufacturers: Ozite and the brand manufactured by Monsanto) makes a pleasing alternative to paper. It can be cut to fit the cage's dimensions, and is easily cleaned with hot water and disinfectants. Initial expense is moderate, but acceptable, since the useful lifetime is a long one.

Excreta, both fecal and urinary, must be removed promptly. It should be part of the daily routine to inspect each cage for stools or solid urinary wastes — these materials will be kept from accumulating, and the owner will be able to notice any abnormal condition. Keeping track of elimination is just as important as keeping track of feeding in monitoring life processes.

Snakes and turtles frequently defecate into their water containers. Turtles should never be housed in the same cage, or in any way share a common water supply, with snakes or lizards. The parasitic amoeba *Endamoeba invadens*, a common, apparently harmless organism in most turtles' intestinal tracts, is quite dangerous to these other species.

HUMIDITY. A reptile thrives at a humidity level that matches its native habitat. Obviously, tropical reptiles, which live naturally in a rain forest, will require a higher relative humidity than desert-dwelling reptiles. Temperate-zone species will usually thrive at about 70 percent relative humidity. Placing the water container over a mild heat source may be sufficient to raise the level of moisture in the air.

TEMPERATURE REQUIREMENTS. There are specific optimum and preferred temperatures for almost all reptiles. They might remain active above and below these temperatures, but their metabolic processes might not operate efficiently. Biological processes are governed by enzymes, each of which has its own optimum temperature.

REPTILIAN TEMPERATURE RANGE

	RANGE OF ACTIVE REPTILES	PREFERRED OPTIMUM	CRITICAL HIGH*
American alligator	26.0° – 37.0°C (78.0° – 98.0°F)	32.0° – 35.0°C (89.6° – 95.0°F)	38.0° – 39.0°C (100.4° – 102.2°F)
Garter snake	16.0° – 34.6°C (60.8° – 94.0°F)	22.0° – 31.0°C (71.6° – 87.8°F)	40.5°C (104.9°F)
Painted turtle	8.0° – 30.2°C (46.5° – 86.0°F)	23.0° – 27.8°C (73.5° – 84.0°F)	39.0° – 41.0°C (102.2° – 105.8°F)
Green iguana	26.7° – 42.4°C (79.7° – 108.5°F)	20.5° – 39.5°C (85.1° – 103.1°F)	46.1°C (114.8°F)
Desert tortoise	19.0° – 37.8°C (66.2° – 100.4°F)	26.7° – 29.4°C (80.6° – 85.1°F)	39.5° – 43.0°C (103.1° – 109.0°F)

*Temperature at which an animal will die from overheating if exposed too long.

These data can also be used to determine temperature ranges for species other than those mentioned: alligators, crocodiles, caimans, and gavials can be compared with the American alligator; temperate lizards and snakes with garter snakes; turtles and terrapins with the painted turtle; tropical lizards and snakes with iguanas; and tortoises with the desert tortoise.

HEATING INDOOR AND OUTDOOR CAGES. When the temperature is not high enough, additional heat can be provided in several ways. Heating cables, available from aquarium suppliers, may be buried within the floor substance of the cages, where the animals will not be in direct contact with them. Since heat tends to rise with air currents, these are more useful than overhead heating devices. Thermostatically controlled, self-contained water-heater-type devices may be more appropriate for larger enclosures.

PHOTOPERIOD. The photoperiod is the light:dark cycle to which an animal (or plant) is exposed. From research conducted with many species, including man, it has been found that each species is best adapted to live under a specific photoperiod that may not be optimum for another species. Exceptions are animals that live underground or in caves and never venture into the light at all — and those that, through evolutionary processes, have lost their eyes.

A general rule can be stated to help determine the proper photoperiod: for equatorial reptiles from tropical zones, an equal day:night cycle of about 12 hours light and 12 hours dark is desirable. For temperate-zone-dwelling species, about 14 to 16 hours of light and 8 to 10 hours of dark would be more appropriate. Since the seasons change, there should be some variation in these periods of light and dark — there should be a gradual increase in light from spring to summer, and it should reduce from fall to winter. A good device for this is an inexpensive electric timer to control the light source. Natural, unfiltered light is sufficient if the photoperiod is correct — but since window glass filters out much of the ultraviolet light, fluorescent light should be used for indoor cages. The lights are usually kept about 20 inches from the animals, and one or two are used, depending on the size and shape of the cage. *Never* light the environment constantly. This imposes a severe stress, and captive animals confined in such an atmosphere will almost invariably cease feeding, refuse to mate, and, eventually, decline in health.

FEEDING

The tables that follow (pages 168–170) include diets for many captive species that can be easily obtained all year long. The insects and animal foodstuffs are usually eaten alive. Some of those recommended — mealworms, corn grubs, earthworms — can be stored in the refrigerator for a limited time.

Although reptile diets vary greatly, some generalizations can be made: young, vigorous, and actively moving snakes, lizards, turtles, and alligators can be fed one to three times a week. Older, more sluggish animals require fewer feedings. Large snakes (large pythons and boas, for instance) can be maintained on a feeding schedule of once every three or four weeks or longer. The larger lizards and crocodilians should be fed twice weekly and the larger chelonians every other day. Tortoises regulate their own daily feeding if vegetation is available. Living food items (animals) should usually be removed if uneaten after an hour or so.

For all reptiles, except those with very restricted diets, variety is desirable to avoid nutritional deficiencies. It is also often wise to supplement their diet with a balanced preparation yielding calcium, vitamins A, B-complex, C, D_3, E, and K (such as Squibb's Vionate, available from most pet shops and veterinarians).

Fasting may be quite prolonged in some reptiles without serious effects if water consumption is adequate to allow for normal kidney function. Reptiles have been reported to fast for as long as thirty-six months without suffering ill effects, but this long a period of fasting is most unusual.

FOOD PREFERENCES

SNAKES. Boas, pythons, rat snakes, gopher or bull snakes, and vipers all prefer warm-blooded prey such as rodents or birds of the right size.

Garter snakes and water snakes will usually take fish, frogs, toads, earthworms, and slugs. Frequently, dead food will be accepted. Often these spe-

FOOD PREFERENCES OF SNAKE SPECIES

SNAKE	SMALL MAMMALS	BIRDS	OTHER SNAKES	LIZARDS	EGGS	FROGS, TOADS, SALAMANDERS, TADPOLES	FISH	INSECTS	WORMS	SLUGS
Anaconda	X	X					X			
Boa, python	X	X								
Boomslang	X	X	X	X						
Coachwhip	X	X	X	X						
Cobra (except king cobra)	X		X	X						
Coral			X	X						
Copperhead	X	X		O		O				
Dekay's									X	X
Egg-eating					X					
Garter	X		X	X		X	X	X	X	X
Gopher, bull, pine	X	X		O	O					
Green				X				X		
Hog-nosed						X				
Indigo	X	X	X	X		X				
King snake	X	X	X	X						
King cobra	O		X							
Krait	X		X	X		O				
Mamba	X	X								
Mangrove	X	X		O						
Marine or sea							X			
Night			X	X						
Racer	X	X	X	X	O	O				
Rainbow						tadpoles				
Rat or chicken	X	X			X					
Rattlesnake	X	X		O						
Ribbon						X	X			
Ring-necked						salamanders			X	
Vine snake				X						
Viper, miscellaneous	X	X	O	O						
Water moccasin	X	X	X	X		X	X			
Water snake	O		O	O		X	X		X	O

X = usual food   O = occasional food

cies will accept mice if fish or worms are rubbed on their fur, leaving a coating of slime.

Indigo snakes and king snakes usually will eat both warm-blooded and cold-blooded prey.

The smaller ring-neck, or brown, snakes and their kin usually confine their diet to earthworms, small salamanders, and snakes or lizards.

Racers and vine snakes usually will accept lizards. These need not be alive and can be provided from a frozen supply in the off-season when they are not readily available.

Some snakes, such as the king cobra, are almost strictly snake eaters; again, these may be frozen and thawed.

FOOD PREFERENCES OF
SELECTED LIZARD SPECIES

LIZARD	SMALL MAMMALS	BIRDS	INSECTS	EGGS	CHOPPED MEAT	MOLLUSKS	FRUIT	VEGETABLES
Alligator	X		X		X			
American anole			X					
Basilisk	X		X					
Beaded, Mexican	X	X		X	X			
Bearded	X		X		O			
Caiman						X		
Chameleon			X					
Chuckwalla			O				X	X
Collared	X		X				X	X
Gecko, miscellaneous	X		X					
Gila monster	X	X		X	X			
Glass "snake"	X		X	X	X			
Horned lizard ("horned toad")			ants, tiny crickets					
Iguana, common	X	X	X		X		X	X
Iguana, desert			X				X	X
Iguana, marine								marine algae, kelp
Lacerta, miscellaneous			X					
Monitor, miscellaneous	X	X	X	X				
Night			termites, tiny grubs					
Skink, miscellaneous	X		X		X			
Spiny	X		X					
Spiny-tailed	X		X					
Swift, fence			X					
Tegu	X		X	X	X		O	
Whiptailed			X					
Worm			X					

X = usual food   O = occasional food

LIZARDS. Horned lizards dine almost entirely upon ants, though some will accept small crickets or mealworms as substitutes.

Night lizards, "worm" lizards, and the like usually limit their fare to termite and ant eggs.

Common green iguanas, usually sold in pet shops, thrive on dandelion flowers and leaves, frozen mixed vegetables (thawed but uncooked), crickets, baby mice, cooked eggs, mealworms, a small amount of dog food, and trout chow slightly moistened with water.

Tegus, Gila monsters, and Mexican beaded lizards usually do well with a diet of raw eggs, chopped lean meat, baby mice, and a multivitamin–mineral powder supplement such as Vionate.

FOOD PREFERENCES OF SELECTED TURTLES, TERRAPINS, TORTOISES

CHELONIAN	MISCELLANEOUS MEATS	FISH	INSECTS, WORMS, SLUGS, DOG FOOD	FLOWERS	FRUITS	OTHER VEGETABLES
Aldabra tortoise				X	X	X
Alligator snapping turtle	X	X	X			
Blanding's turtle	X	X	X			water plants
Box "turtle"	X		X	X	X	X
Chicken turtle	X	X	X			water plants
Desert tortoise			O	X	X	X
Diamondback turtle	X	X	X			water plants
Galápagos tortoise				X	X	X
Gopher tortoise, miscellaneous			O	X	X	X
Greek tortoise			O	X	X	X
Green turtle, marine, juvenile	mollusks	X				marine plants
Green turtle, marine, adult		O				marine plants
Hawksbill turtle, juvenile	mollusks	X				marine plants
Hawksbill turtle, adult		O				marine plants
Herman's tortoise			O	X	X	X
Hingeback tortoise			O	X	X	X
Leatherback turtle, juvenile	mollusks occasionally	X				marine plants
Leatherback turtle, adult		O				marine plants
Leopard tortoise			O	X	X	X
Map turtle	X	X	X			water plants
Matta matta		X	O			
Mud turtle	X	X	X			water plants
Muhlenberg's turtle	X	X	X			water plants
Musk turtle	X	X	X			water plants
Painted turtle, miscellaneous	X	X	X			water plants
Pond turtle, miscellaneous	X	X	X			water plants
Radiated tortoise			O	X	X	X
Red-eared slider	X	X	X			water plants
Red-legged tortoise			X	X	X	X
Side-necked turtle	X	X	X			water plants
Snapping turtle, miscellaneous	X	X	X			
Soft-shell turtle	X	X	X			
Star tortoise, miscellaneous			O	X	X	X
Yellow-legged tortoise			O	X	X	X
Wood terrapin	X	X	X			water plants

X = usual food   O = occasional food

Monitors, depending on their size (a few inches to several feet in length), will eat much the same diet as the tegus, with bigger rodents and birds added for the larger species.

Fence lizards, skinks, alligator lizards, anoles, and chameleons do well on a diet of appropriately sized insects, from tiny fruit flies (genetic wingless strains are especially useful for baby chameleons) to large crickets.

Specialized species, such as marine iguanas, eat only marine algae or kelp. The caiman lizard, with its powerful jaws and flat-cusped teeth, is superbly adapted to a diet of shelled mollusks.

CHELONIANS. Turtles and terrapins usually will eat earthworms, small whole fish, mice, green leafy vegetation (watercress, Swiss chard, or aquarium or pond weeds available in any pet store), and trout chow.

Tortoises usually thrive on flowers, succulents, grass, Swiss chard, cucumbers, frozen mixed vegetables (thawed but uncooked), fresh fruit, and a small amount of bread or dog food.

CROCODILIANS. Alligators, crocodiles, and caimans all eat whatever they can catch or come upon. In captivity, rodents, fowl, whole fish, and raw meat are food substitutes. There should be some variety to help prevent dietary deficiencies or imbalances.

Gavials, like these others, eat whatever they come on, in the wild, but they prefer fish.

CANNIBALISM. In the strictest sense, some degree of cannibalism is normal feeding behavior in some of the reptiles. Many snakes are ophiophagous — that is, they eat other snakes. But it is abnormal for an animal to consume members of its own species. Overcrowding is probably the major cause of cannibalism. Reducing the population and providing hiding places will usually eliminate this problem.

first aid

INJURIES

In clinical practice, a veterinarian sees a wide variety of traumatic injuries to captive reptiles. Most of these wounds are the result of feeding live rats to boas and pythons. Amateurs often forget that rats have a far higher metabolic rate and intelligence than snakes. If the snake does not eat the rat within a short time, the rat soon becomes hungry. It will actively seek food and if the snake is the only source present, the predator will become the prey. Many rat bites require surgical treatment and closure by suturing, and any wound causing loss of tissue or severe laceration should be seen by a veterinarian with an expertise in exotic animal medicine. Minor wounds can be cleaned with hydrogen peroxide (3 percent by volume). The best way to prevent this kind of injury is to remain in attendance when feeding live rats to snakes. Most hungry snakes will attack their prey almost immediately. Don't leave rodents with snakes for a long time or unattended.

Another common injury is the fracture of turtle and tortoise shells caused when they are dropped from some height, run over by automobiles, or attacked by dogs and raccoons. In most cases these injuries should be kept clean and covered by a dry, sterile gauze or dressing until you can get veterinary help. Fractured shells can be repaired by various methods, such as splinting and stabilizing the shell fragments with fiberglass and epoxy resin.

Occasionally, if several aggressive crocodilians or turtles are housed in overcrowded conditions, fights over food or sexual partners will result in severe injuries. Entire limbs may be lost and the victim may die as a result of blood loss or shock. Often, immediate professional care will be necessary if the animal is to be saved.

ABRASIONS FROM RUBBING AGAINST CAGE SURFACES

Many captive reptiles, particularly snakes, are slow to accept captivity, and some never settle down to the point where they stop attempting to escape from their cage. If the cage has sharp edges or rough surfaces, the reptile will soon mutilate its nose from constant rubbing and pushing. There should not be any wire screen in the cage of a reptile that attempts to escape.

BURNS

The use of unguarded electric light bulbs to furnish additional heat in a cage is unwise. Besides being inefficient, expensive, and providing too much light to properly maintain a suitable photoperiod, incandescent bulbs can seriously burn snakes and lizards that climb onto them. Surprisingly, the animals will not always move from the source of heat that is burning them. Minor burns can be treated as they would be on humans, by applying burn ointment. Furacin, which is water soluble, and Neosphorin are good household burn ointments. More serious burns — a burn that blisters, for instance — should be seen by a veterinarian immediately.

Fluorescent bulbs will not burn the animals — but overexposure to them could cause eye damage.

SHEDDING PROBLEMS Properly called dysectysis, failure to shed all or part of the old epidermis is a frequent problem with captive reptiles, especially snakes. This may be due to improper nutrition or dehydration, parasites (especially mites), or a lack of sufficiently abrasive branches or stones in the cage on which the animal can rub to initiate shedding. In trying to free itself of the increasingly dry skin, the reptile may injure itself.

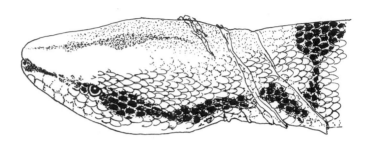

incomplete sloughing

The most effective treatment is to soak the animal in warm water (no warmer than 86°F.) for about fifteen to thirty minutes and gently peel off the adhered old skin with your fingers or a washcloth. Another method is to soak the animal for about thirty minutes, then sandwich it between heavy towels moistened with warm water. As the snake crawls around between the moist toweling, the skin will be gently removed.

EYE INJURIES Fortunately, serious eye injuries are rare in well-managed captive reptiles. Possibly the most common are the result of overzealous attempts to remove retained lens shields over the eyes of snakes, which are normally replaced when the snake sheds its skin. The uninformed amateur may try to pull these caps off with sharp instruments without first soaking them loose for a few minutes in warm water, and the result is permanently damaged corneas.

parasites Reptiles are afflicted with both internal and external parasites. The most common in captive lizards and snakes are mites and ticks. These can be treated in a number of ways, but the easiest and one of the safest is to hang a piece of Shell No-Pest Strip above the cage where the reptiles cannot reach it but it will give off sufficient vapor to kill the parasites. A ¼-inch strip per 10 cubic feet of cage has proved safe and effective. The strip should be left in place for about four or five days and then removed.

Turtles and crocodilians occasionally are bothered by leeches — which can be killed by immersing the reptiles in a salt solution for about thirty minutes. Use approximately 1 tablespoon of table salt (sodium chloride) per quart of water — it doesn't matter whether or not the salt is iodized.

Flies frequently lay their eggs in or near wounds or natural body openings of reptiles, particularly tortoises. These eggs soon hatch into maggots, which

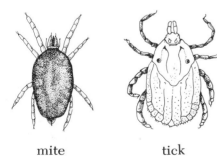

mite   tick

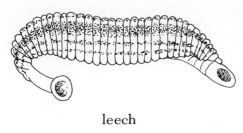

leech

feed on the tissues of their unfortunate victim. Sometimes the resultant wound can be treated adequately at home with one application of a 3 percent hydrogen peroxide solution, but a veterinarian should be consulted to make sure that the damage done by the maggots is confined to the exterior surfaces.

Reptiles may be infested with various internal parasites. Symptoms are loss of weight, failure to gain weight and/or blood in the stools. There are no universal parasiticides which can be used indiscriminately to treat these animals. A veterinarian should be consulted, and stool specimens examined microscopically to determine what the parasites are and how best to treat them. If you are in doubt about whether your reptile has internal parasites, submit a fresh stool specimen to a veterinarian for a laboratory diagnosis.

diseases

Many of the diseases of captive reptiles must be diagnosed and treated by a veterinarian who is trained and experienced in exotic animal medicine and surgery. However, you should be aware of some of the more commonly encountered problems and of the signs of ill health so that you will be able to recognize when your reptile is unwell.

Most of the disease problems seen in captive animals come from their unnatural habitat, with crowding or poor sanitation. Nutrition also plays a major role — many of the actual diseases in captive reptiles are the result of improper diet.

nutritional disorders
STARVATION AND DEHYDRATION

Ignorance of the natural or suitable artificial diet and specific water-drinking habits is the usual cause of starvation and dehydration in captive reptiles. A mammal-eating species will not eat insects and a fish eater will not touch mammals. It is vital to feed your reptile exactly what it needs.

Many of the sick reptiles a veterinarian sees are starved and dehydrated — literally. The animal's stores of body fat and muscle are depleted, its eyes

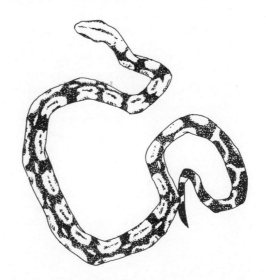

sink, its skin shrivels, and its bones become prominent. At best, these animals are extremely unstable. Many have not eaten voluntarily in months and their resistance to stress is almost nil. As dehydration progresses, the entire circulatory system is placed under massive stress, the kidneys don't clear nitrogenous wastes from the blood, and death soon ends the animal's suffering. Reptiles may survive for months without eating but, eventually, their stores of reserve tissue are exhausted and they decline rapidly. A veterinarian should be consulted when an animal that is active and frequently fed fails to eat properly. Gentle handling and a quiet environment are almost as essential as nutritional replacement.

HAND-FEEDING

If a reptile is not eating voluntarily, attempts to hand-feed a natural diet (young mice, rats, baby chicks, and the like) should be made as soon as possible by or under the guidance of a veterinarian. It takes a great deal of practice to learn how to do this without being bitten. Food for snakes should be lubricated with beaten whole egg. Lizards and chelonians also may be hand-fed appropriate materials (see Feeding, pages 167ff.). The mouth is opened and a small amount of food is passed down the esophagus with a smooth-tipped flexible probe. *Gentleness is essential:* a snake's body should be well supported during handling.

TUBE-FEEDING

If hand-feeding fails or is inadequate, the quickest, most efficient method to restore body fats, protein, and vitamin balance is tube-feeding with a nutritional-replacement product that has a high-calorie, low-bulk formula designed for convalescent animals (Pet Kalorie from Haver-Lockhart; Nutrical from EVSCO; both are available from a veterinarian and should be administered only under guidance). These products may be mixed with pureed infant-food meat diets. A urethral catheter of the proper size or an infant feeding tube (a rubber catheter prescribed by a veterinarian or physician) works well for force-feeding, and both will fit a syringe with a Luer tip. A good tube-feeding formula is:

> 3 parts strained or finely chopped meat
> 1 part beaten whole egg
> ½ part prepared Nutrical or Pet Kalorie or high-potency multi–B complex vitamins
> 1 part warm water

OBESITY

Although most nutritional problems in captive reptiles are directly associated with malnutrition, a lack of totally digestible nutrients, or vitamin/mineral deficiencies and imbalances, some of these animals suffer the effects of too much caloric intake for their particular needs. It is not uncommon for zealous amateur herpetologists to overfeed their pets in order to see how fast they can be made to grow. Without sufficient energy demand, excess food energy is stored as fat deposits. If this continues long enough, certain internal organs, particularly the liver, will accumulate fat.

NUTRITIONAL DEFICIENCIES

The most common nutritional deficiencies in captive reptiles, listed below, are the result of being fed an improper diet. Although a natural diet can, thus, prevent these conditions, once the symptoms occur the animal should be taken immediately to a veterinarian for treatment. This usually consists of injections of the missing vitamin and a supplement to the diet, at least temporarily, in the form of pills or drops. In some cases you may be able to administer these yourself, under the guidance of the veterinarian; otherwise they can be mixed in with the animal's food.

CALCIUM:PHOSPHORUS. This ratio in a reptile's diet is of great importance. The most common imbalance in turtles and iguanas results from a diet containing too much lean meat or lettuce; the condition may be aggravated further by a vitamin D deficiency from not receiving sufficient ultraviolet radiation. GroLux or other synthetic lights provide the needed ultraviolet radiation.

The bony tissues become so depleted that skeletal deformities result. Frequently, the turtle's shell and limbs suffer fractures from bearing weight. Later, it becomes very soft. If the turtle survives, the shell tends to curl and the internal organs become crowded. The outward symptoms in the iguana are markedly firm swollen limbs and tail: the general appearance is that of a well-fed, chubby lizard.

Calcium-phosphorus imbalance is also found in captive caimans fed a meat diet without additional calcium.

THIAMINE DEFICIENCY. Reptiles with a thiamine (vitamin B_1) deficiency often show bizarre neurologic signs from twitching to severe convulsions or paralysis. Frozen fish not recently killed may contain the enzyme thiaminase. Therefore, if thiamine deficiency is to be avoided, thiamine should be added to this diet. Thiamine is available in green vegetables, meat, and grains. In the case of most deficiencies, a veterinarian will prescribe tablets for supplementation.

HYPOGLYCEMIA. Crocodilians are particularly subject to hypoglycemia, caused by fasting and stress (of captivity, handling, adverse temperature, and so on). Typical signs are tremors, slow or absent righting reflex, torpor, and widely dilated pupils. Prevention depends on a high protein diet, and particularly on avoiding stress. Diagnosis of hypoglycemia can be made by a veterinarian, who will prescribe something to correct it.

VISCERAL GOUT AND "RENAL CONSTIPATION." These problems are frequently found in captive iguanas, tegus, tortoises, and crocodilians. The result is usually death — which may be rather sudden. The cause is usually a diet that is too high in protein or contains too much organ meat. Water deprivation, with resultant incomplete clearance of uric acid, also has been suggested as the principal cause of constipation. An adequate balanced (natural) diet and a constantly available source of fresh water will prevent uric acid accumulation.

VITAMIN A DEFICIENCY. This problem is seen frequently in aquatic turtles, especially during the first year or two of life. Commercial turtle food lacks usable vitamin A and should not be used. Frequently, the earliest signs are puffy, swollen eyelids, open-mouth breathing, wheezing, and nasal discharge. In chronic cases, the horny mouth parts and the cornea may be overgrown. While quite alarming, this is reversible once replacement therapy is initiated; and much of the keratin accumulation can be removed by a veterinarian with an appropriate-size curette or spatula.

VITAMIN K DEFICIENCY. In alligators, crocodiles, caimans, and gavials, the first sign is severe bleeding of the gums. As the deciduous teeth are shed, there is excessive bleeding, which may continue for days. The veterinarian can prescribe additional vitamin K for the animal.

VITAMIN C DEFICIENCY. This problem has been found to occur in snakes and lizards. It is thought that most of the vitamin C in a snake's diet is contained within the intestinal contents of its prey. If such prey species (for example, mice) are not fed prior to being presented to the snakes, they might be deficient in this essential vitamin. The signs may be lowered resistance to infection, oral bleeding, and abnormal shedding of teeth.

HYPOTHYROIDISM. Aquatic turtles that are fed only raw meat and lettuce do not get enough trace minerals — which can cause hypothyroidism. Captive tortoises (particularly those from the Aldabra and Galápagos Islands, as well as the more common gopher and box tortoises kept as pets) are also affected with hypothyroidism; in these animals, the condition results from eating goitrogenic vegetables, particularly of the cabbage and kale family (cabbage, kale, Brussels sprouts, broccoli) and soybean sprouts.

The symptoms of hypothyroidism are loss of appetite, lethargy, fibrous goiter, and, often, swelling of the tissues under the skin.

STEATITIS. This inflammation of fat is thought to result from the excessive consumption of unsaturated or rancid fatty acids over a long period of time. It occurs particularly in caimans, alligators, and crocodiles that are fed oily fish exclusively. It also has been found in snakes fed obese laboratory rats. The affected animal may appear totally healthy, or may develop firm swellings of variable size. Yellow-to-brown nodular growths appear under the skin and in the abdominal cavity, and the abdominal organs are frequently found to be a solid mass of discolored tissue with little or no separation of identifiable structures.

SODIUM CHLORIDE DEFICIENCY. Most marine reptiles should be maintained in salt water, but if they are kept in fresh water, they will need additional sodium chloride in their diets. These animals have salt glands that secrete the excessive sodium chloride ingested with food. Even with the ingestion of nonsaline water, the secretion of salt by this mechanism does not cease entirely. A small amount of iodized table salt added to the diet will ensure sufficient turnover of sodium chloride.

There is usually sufficient sodium chloride in the diet of nonmarine species. Though salt deposits often are seen around the nostrils of desert-dwelling lizards, this is not dangerous, but a normal consequence of their excretory system. Reptiles have evolved specialized glands to concentrate and secrete sodium and potassium — if they had not, they would need to pass enough urine to rid their bodies of excess salts; this specialized method conserves water.

bacterial diseases

The three major infectious diseases in captive reptiles are abscesses, infectious stomatitis ("mouth rot"), and pneumonia. All may be caused by the same organisms. These diseases must be treated by a veterinarian because the antibiotics used are under strict drug controls and available only through licensed professionals.

ABSCESSES

Swellings under the skin that slowly increase in size over a period of several weeks may be a sign of abscesses. Most contain semidry pus, which has the consistency of cheese. After incision and drainage, the cavity will be cleansed and packed with an appropriate antibiotic.

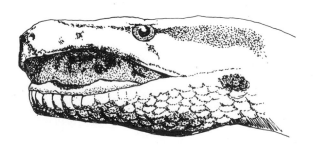

INFECTIOUS STOMATITIS, OR MOUTH ROT

Infectious stomatitis ("mouth rot") is common in captive snakes and lizards and less frequently found in tortoises. The size of the lesions depends on when it is diagnosed. The gums and oral membranes will be ulcerated and often hemorrhagic. Shreds of diseased tissue and shed teeth are also often mixed with the discharge. Initial treatment by an amateur should be a thorough cleansing of the mouth and surrounding areas with a 3 percent solution of hydrogen peroxide. The snake should be restrained gently and its mouth opened with a cotton-tipped applicator stick dipped in the solution. Sweep the stick toward the back of the mouth to avoid snagging the snake's teeth, which lean in a rearward direction. The animal should then be given antibiotic injections by a veterinarian.

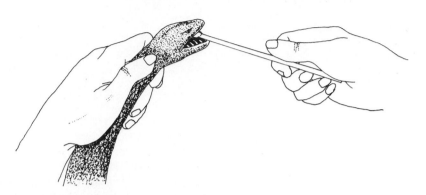

PNEUMONIA   Pneumonia and upper respiratory infections are very common in a captive reptile, and the other reptiles you have are easily infected. Any reptile showing signs of a respiratory disease — nasal discharge, open-mouthed breathing, rapid breathing, an audible wheezing or sneezing — should be quarantined immediately to halt transmission. Immediate antibiotic therapy should be started by a veterinarian and continued long enough to ensure that relapse will not occur.

reproduction

The small snake, lizard, turtle, and tortoise species can be bred in captivity — but it usually takes experience and great care, and even experts have trouble. But if temperature, photoperiod, nutrition, and general husbandry are all satisfactory, an amateur may be blessed occasionally with eggs and/or baby reptiles.

Most female reptiles that lay eggs do not take special care of them after they are deposited and covered. There are exceptions, but they are few.

If you are lucky in having either eggs or live young produced by your reptiles, consult your nearest zoo for specific advice applicable to those species. There are no general rules — the incubation temperature, humidity, and nesting media are quite variable. The same is true with respect to the proper diet for many newborn reptiles.

further readings

CONANT, R. A Field Guide to Reptiles and Amphibians of Eastern North America. Boston, Houghton Mifflin, 1975.

FRYE, F. L. Husbandry, Medicine, and Surgery in Captive Reptiles. Bonner Springs, Kansas, V. M. Publishing, 1973.

GOIN, C. J., AND GOIN, O. B. Introduction to Herpetology, 2nd ed. San Francisco, Freeman, 1971.

HOKE, J. First Book of Turtles and Their Care. New York, Watts, 1970.

MARTENS, R. The World of Amphibians and Reptiles. New York, McGraw-Hill, 1960.

OLIVER, J. A. The Natural History of North American Amphibians and Reptiles. Princeton, New Jersey, Van Nostrand, 1955.

PORTER, K. R. Herpetology. Philadelphia, W. B. Saunders, 1972.

STEBBINS, R. C. A Field Guide to Western Reptiles and Amphibians. Boston, Houghton Mifflin, 1966.

Amphibians
frogs, toads, salamanders, and caecilians

FREDRIC L. FRYE, D.V.M.

The class Amphibia includes frogs, toads, salamanders, and the lesser-known caecilians — many of them make fascinating and convenient pets. They require a small living space, are essentially odor-free and — except for over-amorous bellowing bullfrogs — quiet. Although amphibian life spans vary, toads are long-lived: they may be with you for over two decades.

Often, amphibians superficially resemble reptiles but do not have a scaly skin. Glands distributed over most of their body surface secrete moist, often mucoid substances, which help to prevent the skin from drying out when they are away from their usual watery environment. Some frogs and toads and a few salamanders produce poisonous secretions from certain skin glands as a defense against predators. These poisons may cause irritation in humans if they are absorbed through cuts or the membranes surrounding the eye.

Like reptiles (and unlike mammals and birds), amphibians are poikilothermic — their body temperatures are largely determined by the environmental temperature — though they prefer far cooler temperatures than do most reptiles.

There are about 3,500 species of amphibians, which are assigned to three major orders:

ORDER APODA (Without legs.) These are slender, wormlike creatures called caecilians, which live most of the time entirely buried in forest litter. They range from a few inches to approximately three feet long. Most are from tropical countries and are rarely available from exotic animal dealers in the United States.

ORDER CAUDATA (With tails.) These are the tailed amphibians, commonly called salamanders, which include hellbenders, sirens, mud puppies, newts, congo eels, mole salamanders, and lungless salamanders. They are from a few inches to over three feet long. Salamanders usually have well-developed forelimbs and hind limbs. Sirens have only poorly developed forelimbs, and the minuscule forelimbs and hind limbs of congo eels are easily overlooked.

ORDER ANURA (Without tails.) The adults of this order, which includes frogs and toads, have both forelimbs and hind limbs. Many weigh less than half an ounce and are just a few inches long, but the giants of the frog and toad world grow to 10 inches, sometimes, and weigh 2 to 3 pounds. In the United States frogs are jumpers with a relatively smooth, moist skin, while toads are hoppers with a dry, warty skin. The distinction between frogs and toads disappears, though, when they are studied on a worldwide basis.

Perhaps the greatest difference between reptiles and amphibians is that amphibians undergo a major metamorphosis during their early life. Meta-

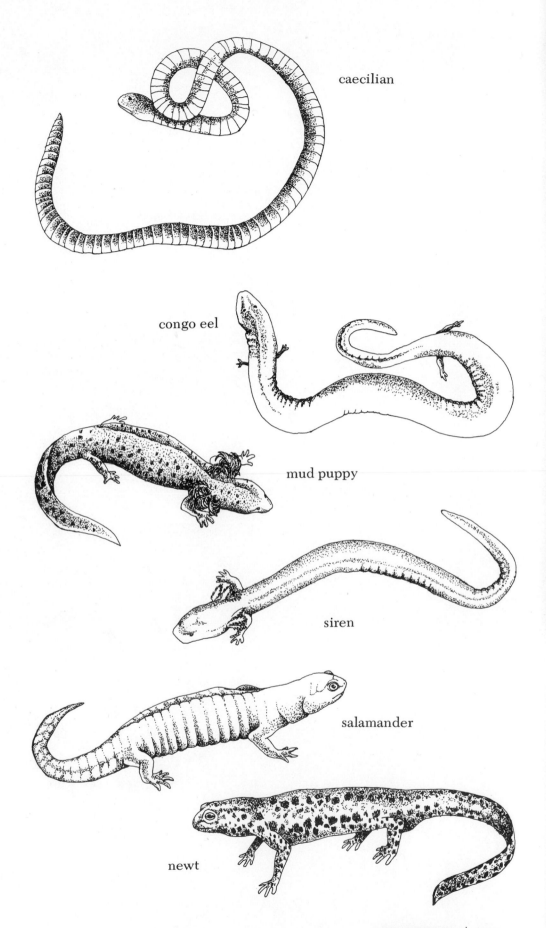

caecilian

congo eel

mud puppy

siren

salamander

newt

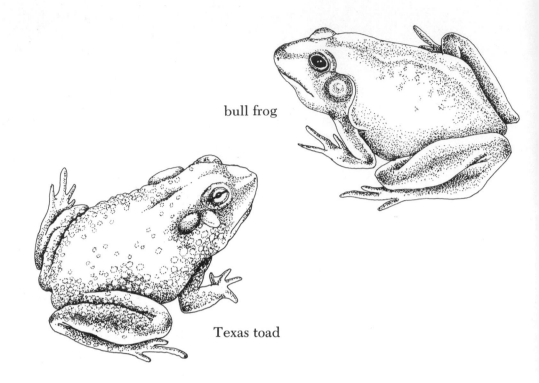

bull frog

Texas toad

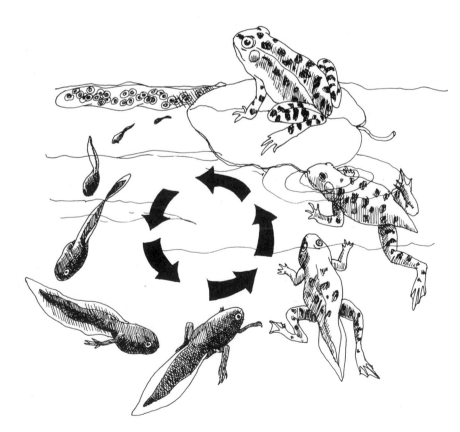

life cycle of the frog

morphosis may require from only a few weeks to several years, depending upon the species, the temperature of its environment, and the availability of food during the larval period. The eggs of most frogs and toads are laid in water where they are fertilized, develop, and hatch out as tadpoles, or "pollywogs." As the tadpoles develop, most grow legs — first hind legs and then forelegs — and the tail is gradually resorbed and disappears. The gills, which exchange needed oxygen and carbon dioxide in the aquatic environment, disappear in most species and are replaced with air-breathing lungs. Most adults live on land, though some frogs and toads, such as the African clawed frog, are entirely aquatic and rarely if ever venture from their water milieu.

Some salamanders and a few frogs and toads lay their eggs on land, in damp places and under logs. The transformation of the salamander is less dramatic than the frog's because it is not a complete change in form; the hind limbs develop before the forelimbs and in some cases are present before birth, the gills shrink, and the tail lengthens. A few species, such as the lungless salamander, have no free larval stage at all. The metamorphosis takes place in the egg and, at hatching, a miniature adult emerges. Some species, such as mud puppies and axolotls, develop lungs but retain gills throughout their lives. Others, including lungless salamanders, breathe through their skin (transpiration).

OBTAINING AMPHIBIANS   You can acquire amphibians either by catching them yourself or by buying them. Often the woodlands surrounding a major urban center will yield a variety of species, and a search in streams, ponds, under rocks, fallen trees, or loose bark may turn up members of the order Anura or Caudata. Be sure to follow local conservation regulations and take only one or two amphibians from a particular site — there is no excuse for greed.

Take a careful look around you when you catch an amphibian in the wild — for two reasons. One is that you will want to reproduce its natural habitat as faithfully as possible in its new home (see Housing, page 182). The second reason is that many amphibians, when it is their turn to breed, return to the exact geographical area where they hatched and matured through their metamorphosis. If and when you decide to release your wild-caught pets, try to do so exactly where you found them.

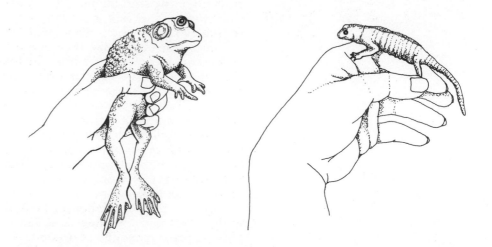

Many newly caught animals, including amphibians, suffer some degree of shock due to the stress of being captured and confined. Always try to handle the animal as little and as gently as possible, and provide some shelter in which it can find privacy and darkness. Small aquatic amphibians should be handled in a small net — picking them up by hand is likely to cause harm. Large frogs should be grasped under the chest and held upright. Large salamanders can be placed on top of the forefinger, and held gently by a hind leg. Eggs, which are found in clusters or strings, and larvae should be transported in well-insulated jars or thermos jugs to prevent overheating.

Exotic or foreign amphibians are sometimes available in pet shops or through trades with other collectors. There are many herpetological societies whose members cooperate in developing husbandry, breeding, and morphological data, and are willing to trade specimens.

Amphibians purchased from commercial sources have often been kept in crowded communal cages or tanks where exposure to bacterial, fungal, and parasitic disease organisms is greater than in the wild. They have undergone the multiple stresses of capture, shipment (perhaps several times), dietary changes, and disease agents. Strict quarantine for four to six weeks is recommended before a new animal is introduced into the resident population. As with specimens caught in the wild, they should be treated very gently and handled only when absolutely necessary, for their skins are extremely fragile.

preventive medicine
HOUSING

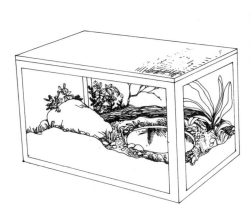

Most amphibians live in a moist, relatively cool environment and, depending on whether the specimen is terrestrial or aquatic (whether you found it on land or in the water), small terrarium or aquarium tanks serve well as captive homes.

Amphibians should never be housed with reptiles, birds, or mammals. Large predatory amphibians should not be kept in the same enclosure with smaller, more delicate species. Bullfrogs and giant salamanders are cannibalistic and will reward the unheeding pet owner with a steadily diminishing collection.

If you intend to keep woodland species such as most toads, terrestrial frogs, tree frogs, salamanders, or newts as pets, a well-planned terrarium setting should be prepared *before* getting the animals. Choose a suitable tank or cage large enough to allow free movement — depending on the size of your amphibian, you will need a 3 to 5 gallon tank. The minimum would be 3 gallons. Discuss it with the owner of the pet store where you buy the tank.

The tank should be partially filled with slightly moistened sand, fine gravel, potting soil, humus, leaf mold, and so on. Use rocks, pieces of heavy, *nonresinous* tree bark, moss, and either natural or artificial plants to create a setting pleasing to both the inhabitants and human observers.

Since some amphibian species are only semiaquatic or semiterrestrial, you must provide not only bathing facilities but a way for the animals to "haul out" and leave the water entirely. A small pond or pool made from a glass dish or glazed flowerpot saucer embedded in the soil can be removed or drained easily for routine cleaning every two or three days without disturbing the entire habitat or its lodgers. A plain rock or float may be provided in a more aquatic setting so that amphibians which leave the water only occasionally may crawl out at will (sterilize the rocks before you put them in the tank). With the available field guides to the amphibians of various regions of the United States, it is easy to identify the specimen and read of its particular habits and food preferences.

As they near completion of their metamorphosis, larvae breathe increasingly with their new lungs and less with the now-disappearing gills. At this point, a place to climb out becomes essential to survival.

Eggs found in the water should be kept in a jar of water; eggs found on land should be kept moist but not immersed in water.

THE AQUARIUM. For the more aquatic species, the water must be kept clean and purified between total changes. Aquarium filters often are suitable if the volume is not too great, and can be purchased from a well-stocked aquarium shop or pet supply store (see "Fish," pages 146ff.). Snales, freshwater clams,

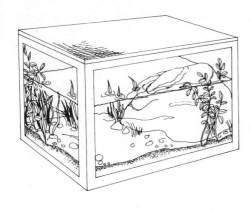

crawfish, and small catfish serve as biological filters, but often end up on the amphibians' menu.

Since most municipal water supplies have chemicals added to make the water safe for human consumption, it is generally advisable to allow it to stand for a day or two in an open jug or gallon pickle jar before use, in order to dissipate the chlorine. Bringing the water to a boil will hasten removal of chlorine — of course, it has to cool to around room temperature before you use it. (See Temperature Requirements, below.) Dechlorinating drops and tablets are also available from aquarium and pet shops. Distilled water may be used immediately.

Much of the waste material excreted by amphibians is rich in compounds containing nitrogen, particularly ammonia. Great care must be taken to ensure that an adequate rate of flushing or exchange of water is provided to prevent an accumulation of these compounds, which can reach toxic levels for captive amphibians. Dangerously large amounts of ammonia may also be produced by bacterial action upon nitrogen-rich wastes. Never allow the water in your tank to get cloudy, murky, or foul-smelling.

Aquatic salamanders and frogs shed their skins frequently — unless the shed skin is removed from the water (with small tweezers), it may block your filtering system.

When changing the water in a tank, be sure to dispose of the old water in a toilet or other wastewater system. It is teeming with bacteria and should not be poured into a kitchen sink or any other area where food is prepared.

Gill-breathing amphibians need an adequate supply of oxygen-rich water in which to swim. Normally, if there is sufficient oxygen to support living fish, it should be adequate for a small number of gill-breathing amphibians. A professional aquarist or dealer can help in the selection of suitable aquarium plants, air pumps, and air stones (see "Fish," pages 146ff.).

pH MAINTENANCE. A pH of 6.5 is ideal for most aquatic amphibians, although they can tolerate a range of up to 8.5.

The acidity or alkalinity of a particular water sample can be tested easily with pH-indicating paper strips, which show the hydrogen-ion concentration by color. It is available from aquarium stores, chemical supply stores, and pharmacies. More accurate results can be obtained with an electronic pH meter.

You can safely raise the pH value of a water sample by adding sodium hydroxide or lower it with calcium sulfate. Acetic acid can be used to lower the pH of particularly alkaline water even further, but if this is necessary, you probably would be wiser to use distilled water from the start.

WATER REQUIREMENTS. Almost every woodland amphibian gets moisture directly through its skin and, unless direct access to a pool or pond is available, a sprinkle or shower once a day is imperative. A spray bottle is ideal for this purpose. Be sure that the water does not contain toxic levels of chlorine.

TEMPERATURE REQUIREMENTS. Most authorities recommend a room and water temperature of 65° to 68°F. For some larvae, 68° to 72°F. is advised. For actively feeding frogs (which eat at least once a day) from the more temperate climates, a room and water temperature of 72° to 78°F. is appropriate, while tropical species would find 78° to 86°F. more to their liking. Some of the aquatic salamanders are more comfortable in water cooled to 45° to 55°F. If a heater is necessary, see "Fish," pages 146ff.

If they are too cold, amphibians will be inactive and won't eat. If they are too hot, they will be overactive and may die.

LIGHT REQUIREMENTS. While specific photoperiod or light-dark cycles are not determined for all species of amphibians, a general rule can be stated: in species from the tropics, an equal day:night cycle of about 12 hours each is desirable; for species from the temperate zone, a photoperiod of about 14 to

16 hours of light and 8 to 10 hours of dark is better. Since the seasons change, some variation in the amount of light is desirable. Light should be gradually increased from spring to summer and decreased from fall to winter. At no time, however, should there be a constantly lighted environment.

FEEDING   The larvae of frogs and toads, in their natural environment, eat algae and other plant life, while salamander larvae eat simple water animals and, accidentally, decaying organic material. As metamorphosis progresses, the digestive system changes, and more complex animal material can be assimilated: adult amphibians eat earthworms, slugs, insects, fish, and smaller amphibians.

Amphibians eat only what they need. The correct amount to feed them is whatever is consumed in ten to fifteen minutes. Uneaten food should be removed — it will spoil and foul the water.

MOST TOADS AND FROGS. Larvae may be fed romaine lettuce, ground rabbit or guinea pig pellets, small crumbled pieces of dry dog food, finely minced hard-boiled egg yolk, brewer's yeast, finely ground raw beef liver. A diet that appears to be nutritionally sound and also creates the fewest problems in maintaining water quality is ground rabbit or guinea pig pellets as a main food source, plus small amounts of crumbled dry dog food and supplemental feeding of egg yolk or meat once or twice weekly. Larvae should be fed daily to three times a week depending upon age and size — young larvae eat more frequently because they are growing rapidly.

Most adults can be fed earthworms, corn grubs, crickets, and sow bugs, three times a week. For tree frogs, which usually are somewhat smaller than other species of terrestrial frogs and toads, wingless fruit flies are very useful and can be obtained from the genetics department of a university or college. They can be bred easily in small culture bottles, and have the decided advantage (in case of escape) of being flightless. Baby crickets also are an excellent diet for smaller frog and toad species. It must be remembered that most terrestrial frogs and toads are "sight" feeders and will respond only to moving bait.

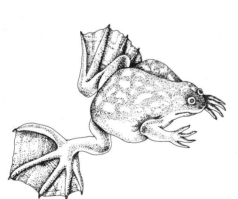

CLAWED FROG (Xenopus). The recommended diet for the larvae of these interesting creatures is finely ground dried green peas, finely ground dried split peas, finely ground rabbit pellets (with all these, you do the "fine grinding" yourself, in a blender or by pulverizing in a mortar), or *unseasoned* dried split pea soup base, which has the consistency of flour. Mix this before their daily feeding with enough water to produce a thin paste. As the larvae grow larger, finely ground or crushed rabbit or guinea pig pellets should be substituted. When they begin to form rear limbs, the larvae should have a mixture of finely ground lean beef and powdered milk added to their diet. They can also be fed tubifex worms and daphnia.

The adult clawed frog is perhaps the easiest of the anurans to feed. These aquatic frogs, by the way, were first brought to the United States from Africa to be used for pregnancy diagnosis. They will eat earthworms, raw beef, beef heart, small live fish, and commercial trout chow (a well-balanced ration that contains the required vitamins and minerals and is rich in protein). If beef, heart, or raw liver is used exclusively, a small amount of powdered vitamin-mineral supplement should be mixed with it to prevent deficiencies: about ¼ teaspoon of supplement to 4 ounces of meat. A natural diet — earthworms — is recommended; it is the simplest, is well balanced, and causes the least problem with water fouling. Adult clawed frogs should be fed three times a week.

AXOLOTLS, MUD PUPPIES, AND OTHER SALAMANDERS. The larvae can be fed brine shrimp, tubifex worms, and daphnia. As growth progresses, earthworms, beef heart, and raw beef liver cut into thin strips will be taken. Later, as growth increases, earthworms, corn grubs, mealworms — any worms you can buy in a pet store for this purpose — or commercial trout chow can be used. These larvae should be fed three to four times weekly.

For adults, earthworms, corn grubs, and crickets provide a simple, stable, well-balanced diet. They should be fed about three times weekly, that is, about every other day.

CAECILIANS. These secretive, legless creatures feed well throughout their lives on earthworms and small grubs, both as larvae and adults. They should be offered food at least three times weekly.

Special note on commercial trout chow. If any of the pellets remain un-eaten, they will disintegrate and foul the water. You can prevent this by feeding only enough so that nothing is left behind or by mixing a binder, such as unflavored gelatin, in with the pellets. Mix one package of gelatin according to the instructions on the package, stir in 2 cups of trout chow; after the mixture sets thoroughly, cut it into pieces. In this form, the trout chow can be fed as needed and the unused portion stored in the refrigerator for about two weeks. Frozen, it lasts for several months; thaw before feeding.

first aid
INJURIES

When the more aggressive frog, toad, and salamander species are housed with smaller, more timid members of their own kind, there will occasionally be injuries and wounds. Overcrowding may also stimulate antisocial behavior and result in traumatic injuries. Rivalry over food, shelter, or sexual partners may result in fights and attempted cannibalism. Abrasions, lacerations, and lost digits or entire limbs are ample evidence that some drastic housing changes are necessary.

Topical antiseptics can be dangerous — they should be used only under the direction of a veterinarian. They may be absorbed through the skin, and thus harm the amphibian.

Bleeding from a wound will normally stop spontaneously, and the limbs and tails of some amphibians can be regenerated, though this depends on the severity of the trauma and the age and health of the victim. To prevent infection, an injured amphibian should be moved into a clean environment. If it has been so severely wounded that you decide to put it to death, the most humane and painless method is to place it in the freezer.

THERMAL SHOCK

An amphibian exposed to thermal shock will exhibit signs of distress or suddenly die. Thermal shock occurs when an animal is allowed to become overheated or is suddenly chilled. Both causes can be eliminated by careful attention to the animal's habitat needs and *gradual* changes to cooler or warmer water. If ice is used to help cool an aquatic environment, be certain that it is made from chlorine-free water.

diseases

Many of the diseases affecting captive amphibians must be diagnosed and treated by a veterinarian with an expertise in exotic animal medicine and surgery. But you should be aware of the most common medical problems and be able to recognize the general signs of illness: lack of appetite, lethargy, obvious skin lesions (ulcers, swellings, and discolorations).

STARVATION AND DEHYDRATION

Unfortunately, all too frequently, pet amphibians starve and become dehydrated simply because their owners are ignorant of the general care and feeding needed by a particular species. Obviously, to persist in trying to feed an animal the wrong food will result in disaster for the pet and disappointment for the owner. And, if you don't provide a terrestrial species with sufficient water in a way the animal can absorb it, eventually it's going to die from dehydration and kidney failure. Always try to find out as much as you can about the needs of your particular amphibian — field guides are available, and a librarian can help you find them.

VITAMIN-MINERAL IMBALANCES AND DEFICIENCIES

Vitamin-mineral imbalances and deficiencies usually are caused by an artificial diet. For instance, a diet of raw beef or heart without supplemental calcium-vitamin D_3 will result in developmental bone diseases such as rickets and fibrous osteodystrophy. Raw liver alone will produce multiple vitamin and mineral imbalances.

The use of natural food such as earthworms, corn grubs, crickets, tubifex worms, and fruit flies will aid greatly in preventing such problems.

VIRAL, BACTERIAL, FUNGAL, PROTOZOAN, AND METAZOAN PARASITIC INFECTIONS AND INFESTATIONS

Many of the infections and infestations that occur with captive amphibians can be traced to overcrowded conditions and poor sanitation. Often a frog, toad, or salamander might not appear to be sick but will exhibit subtle signs such as appetite loss, sluggishness, and abdominal distention or bloating that could easily be overlooked or misinterpreted.

The diagnosis and successful treatment of such animals is very specialized. Most parasites, for instance, are rarely visible to the human eye, and must be identified under the microscope in a sample of feces; specific remedies for various disease conditions must be determined by a veterinarian.

Amphibian owners should know, however, about the correct use of tetracycline hydrochloride. There is a widely held belief that tetracycline hydrochloride may be added to the water of aquatic amphibians as a means of treating bacterial diseases, especially "red leg." This drug may cause more harm than good, though, if used improperly. The amount that could possibly be absorbed through an amphibian's skin would be totally inadequate to serve as an effective antibiotic — and in significant concentrations it will induce severe toxic skin reactions. The *only* effective means for administering tetracycline hydrochloride to amphibians is by a carefully inserted gastric tube, at a dosage of 5 milligrams per 30 grams of amphibian. This should be repeated twice daily for about one week — the pet will need to be left with the veterinarian for treatment.

Because of the amphibians' delicate and highly absorptive skin, topical antiseptics, antifungal agents, and the like may be of limited usefulness and, like tetracycline, should be administered only under the guidance of a veterinarian.

There is a great deal the owner can do, however, both to prevent illness and to aid recovery. The owner should vigilantly check over, and perhaps improve, the conditions in which the amphibian is living — which can make, in prevention, a life-or-death difference.

breeding and reproduction

Many amateurs have been successful in rearing amphibians from fertilized eggs found in the wild or have managed to get animals to mate in captivity, observing the entire sequence of ovulation, fertilization, and metamorphosis. Doing this requires a high standard of animal care and optimum nutrition. Eggs and/or larvae that are either found in the wild habitat or produced in captivity should be cultivated in a separate aquarium or terrarium. This will allow for a proper quarantine to be established and will also prevent cannibalism.

It is extremely difficult to determine the sex of an amphibian, and much easier to let the amphibians settle the question themselves. The best way to ensure that breeding will occur is to capture a mated pair, place them in your aquarium, and leave them alone until the female lays her eggs.

further readings

BROWN, A. L. *The African Clawed Toad.* London, Butterworth, 1970.

BUTERENBROOD, E. L. "Newts and Salamanders," chap. 52, pp. 867–892, in *UFAW Handbook on the Care and Management of Laboratory Animals,* 3rd ed. London, Livingston, 1966.

COCRAN, D. M. *Living Amphibians of the World.* Garden City, New York, Doubleday, 1961.

COMMITTEE ON ANIMAL NUTRITION, National Research Council. No. 10: *Nutrient Requirements of Laboratory Animals,* 2nd ed. Washington, D.C., National Academy of Sciences, 1972.

CONANT, R. *A Field Guide to Reptiles and Amphibians of Eastern North America.* Boston, Houghton Mifflin, 1958.

CULLUM, L., AND JUSTUS, J. T. "Housing for Aquatic Animals," vol. 23, pp. 126–129, in *Laboratory Animal Science,* 1973.

FRAZER, J. F. D. "Frogs and Toads," chap. 51, pp. 853–866, in *UFAW Handbook on the Care and Management of Laboratory Animals,* 3rd ed. London, Livingston, 1966.

FRYE, F. L. *Husbandry, Medicine and Surgery in Captive Reptiles.* Bonner Springs, Kansas, VM Publishing, 1973.

GOIN, C. J., AND GOIN, O. B. *Introduction to Herpetology,* 2nd ed. San Francisco, Freeman, 1971.

MERTENS, R. *The World of Amphibians and Reptiles.* New York, McGraw-Hill, 1960.

NATIONAL ACADEMY OF SCIENCES. *Amphibians: Guidelines for the Breeding, Care, and Management of Laboratory Animals.* Washington, D.C., Printing and Publishing Office, National Academy of Sciences, 1974.

OLIVER, J. A. *The Natural History of North American Amphibians and Reptiles.* Princeton, New Jersey, Van Nostrand, 1955.

PORTER, K. R. *Herpetology.* Philadelphia, W. B. Saunders, 1972.

STEBBINS, R. C. *A Field Guide to Western Reptiles and Amphibians.* Boston, Houghton Mifflin, 1966.

In cages — and out

Caged birds

W. J. MATHEY, V.M.D.

There are about 8,700 species of living birds, grouped into about 170 families within about 30 orders. Not all of these are the small, feathered, flying creatures we usually think of as birds. The ostrich weighs ⅙ ton, and the recently extinct elephant bird of Madagascar weighed ½ ton; the cassowary and the kiwi have what seems to be hair; the penguin, along with these, cannot fly. The features all birds do share, however, are: a horny bill or beak (all modern birds lack teeth); a scaly or horny covering of the lower portion of the legs; a feather coat (cassowary and kiwi "hair" is really fine feathers); fusion of the vertebrae of the lower back; a system of air sacs within the body cavities and in some bones; reproduction through eggs protected by a calcareous shell; oval red blood cells containing nuclei; and a constant high body temperature. With good care, most small caged birds should live for about seven years. Larger psittacines may live as long as a human being.

Two zoological orders, Psittaciformes and Passeriformes, include most of the more common pet cage bird species. The second contains also most of the commonly seen birds of city and suburb.

THE PSITTACIFORMES

The Psittaciformes are the parrotlike birds. They all have a rounded body with short legs, broad rounded wings, a short neck, and a large head. Their powerful hooked bill has a cere (a fleshy swelling into which the nostrils open) at the base of the upper beak. They walk well on their strong feet, with two toes forward and two back, and can climb with the aid of the beak. They cannot swim; and most do not migrate. The young are hatched naked in hollows of trees, banks, and similar locations — their eyes are closed, and they are incapable of locomotion — where they stay for a long time dependent on their parents to feed them by regurgitation. Most species live in flocks, roosting in trees. Their disposition depends mainly on being acquired very young and being treated kindly. Many of the psittacines establish a close personal relationship with an owner, much like that of a dog, and like a dog, require personal attention to be happy. Male parrots usually prefer women, and female parrots prefer men.

THE PASSERIFORMES

The Passeriformes are the "perching" birds, which include about 60 percent of known living bird species. The common characteristic of the order is the perching foot, with all four toes at the same level and never webbed. The hind toe is very well developed, and always projects to the rear. Many of the passerines are noted for their singing ability.

In other respects, passerines vary greatly. Bills vary from the slender one of the tiny gnatcatcher to the heavy bill of the raven. Most passerines cannot walk — they hop. Many passerines are migratory, sometimes over long distances (the black-poll warbler travels from northern North America down to central Chile). Most cannot swim, although the dipper can walk under water.

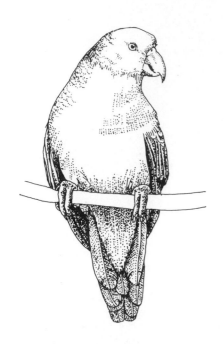

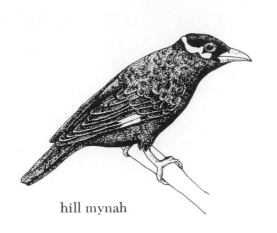

hill mynah

blue and gold macaw

Mexican double yellow-head parrot

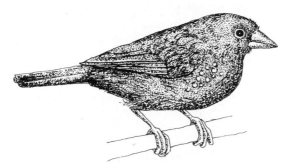

common fire finch

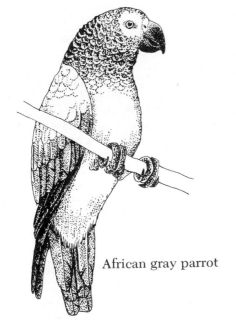

peach-faced love bird

African gray parrot

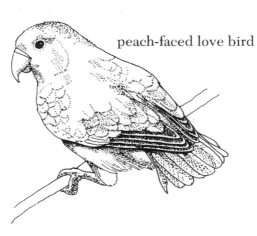

Java sparrow

Nesting sites vary tremendously, from the grass-lined ground nest of the horned lark, through the mud nest of the swallow, to the hole nests of bluebirds. The young are hatched naked, with their eyes closed, incapable of locomotion, dependent on their parents for food (insects, worms, fruit); they remain in the nest for a long period. Some passerines are solitary, a pair living isolated from others of the species, except at migration time. Other passerines live in flocks — the starlings and the blackbirds are examples.

The following chart gives the characteristics of some of the more commonly kept pet birds. The smaller birds require less space and less feed.

CHARACTERISTICS OF COMMON PET BIRDS

PSITTACINES	SIZE	ORIGIN	DISPOSITION	DIET*
Budgerigar (c.v.) *Melopsittacus undulatus*	6 inches	Australia	Mild	Budgie mix
Cockatiel (c.v.) *Nymphicus hollandicus*	13 inches	Australia	Mild	Budgie mix and small sunflower seeds
Petz' conure (half-moon parrot) *Aratinga canicularis eburnirostrum*	10 inches	South America	Mild†	Sunflower seeds and budgie mix and peanuts
Blue and gold macaw *Ara ararauna*	36 inches	South America	Mild‡	Sunflower seeds and budgie mix and peanuts
Peachface lovebird *Agapornis roseicollis*	6 inches	Africa	Mild†	Sunflower seeds and budgie mix and peanuts
African gray parrot *Psittacus erithacus*	13 inches	Africa	Mild	Sunflower seeds and budgie mix and peanuts
Mexican double yellow-head parrot *Amazona ochracephala oratrix*	15 inches	Mexico	Mild	Sunflower seeds and budgie mix and peanuts

PASSERINES	SIZE	ORIGIN	DISPOSITION	DIET*
Canary (c.v.) *Serinus canarius*	5 to 7 inches	Canary Islands	Mild	White millet and canary seed
Zebra finch (c.v.) *Taeniopygia castanotis*	4 to 5 inches	Australia	Mild	Finch mix
Gouldian finch (c.v.) *Poephila gouldiae*	5 to 7 inches	Australia	Mild	Finch mix
Java sparrow (temple bird) (c.v.) *Padda oryzivora*	5 inches	Indonesia	Pick on smaller birds	Finch mix
Society finch (Bengalese) (c.v.) *Uroloncha domestica*	3 to 4 inches	China and Japan	Good foster parents	Finch mix
Common fire finch *Lagnosticta senegala*	3 inches	Africa	Mild	Finch mix
Greater hill mynah *Gracula religiosa*	10 inches	India	Pick on smaller birds	Mynah mix (feed cracked or milled versus whole seeds); supplement with fruit, cooked egg, and moistened puppy food (proportion, depending on appetite: ⅓, ⅙, ½)

c.v. = color variants produced by breeding.
*See also Nutrition, pages 198ff.
†Noisy.
‡Ear-shattering.

THE BIRD'S PSYCHOLOGY

The bird begins to react to other birds — its parents and its hatch mates — even before it leaves the egg. Chicks can be heard cheeping before they start to break the shell. Apparently the cheeping and the shell-tapping stimulate other chicks to do the same.

Chicks are imprinted with the image of the bird or person who cares for them when they hatch — which results in breeding difficulties: a bird hand-reared by a human being seems to think it is a human being, too. A zebra finch brought up by Bengalese finches will prefer to mate with Bengalese finches.

Some songbirds need to be exposed to the song of their species while they are still young. If they are reared away from their own species, they do not develop the typical repertory of songs. The talking birds (the psittacines, the mynahs, and some of the corvids) learn to talk by being kept by themselves with human speech as their only model from their earliest days.

Young birds are equipped with physical and behavioral signals that let the adults know they are babies and need to be fed — feather coat color, beak color, wing fluttering (begging), gaping mouth, mouth coloration, and specialized nodules inside the mouth. Some species of birds know by instinct what their young should look like, but other species, for example, the lovebirds, learn from their first brood. If eggs of another species are substituted for the first eggs of lovebirds, the appearance of the resulting young becomes the parent lovebirds' standard; they will reject their own young that hatch in later broods.

Birds distinguish between types of possible enemy. Birds of prey are a potential danger to any bird that draws notice to itself, and the call that warns that a hawk is near is a shrill "see-see" sound, the source of which is difficult to locate. Land predators are not so dangerous, and a dog or a human brings forth traceable loud warning calls.

Birds usually relate to each other in a peck order based on aggressiveness, and life can be chaotic for them while the order is being established. Accidents and changes in hormonal status can change the peck order dramatically — so can the addition of new birds to a group. In a straight-line peck order, Bird A is dominant to Birds B, C, and D. A "circular" peck order can exist with Bird A being dominant to Bird B, Bird B to Bird C, Bird C to Bird D, but Bird D dominant to Bird A. The low members in a straight-line peck order are better removed to separate cages, since they may become semistarved.

Between species, a similar peck order exists, based on size and aggressiveness. Some species of caged birds are very aggressive and will kill other species kept in the same cage or aviary with them. Java sparrows, for example, should be kept with birds their own size or larger. Cockatiels, on the other hand, are very peaceable, and it is safe to keep them with species of smaller birds.

FEDERAL REGULATIONS

The importation and possession of birds are controlled by federal regulations. As a result of a disastrous problem with Old World Newcastle disease brought into southern California with imported pet birds in the early 1970s, the federal government requires inspection and quarantine of all birds imported from any part of the world. Certain foreign birds, like the English sparrow and the starling, become pests when introduced into a new territory, and are banned from import as "injurious species."

Concern over endangered wildlife has brought about regulations making it illegal for an unauthorized person to possess any wild bird except the English sparrow or the starling. If you pick up sick and injured birds to care for them and rehabilitate them, you should apply for the necessary state and federal permits to cover your activities, though it is unlikely that you would be arrested for helping a sick robin without a permit.

The care of wild birds is much the same as that of the more or less domestic caged birds. One of the greatest problems is finding acceptable feed materials. A second problem is the likelihood of wild birds having external parasites.

preventive medicine
THE FEATHER COAT

The feather coat, formed by the feather follicles, is renewed at least once a year in a molt. The old feathers are shed and new ones develop to take their place. In most birds, the wing feathers are shed one at a time, so that the bird never loses its power of flight.

Feathers are sensitive in the formative stage and will bleed, sometimes profusely, if injured. Young birds just getting their first feathers, and older birds going through a molt, should be handled as little as possible to avoid pain for the bird and to prevent damage to the forming feathers. If bleeding does occur, use a styptic pencil on the follicles. Once the feather is fully formed it is no longer alive; it is then like a human hair.

Feathers serve to insulate the bird, to signal sex differences, and to communicate its moods. An angry cockatoo, for instance, raises its crest. They are needed for flight, of course: the wing feathers, attached to the bones of the wing, allow the bird to lift itself with the flapping of the wings, cupping to hold the air on the downstroke, and opening like a venetian blind on the upstroke to let the air pass. They are controlled by muscles, which can turn them and spread them in various patterns to suit the needs of flight.

Birds work on their feathers, preening, to rearrange any disturbance in their complex arrangement (a study in itself). At the same time, the bird usually dresses the feathers with a fatty material from the uropygial gland (located over the base of the tail).

THE BEAK

The beak is an essential tool for the bird. It is used to grasp food, to separate edible from inedible parts of the food, to dress the feathers, feed the young, and fight rivals or enemies. Its size and proportions vary with the species of the bird, and the color may even vary from young bird to adult. The beak is a hard protein (keratin) formed by living cutaneous cells (like those forming our fingernails) and supported by underlying bone.

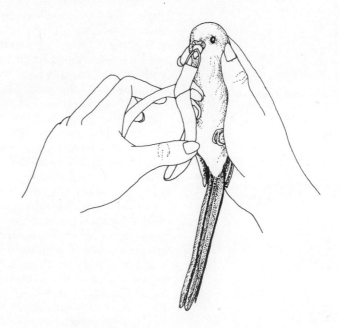

TRIMMING. If a bird's environment lacks abrasive materials, its beak may become overgrown. This is particularly true for the psittacines. The beak may be trimmed with a sharp knife or toenail clipper — very carefully, for there is living tissue just underneath, except at the tip. (See illustrations on page 200 on how to hold the bird.)

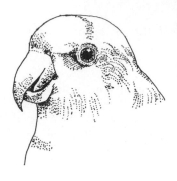

ABNORMALITIES AND SPLITS. If there is any abnormality of the beak's color or consistency, the overgrowth may be due to infectious or parasitic problems and the bird should be taken to a veterinarian for diagnosis. (See Tuberculosis, page 209, and Ticks and Mites, page 207.) If the beak splits, like a fingernail, it is best to have your veterinarian wire the split with fine stainless steel wire. If you want to take the time to hand-feed your bird, the split will usually heal without the wiring.

Injury can cause a hemorrhage between the keratin layer and the underlying living tissue. The result will be imperfections of the beak structure, with flaking and discoloration, for which there is no remedy.

THE CLAWS   Like the beak, the claws are keratin formed by living tissue and supported by bone, and are constantly growing to replace what is lost by wear. If insufficient wear takes place, the claw becomes overgrown, sometimes so overgrown it interferes with the use of the foot. In extreme cases, the claw curves around and injures the flesh of the foot. If your bird has long claws, trim them carefully with a sharp cuticle scissors (small birds) or dog toenail trimmers (large birds). A small bird should be restrained by cupping it in your hand on a tabletop, holding the leg to be trimmed between your thumb and forefinger. A larger bird should be wrapped in a towel, as in beak trimming. Try to prevent further overgrowth by replacing the bird's perch with one of larger diameter or one covered by sandpaper. Claws can also be deformed by scaly-leg mites. (See Ticks and Mites, page 207.)

CAGES AND AVIARIES   Cages for birds date back to Greek and Roman times. These ancient cages were usually small fabrications of wood or wicker, but some wealthy people had large aviaries with hundreds of birds restrained by hemp netting.

Flight cages or aviaries have advantages and disadvantages. They give birds valuable exercise, and allow them to be displayed to advantage. On the other hand, birds often get serious injuries from flying full tilt into the walls of the cage. This is especially true of aviaries with glass walls.

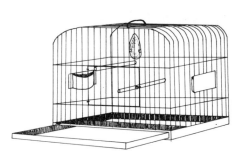

The cage should be of a size to suit the bird. Don't put a Great Dane in a Volkswagen. As a rule of thumb, the smallest dimension should be twice the wingspread of the bird. Males and females can be kept in the same cage, and species can be mixed if they are the same size. In general, it is not safe to mix small and large birds, because some species become aggressive during the breeding season. Most of the small finches and the budgerigars like company. Gregarious birds can be kept together — the only limiting factors would be perch space and, for some breeds, flying space. Remember, too, that feeders and waterers must be adequate for the number of birds. If a bird is to be a talker, it should be kept by itself.

A bird's cage should have few joints (which harbor mites). You should be able to disassemble it for easy daily cleaning. Metal cages are usually the best choice. Psittacine birds tend to destroy wood or bamboo cages, and, as well, they become stained with droppings.

If you are an amateur craftsman, you can make your own cage, using wood or metal. Make the cage bottom the size of a full or half newspaper page (it saves trimming time). If you make a metal cage, do not solder the joints, because lead is poisonous to birds — braze or weld instead.

The droppings pan should be at least as large as the cage, and should slide in and out easily — otherwise your Oriental rug may serve as the droppings pan. The lower section of each side of the cage should have a transparent shield to reduce the amount of seed husks and other debris thrown out by

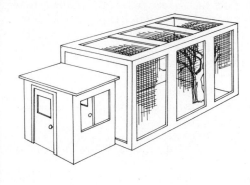

the birds. Some owners use a cloth strip hung out horizontally all around the bottom of the cage to catch such debris.

Waterers and feeders should be designed to be easily removed for cleaning and refilling. A cover of some sort should be used to prevent the bird's escape when they are not in place.

Since the smaller birds can squeeze through a narrow space, the spacing of the bars is a consideration. Finches require ⅜-inch spacing. Budgies and canaries can be contained by ⅝-inch spacing.

Every cage should have fixed or swinging perches at various levels. The diameter should suit the size of the bird's foot, ranging from a ¼-inch dowel for very small birds to a 2-inch rod for large birds. If you use tree prunings, remove the bark, where mites and ticks from wild birds may be hidden. Look the perches over carefully for possible booby traps where a bird might snare its toe.

Occasionally furnish your birds with a bath. This can be a saucer of water placed in the cage once a week or so, or a spray or shower bath (which parrots like).

The bird cage should be in a room that does not have a door opening directly to the outside. Despite all precautions, the bird is likely to get out of its cage at just the wrong time and can easily be lost when the outside door is opened. Similarly, outside aviaries should have a double entry, so that the outer door may be closed before the inner door is opened.

INSECT SCREENS. Birds are prey for mosquitoes, deerflies, horseflies, stable flies, and all the other bloodsucking parasites that can make outdoor life miserable. These can take enough blood from a small bird to kill it. Perhaps even more serious is the fact that they act as carriers for various infectious diseases. Bird malaria is especially serious in the canary, which is susceptible to many kinds of plasmodium from wild birds. Avian pox viruses, as well as other viral and bacterial agents, can be carried by the bloodsuckers.

Birds should always be protected from insects. A bird cage outdoors should be covered with mosquito netting (a fine-mesh nylon window curtain will do). An outdoor aviary should have insect screening, in removable panels to facilitate cleaning, as well as heavier wire netting.

TEMPERATURE
REQUIREMENTS

Since most pet birds are small, they can easily be chilled or overheated, just as a thimbleful of water can be easily boiled or frozen.

The best temperature for most caged birds is 60° to 70°F. The bird's cage should not be kept in direct sunlight for very long — always have part of the cage in shadow. An overheated bird pants rapidly, and holds its wings out from the body to allow air currents to help remove some of the heat. An extremely overheated bird may lose consciousness. If this happens, cool its head by moistening the feathers with a damp pledget of cotton. If it does not revive, take the bird to your veterinarian.

Adult birds, even tropical ones, can often be kept in outside aviaries in cold climates, *if they are protected from the wind.* Young birds are much more susceptible to temperature changes, either chilling or overheating. Air currents (wind, drafts) take heat away from the bird rapidly, reducing the insulating value of the feather coat.

A chilled bird fluffs out its feathers, and huddles together with other birds if there are several in a cage. A bottle of hot water in or next to the cage (or a small electric light left burning), with a cloth cover over both the cage and the heat source to conserve heat and protect against drafts, will keep birds comfortable even in very cold weather.

ENVIRONMENTAL HAZARDS

Expanded metal screening, with its diamond-shaped holes, or any other screening whose elements cross at less than 90-degree angles, can catch the toes of a bird and trap it.

Bits of string in the cage or anywhere the bird can reach can entangle the legs or wings, and can cause severe digestive trouble if eaten.

Lead paint — if you buy an old cage that has been painted, assume that the paint may have been lead-based. Remove the paint with paint remover, and repaint with lead-free paint.

The kitchen — birds are easily killed by fumes from overheated fats or from overheated Teflon. They are also sensitive to cooking gas.

Solvent-based paints or varnishes, paint thinners, paint removers, solvent rug cleaners, or similar products in the room where you keep the birds — when painting, remove the birds to a well-ventilated room. Make sure all odor of solvent is gone before you replace the birds.

Fans — place ¼-inch mesh netting protectors over all fans.

Unguarded fireplace openings — a bird can fly into a fire. Even if there is no fire, the bird can be lost up the chimney.

Unguarded electric heaters — a bird can fly into a heater and be killed.

Ultraviolet radiation, such as from the special fluorescent lights used for house plants, may damage the bird's eyes and should be kept at least six feet away.

NUTRITION

WATER. A supply of fresh water is essential to a bird's life. It should be changed at least daily, and more frequently if it is fouled by droppings, especially in warm weather. Stale water, standing in a waterer for some time, may have bacterial or fungal growth in it, which will cause digestive troubles. The water also should not be extremely cold, for birds are likely to refuse to drink anything under 40°F.

Birds drink more water in warm weather, for they rid themselves of excess heat by panting and evaporating water from the lungs. Desert birds, like the budgerigar, are able to get along with less water than birds originating in humid climates.

DIET. The caged bird's basic diet should consist of the prepared mixes available in pet stores (see chart, page 193). The mixture ensures a balanced diet, since oil seeds (flax, sesame, poppy, peanut, hemp, rape, and niger) and cereal or grass seeds (millet, canary seed, wheat, oats, rice, milo, corn) vary in their ability to provide the different amino acids that make up the proteins a bird needs. A budgerigar will eat one to two teaspoonsful of seed daily, depending on its size, activity, and the season of the year. Smaller species will eat slightly more than would be expected in proportion to their body weight, especially in winter.

This diet should be supplemented with green foods and fruit, the amount depending on the bird's appetite, and a vitamin-mineral mix, which includes the iodine that is likely to be missing from seeds grown in the iodine-deficient area between the Great Lakes and the Pacific, and Vitamin D_3, since caged birds usually do not get enough sunlight. This mix is generally given daily, unless the directions on the container instruct otherwise. Cuttlefish bone, which contains about 85 percent calcium carbonate and many of the trace minerals needed by birds, should be available in every cage.

It is particularly important that these nutritional needs be satisfied for young growing birds and breeding hens, which use great amounts of calcium and protein. Along with birds in molt, they should be given supplemental animal protein (milk, egg, meat meal, fish meal, insects, and worms).

PRECAUTIONS

If you have a few birds and acquire new bids, quarantine the new birds in a separate room for as long a time as possible, preferably a month, to make sure they are not carrying an infectious disease.

If you wish to put the new birds in with the old birds after the period of quarantine, take the precaution of medicating both new and old birds with a tetracycline drug, available from your veterinarian. This preventive treat-

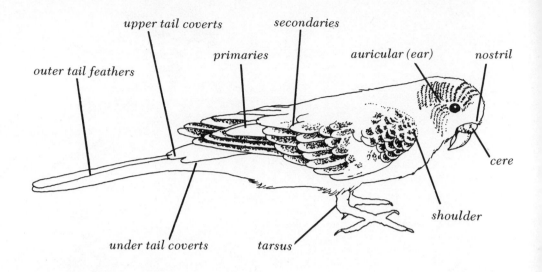

outer tail feathers

upper tail coverts

primaries

secondaries

auricular (ear)

nostril

cere

shoulder

under tail coverts

tarsus

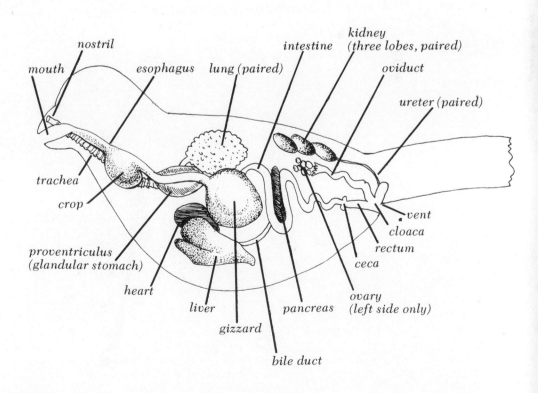

mouth

nostril

esophagus

lung (paired)

intestine

kidney
(three lobes, paired)

oviduct

ureter (paired)

trachea

crop

proventriculus
(glandular stomach)

heart

liver

gizzard

bile duct

pancreas

ovary
(left side only)

ceca

rectum

cloaca

vent

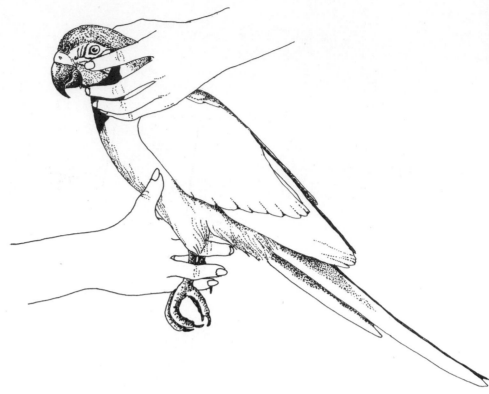

holding a large bird

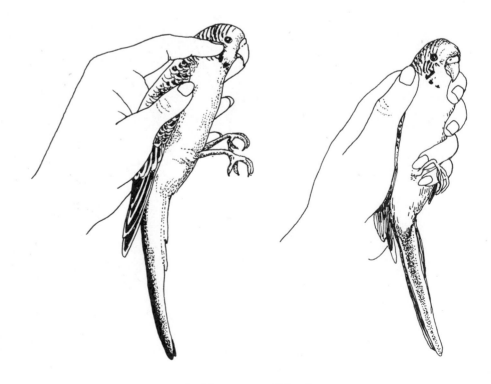

holding a small bird

ment may help to protect both newcomers and residents against contagion from each other.

If you exhibit your birds, use the preventive medication while the birds are away and for a week after they return. Bird shows are prime places to pick up infections. You may also want to vaccinate your birds with B_1 strain Newcastle disease vaccine, equine encephalomyelitis vaccine, which might be advisable if you live or travel along the East or Gulf coasts, and fowl cholera bacterin.

There are also blood tests to determine past infection (or previous vaccination) with various disease agents, which your veterinarian can probably arrange to have done. If you take pet birds out of the country with you and those birds have positive tests for Newcastle disease antibodies, you may have trouble bringing them back into the United States.

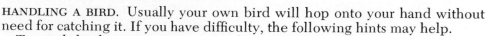

the home clinic
EXAMINATION OF THE BIRD

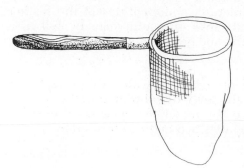

It is important to observe the bird carefully before it is handled. Handling often will stimulate the bird into seeming almost normal even if it is ill. Observe it as it sits, moves from the floor of the cage to the perch and back, as it eats and drinks, and as it preens. Watch its breathing and listen for sounds. Look at the cage-bottom lining. Notice if the droppings are unusually moist for the species (fruit-eaters normally have moist droppings). Observe the color of the droppings.

HANDLING A BIRD. Usually your own bird will hop onto your hand without need for catching it. If you have difficulty, the following hints may help.

To catch birds in an aviary, use a hoop net. It is best to try to do this at night, under a dim red light, which allows human beings to see much better than the birds.

Large psittacines can be distracted by a piece of paper towel spread over one open hand, which can grasp them without offering a target for a nip. Another approach is to use a heavy towel, throwing it over the bird and wrapping the bird in its folds. A heavy leather glove is very helpful, if one is available.

Small caged birds should be grasped with the hand. The room may be darkened to lessen evasive struggling on the part of the bird.

Once you have a small bird in your hand, restrain its head by holding the neck *gently* between the index finger and the middle finger, or by holding the angles of the jaws *gently* between the thumb and the index finger, meanwhile encircling the body with the other fingers. Do not exert much pressure on the body with the encircling fingers.

Restraining larger psittacines is a two-handed job. Get someone to help you. The head and neck are held with one hand — the head is restrained between the index finger and the thumb, at the angle of the jaw, while the other three fingers loosely encircle the neck. The other hand grasps the two legs — one between the ring finger and the middle finger, and the other between the index finger and the middle finger. The thumb is used to restrain the body.

LOOKING FOR CHANGES. Use a bright light to examine the bird. A spotlight or a high-intensity lamp will do, or the beam from a movie or slide projector. This will allow you to detect small external parasites, changes in the eyes, such as cataracts, or swellings and color changes in various parts of the body that might otherwise be missed. The bright light cannot injure the bird, though heat from the lamp would if your examination were very protracted.

Look at your bird while it is in good health, when it is eating well, when it is vocalizing, when it is alert. Then, when it is sick or injured, you may be able to detect an illness or injury by noticing a significant activity or a physical change.

The feather coat is an important indicator of health. If it is unkempt, the

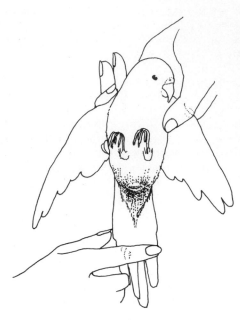

bird is not taking care of it. If it is fluffed out, the bird is feverish. A ragged coat with many missing feathers or whitish masses or yellow to dark brown specks attached to the feathers may be evidence of external parasites. Irregularities of shape of the body or its parts may be evidence of local inflammation or of tumors.

The eyes can also show signs of disorder. Look for discoloration, discharge, or clouding of the pupil. If the pupil does not contract in response to a bright light, there may be nerve damage. (Normal avian pupils contract and expand even though light intensity does not change.)

The beak may be overgrown, or deformed, or of an abnormal texture or color. Look inside the mouth for swellings or deposits on the lining or on the tongue.

Look at the vent — the feathers below it may be soiled or even caked with fecal and urinary discharges. If the vent of a female protrudes, she may be having difficulty passing an egg the final distance from the oviduct through her cloaca.

Spread the wings, looking for parasites and for abnormalities.

Look at the feet and legs. Are the claws long or deformed? Is the scaly part of the leg thickened or scurfy? If the joints are puffy, there may be a bacterial or viral infection.

Run your fingers gently over the body surfaces, back and forth. Take each limb gently between your thumb and forefinger and feel the muscles, the skin, and the bone carefully. Through palpation, you may detect imperfections of the skin, nodules in the musculature, abnormalities of the feather coat, and broken bones. (Bones broken close to a joint may be felt as a grating sensation when the limb is slightly and gently moved.)

ADMINISTERING MEDICINE   Drugs may be given in many ways: in the drinking water, by drops in the mouth or nostrils, by incorporation into the feed, by rubbing into the skin, by intubation (of the esophagus or crop), or by injection. Because of possible danger to the bird, it is best to leave the latter two to the veterinarian.

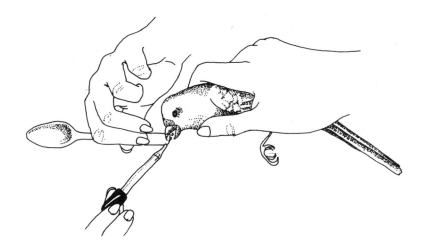

Drugs used to control parasites or infectious agents are two-edged swords. By their nature, they are selective poisons, more poisonous for the parasite or other disease agent than they are for the bird. If the dose is greater than the safe level, or if the use of the drug is continued for too long a time, damage to the bird may result. Remember: *the dose that is safe for one species may be lethal for another.*

Be extremely careful in using liquids by drops into the mouth. Do not drown the bird — give it a chance to swallow between drops. The bird's

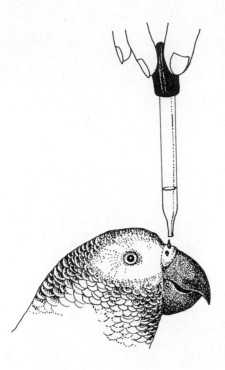

mouth should be opened by inserting a smooth object (the handle of a plastic knife or spoon, for example) and prying the upper and lower beak apart.

When using antibiotics, use them at high treatment levels for several days or longer. Low-level treatment, or too short a period of treatment, tends to build up a drug-resistant population of disease agents in the bird.

DRUGS IN HOT WEATHER. Drugs given in the drinking water during hot weather may cause trouble. The bird drinks more water than usual, taking in the drug with the water, and evaporates the water from its lungs to cool its body. This leaves the drug behind, often in greater concentration than is safe. In very hot weather, take the medicated water away during part of the day and substitute unmedicated water.

CAUTION WITH TETRACYCLINE. Calcium salts (such as are contained in cuttlebone) tie up tetracycline drugs in the bird's system, making them less effective. If tetracyclines are used, take the cuttlebone away for a few days — but don't forget to put it back.

THE USE OF HEAT. A sick bird is using its available stores of energy to do several things: to keep up its body temperature, to power its muscles, to digest its food, and to fight the disease agent that is causing trouble. You can help the bird by giving it additional heat, so that more of its own energies may be used in the fight against the disease agent. This may make the difference between a prolonged sickness (or even death) and a rapid recovery.

Heat may be supplied in the form of a bottle of hot water in the cage, a light bulb, a heating pad, or an electric heater. Be cautious that you do not overheat the bird — give it room to get away from the heat source.

first aid

It is very important to realize that if you don't know what you are doing it is better to do nothing. Well-meaning but inept owners can cause more damage than they correct.

TRAUMA

Birds can be injured by mammals, by objects in the surroundings, or by human agency (BB gun). Penetrating wounds from sharp beaks may lead to wound infections and death. Other common casualties are broken bones, lameness, an inability to walk or fly, or deformity of a limb.

Injury to the skull may be serious, resulting in death from brain damage; but often a bird seemingly near death from a collision with a window will recover if placed in a box and left alone. If the bird is very valuable, or an especially beloved pet, take it to your veterinarian right away.

BROKEN BONES

If a limb is grossly deformed and/or the bones protrude through the skin, go to a veterinarian. If the bones do not protrude and the limb is not grossly deformed, treat as follows:

WING. Immobilize the wing by folding it against the body in its natural position, holding it in place with gauze wrappings in the front and around the wing tips and tail reinforced and anchored by adhesive tape. An elastic stockinette tubing called Petnet* works well for small birds; holes can be cut for the legs. This will usually allow the bird to repair the damage in about a week. Some birds (psittacines especially) will remove the bandages almost as fast as you can put them on.

LEG. In a small bird, make a splint by wrapping the leg first with a layer of tissue paper close around the break, and then wrap several layers of adhe-

* Available from the Petnet Corporation, P.O. Box 451, Carnegie, Pennsylvania, 15106.

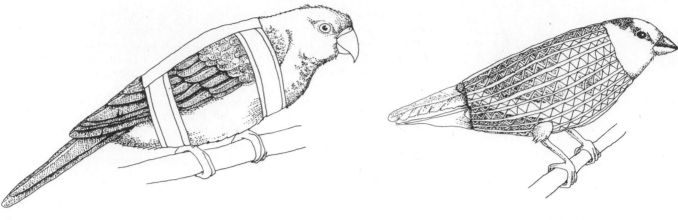

wing bandage

Petnet wing bandage

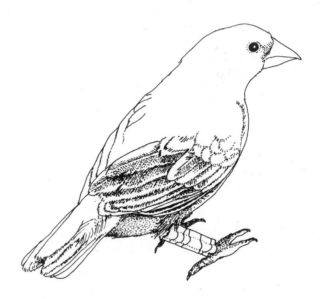

splint on small bird

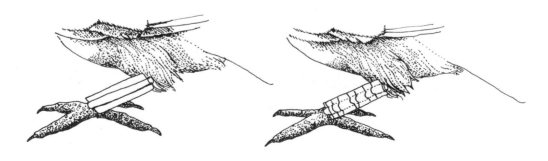

splint on large bird

sive tape loosely around the leg. Squeeze the slack fore and aft with a pliers to make strengthening fins. Remove carefully after a week or so. The tissue paper should aid in removal. Avoid applying to the skin.

In a larger bird, use a wrapping of absorbent cotton or soft plastic foam next to the limb. Hold splints (swab sticks, or pieces of tongue depressor) in place outside this with a wrapping of adhesive tape. Use great care in removing the tape after a week or so. Make sure the splints do not press into the bird.

BLEEDING

EXTERNAL. A pledget of clean (preferably sterile) cotton held firmly for a couple of minutes against a wound will usually stop bleeding in normal birds. Some poisons delay clotting. If bleeding continues, get the bird to a veterinarian.

INTERNAL. Most often internal bleeding results from an injured liver. The signs are pale mucous membranes in the mouth and inside the eyelids. Put the bird in a completely darkened room so that it will remain quiet. This will allow clotting to take place.

BLEEDING FROM INJURED CLAWS. Claws may be caught in crevices or holes, with resultant damage. They may even be pulled off by the struggles of the trapped bird. Control bleeding with a styptic pencil. The loss is not likely to be serious.

FOREIGN BODIES

EYE. Awns of seeds sometimes lodge in the eye of a bird, causing irritation and ocular discharge. These should be removed by the veterinarian.

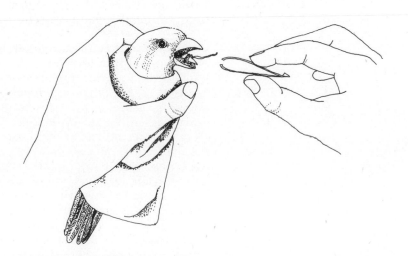

TONGUE. Thread, small rubber bands, small metal washers, and similar objects get wedged on the tongue, interfering with eating and drinking. These can cause discomfort and even kill the bird if not removed quickly. When you detect the object, restrain the bird by wrapping it in a heavy towel. Cut the object with a scissors (if possible), or grasp it with an eyebrow tweezers or a needle-nosed pliers. Use a surgical lubricant (obtainable from the drugstore) to help the object to slide off. Be careful — do not do more harm than good.

LEG OR WING. Sometimes metal wire or nylon fishing line becomes wrapped around a limb. Cut the line or wire with a scissors and remove gently. If the line or wire has been in place long enough for tissue to grow around it, bleeding willl follow removal of the object. Use a pledget of cotton and pressure.

INTERNAL. Birds tend to swallow all sorts of objects, including pins, nails, and sheet-metal trimmings. These usually lodge in the gizzard, penetrating the wall. Birds so affected get gradually thinner. X-ray examination is needed for diagnosis.

NERVOUS DISORDERS

For nervous disorders (fits, tremors, comatose conditions), restrain the bird in a box with cotton or other padding.

PENETRATING WOUNDS

Any wound that is more than skin deep may lead to serious infection, although birds are less prone to casual bacterial infections than are mammals. The pointed beak of an aggressive bird can pierce deeply, leaving little external evidence. Bacteria introduced by the beak can build up in numbers, killing the tissues and producing toxic materials. It is best to take a bird with such a wound to a veterinarian. If that is not possible, flush out the wound with sterile salt solution (boil 1 pint water containing 1 scant teaspoon *noniodized* salt for ½ hour; cool to body temperature before using). Squirt the salt solution into the wound with an eyedropper, and pull it back out of the wound with the eyedropper. Repeat several times, rinsing out the eyedropper each time. If a capsule of a tetracycline drug is available, carefully mix the powder from the capsule in some of the salt solution (about 2 tablespoons salt solution for a 250-milligram capsule), and use the mixture for the last washing. Leave this last mixture in the wound.

POISONING

Birds are susceptible to poisoning from many sources — plants, bacteria, fungi, minerals, man-made chemicals, gases from cooking.

FUMES. Caged birds are generally very sensitive to poisonous gases in the environment. Canaries have been used as monitors for dangerous levels of gases in mines for this reason. The canaries would die before the gas reached really dangerous levels for human beings. Cooking, heavy tobacco smoking, gas or charcoal heating — all these activities may cause sickness and death in caged birds kept in the room where they take place. Fumes from overheated fats or overheated Teflon are very toxic for caged birds.

NICOTINE AND PLANTS. Many plants are poisonous to birds. Tobacco is a prime example. Ingestion of tobacco leaf in cigarette butts or cigar butts will cause nicotine poisoning. Nicotine sulfate is used as an insecticide in the garden, and is also used to control mites and lice on birds; carelessness in its use can poison caged birds, evidenced by depression, coma, and death. Philodendron is a common house plant that is poisonous. The oleander, which is widely planted in the warmer parts of the country, is very toxic. Rhubarb leaves (not the stalks) are deadly.

BACTERIA AND FUNGI. Bacteria produce poisons; their development can be prevented by regular and careful cleaning of cages, feeders, and waterers. Many fungi also produce poisons. Fungal poisoning may be avoided by regular cleaning of cages, feeders, and waterers, and by inspection of feeds to make sure that only clean seeds are fed. The poison is formed by the growth of the fungus within the seed or the feed, which usually causes discoloration and often caking.

IN METAL AND PAINT. Lead and cadmium, both poisonous, are likely to be present in metal objects or in paints. Lead in particular tends to build up to toxic levels in the body from small doses, causing damage to the nervous system. Affected birds may be lame or have drooping wings. They tire rapidly. Soldered joints in cages are especially dangerous for psittacines (who nibble on everything). Although lead paints are rare now, they were formerly widely used, and old bird cages may have coats of lead paint.

OIL SPILLS. Wild birds caught in oil spills have problems with gumming of the feather coat by the oil, and they may be poisoned in various ways depending on the composition of the particular product involved. Generally, it is far kinder to use a painless method of killing oil-spill birds, since only a few treated birds can survive after release, though no one yet knows why.

OTHER POISONS. Insecticides and fungicides are toxic by their nature. Drugs of all kinds may be toxic. Follow the directions on the label of any product you use.

It takes a great deal of detective work to arrive at a confirmed diagnosis of poisoning. The effects of many poisons simulate those of many infectious agents (see chart on pages 212–213). If you suspect poisoning, see your veterinarian, and bring along labels and any other information you have that might help in solving the problem. The veterinarian will use various drugs and physical therapy methods, depending on the nature of the problem. Chances for recovery are usually poor, depending on the poison involved, the dose, the general health of the bird, the promptness with which poisoning is detected and treatment initiated, and even diet and weather.

parasites
ARTHROPODS

Arthropods are jointed-leg invertebrates. They cause trouble in many ways. Some are bloodsuckers, and can cause the death of small birds by their collective drainage of large volumes of blood; others cause irritation and interfere with rest. Some live in the body of the bird and produce toxic substances. Many arthropods serve to spread other disease agents (bacteria, viruses, worms, and even other arthropods) from one bird to another.

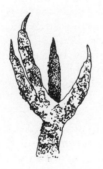

scaly-leg mites symptoms

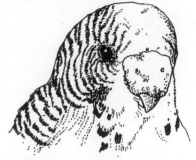

scaly-face mites symptoms

TICKS AND MITES

Ticks and mites are eight-legged creatures. The ticks are large and easily seen; they attach themselves to the skin and suck blood, The mites, on the other hand, are small — most can be seen only with the aid of a microscope — and have a variety of ways of feeding. Larger mites, which often spend part of their time off the bird living in cracks and crevices of the cage or aviary, suck blood. They leave droppings, pepperlike specks, on the surface of the cage or aviary. Other mites live in the skin of birds, absorbing nutrients from the tissue fluids, but do not suck blood. They often cause overgrowth and distortion of the scaly part of the leg (scaly-leg mites) or of the face and beak (scaly-face mites). Scaly-leg mites also often cause sensitive spots on the bird's feet, which make it flinch and fall when landing on a perch. Some mites live inside the quill of the feather, sucking tissue fluids from the wall of the feather follicle. This causes intense itching, and the bird will often cut off or pull at its own feathers. Other mites live on the skin or on the feathers, eating feathers or skin flakes. Among the more dangerous mites are the respiratory mites, which live in the respiratory tract and often give the bird a wheezing cough; they can cause death. The larger arthropods can often be detected by the owner, but the diagnosis of mites is best left to a veterinarian.

LICE   Lice are insects without wings, flattened from top to bottom, usually much larger than mites. Body lice are usually very active, whereas many of the wing-louse species are very slow moving. The lice live on the skin, eating skin debris, chewing on tender feather follicles, and collecting blood and tissue fluid from injuries. Adult lice are usually brown to almost black in color. Louse eggs are attached to feathers.

FLEAS   Fleas are wingless insects, flattened from side to side, which can jump long distances. Though some kinds of fleas will attach themselves very securely to the bird, most move rapidly through the feathers. Since flea eggs are not attached to the bird, they will roll off to the bottom of the cage. The egg hatches, producing a small caterpillarlike larva, which eventually makes a cocoon (a pupal case) and metamorphoses into an adult flea. Fleas, unlike lice, do not care from what animal they get blood, and fleas from cats and dogs can cause trouble in caged birds.

WINGED INSECTS   A number of winged insects — the mosquitoes, the black flies, the buffalo gnats, and the louse flies — are important parasites of birds, spreading such viral diseases as pox and equine encephalomyelitis, such protozoan diseases as the bird malarias, and such worm diseases as filariasis. Deerflies and horseflies are also problems, usually in outdoor aviaries.

INSECTICIDES   The insecticide malathion, which is generally available in garden shops and hardware stores, is fairly effective against arthropods and is safe for many species of birds. It must be remembered that it is a poison, and that possibly some species may be very sensitive to it. Certainly, nestlings are known to have died from doses that do not affect adult birds. Follow the directions on the label of any insecticide very carefully.

HELMINTH PARASITES   Leeches (usually a problem only in waterbirds), tapeworms, roundworms, thorny-headed worms, and flukes are usually internal parasites. Most live in the digestive tract, although some live on the surface of the brain, some in the walls of blood vessels, and some in the air sacs and other parts of the respiratory tract. Being internal, they are detected when eggs are found in the droppings or in swabbings from the esophagus, or when their larval stages are found in the blood. This all requires a microscope and the ability to recognize what you see. Worm problems are usually associated with weight loss. Respiratory tract worms may cause rapid tiring, and respiratory sounds.

See your veterinarian if you suspect worms. A veterinarian will use a drug to kill them, the kind depending on the kind of worm.

Worms are transmitted from an affected bird to other birds either directly as eggs or indirectly as immature stages of the worms that develop in other life forms — intermediate hosts — and are eaten by the bird. Preventive measures include regular cleaning of cages (dropping removal), control of grain pests, ants, and similar vermin through cleanliness and fumigation, and control of bloodsucking arthropods through screening and insecticides.

diseases

VIRAL Viruses are tiny infectious agents that can reproduce only within living cells and can be seen only with an electron microscope. Viral diseases are very difficult to diagnose, even for a trained person with years of experience. Laboratory resources, including cell-culture facilities or embryonated-egg isolation methods, are needed.

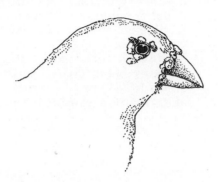

AVIAN POX. This is the only virus the amateur might attempt to diagnose. It is evidenced by thickenings of the skin about the head, usually accompanied by ocular discharge. Nodules may form on the skin in various parts of the body. The more virulent canary pox viruses can kill nearly all the canaries in an aviary. Less virulent strains may cause only temporary sickness.

BACTERIAL Caged birds are susceptible to a wide variety of bacterial agents. As with viral disease, bacterial infections are difficult to diagnose. Laboratory resources are essential.

PSITTACOSIS. Also called parrot fever or ornithosis, this was once a highly publicized disease that, through treatment of pet stock with chlortetracycline-treated seeds, has been all but eliminated from caged birds. There may be respiratory and digestive ailments as well as general systemic disease, or no signs at all.

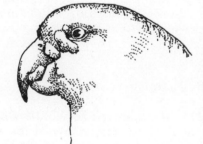

TUBERCULOSIS. This is relatively rare in caged birds. Parrots and other psittacines are susceptible to all three of the bacterial species causing tuberculosis. Most birds are susceptible to *M. avium*. Horny growths on the face or skin of parrots occur with tuberculosis.

ENTEROBACTERIAL DISEASES. These are of more importance to the average caged bird owner. Usually the greatest problem is in nestlings and young birds. Signs are usually diarrhea and weakness. Treatment with tetracycline or other antibiotics usually alleviates the problem temporarily, but the infectious agents are still present. Strict attention to cleanliness of the cage, waterers, and feeders helps to reduce the problem.

PASTEURELLA MULTOCIDA. This disease affects a wide variety of birds and mammals. Caged birds can become infected from dogs, cats, rabbits, or other pets. The disease may be dramatically acute, producing only sudden death; or it can be chronic, with swellings of the joints, nasal discharges, and diarrhea. Laboratory resources are essential for diagnosis. Treatment may include a suitable drug, draining, and irrigations.

FUNGAL The amateur without microbiological training and equipment can only guess in fungal disease diagnosis. Fungal disease may be produced by actual infection or through toxic substances formed in the feed.

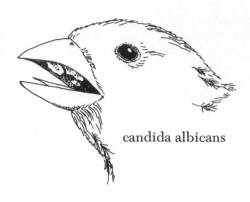
candida albicans

ASPERGILLUS FUNGI. Birds seem especially susceptible to the aspergillus fungi, which most commonly affect the respiratory tract, producing nodular growths in the lungs and air sacs. Sometimes they affect the brain, causing nervous signs as a result of necrotic damage.

CANDIDA ALBICANS. This is a yeastlike fungus that usually affects the upper digestive tract, causing a disease called thrush. This may cause whitish cheesy deposits to form in the mouth and on the tongue. Invasion is fostered by the feeding of honey or other feeds containing simple sugars (hexoses).

FAVUS. The skin may be affected by various fungi, one of the more common diseases being favus, usually evidenced by whitish crusts of featherless areas. In severe cases, the feathered skin is also affected. Other fungi can affect the skin, causing intense itching.

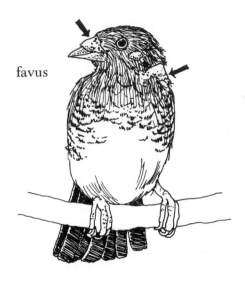
favus

TREATMENT. This is often long, drawn-out, and unrewarding. Prevention — through cleanliness, inspection of feed materials, and, in problem aviaries, the use of preventive drugs for the particular causative agent — is more effective.

PROTOZOAN

The protozoans are microscopic one-celled animals.

TRICHOMONIASIS OR "CANKER." This is often evidenced by whitish thickenings of the mucous membrane of the mouth and other parts of the upper digestive tract. It is spread from bird to bird by infected adults feeding young, or through contaminated drinking water.

COCCIDIOSIS. The coccidia are mostly intestinal parasites, which cause infections that interfere with digestive functions. Young birds may develop deficiency diseases, such as rickets, on a perfectly adequate diet. Regular cleaning of cages or aviaries greatly reduces the danger of coccidiosis.

HAEMOSPORIDIA. The blood protozoans (the "bird malaria organisms") can affect the blood cells, and cells of various organs of the body. They are sometimes evidenced only by death of young birds. Less severe cases are lethargic, often with a puffed-out appearance. Mosquitoes and other blood-sucking flying insects take in infected blood, which in turn infects the insect. Multiplication and development go on in an insect, which then becomes a source of infection for every bird it bites. Screening of aviaries and the use of insecticides protect against the bird malarias.

Diagnosis of the protozoan diseases requires knowledge of the various protozoans, a good microscope, and experience. Drug treatment depends on the particular organism involved.

NUTRITIONAL

Nutritional diseases may be primary (caused by a deficiency of a given nutrient in the feed itself) or secondary (caused by an interference with digestion or absorption of food, or by destruction or increased excretion of the nutrient).

A common example of primary nutritional disease is bone weakness (lameness) in breeding hens or in young birds, resulting from omission of cuttlebone in the diet (calcium deficiency).

An example of secondary nutritional disease is bone weakness (lameness) in young birds resulting from coccidiosis of the intestine interfering with nutrient absorption.

STARVATION. An important nutritional disease in the seed-eating caged birds is starvation due to lack of seeds. Bird-feeders may remain apparently full of seeds — which closer examination would reveal to be merely husks. The inexperienced owner does not add fresh seeds, thinking the feeder is full, and the bird starves in the midst of apparent plenty.

Another important nutritional disease is starvation because the feed is refused by the bird, either because the type of feed is improper for the species (seeds for a meat-eater), or because the bird is accustomed to certain varieties of seeds. Some birds readily adjust to a change in feed and eat what is offered; others will refuse to eat anything but what they have always eaten.

DEFICIENCIES. Deficiencies of several vitamins — vitamin A, riboflavin, pantothenic acid, or biotin — may be indicated by skin troubles. An iodine deficiency will cause enlargement of the thyroid glands, which then press on other structures passing from the neck to the chest. This may cause difficulty in eating or drinking; difficulty in breathing; staggering or other abnormal behavior.

Thiamine deficiency results in paralysis, with spasmodic contraction of the muscles. It can result from destruction of thiamine by yeasts growing in dirty feeders or waterers.

See the chart on pages 212–213 for further signs of nutritional disease.

Since the signs of nutritional disease are much like those of infectious diseases, it is best diagnosed by a veterinarian. Treatment depends on the particular deficiency and usually involves supplying the deficient nutrient in quantity, sometimes by parenteral injection. What the owner can do is to always feed fresh, clean food, containing a mixture of ingredients, along with cuttlebone or other mineral supplement. This should be coupled with regular cleaning of feeders and waterers.

METABOLIC

Metabolic diseases commonly seen in caged birds are obesity, gout, and chronic diarrhea.

OBESITY. This is especially common in budgerigars, but is found in all species of caged birds. Some individual birds are more likely to become obese than are others fed and treated in the same way — such fat-prone birds may be helped by strict rationing of feed. The fat can interfere with movement of the bird and can make breathing difficult. An ever-present danger in obese birds is the development of tumorous changes in the excess fat. The tumors may be felt as firmer nodules within the softer fat. These should be removed promptly, since they may develop to large size and cause great shock to the bird if removed at that time. Early removal also tends to prevent further spread through the body.

SYMPTOMS AND CAUSES OF DISEASE

SIGNS	CAUSES						
	PSYCHOLOGICAL	INFECTIOUS	TRAUMATIC	CHEMICAL	PHYSICAL	TUMOR	NUTRITIONAL
Refusal to eat	not usual food	various	tongue, beak	spoiled feed	blockage		
Comatose condition		various	head	solvents; drugs	chilling	brain	
Wasting away	not usual food	various	tongue, beak	chronic poison		digestive tract	poor feed
Shivering	strange surroundings	malaria; encephalitis	head	poison			calcium deficiency
Soft swellings of breast (budgerigar)						lipoma	overeating
Excess preening (with feather pulling)	boredom	parasites; fungal					
Pupil with white spots, or completely white		various					
Bar across pupil			detached lens				
Red color of lower part of iris		hemorrhage from various infections		hemorrhage from poisons			vitamin K deficiency
Ocular discharge		various	dust	fumes	foreign body		vitamin A deficiency
Panting		various			room too hot		
Wheezing cough		sternostoma mites					
Dry cough		aspergillosis					
Swelling under eye		sinusitis (various)					
Soiled vent		enteritis (various)		various			

Symptom					
Nasal discharge	various		various		
Wet droppings	enteritis (various)		various		
White cheesy material on mouth lining	candidiasis (thrush)				
Beak "moth-eaten," thickened	scaly-face				
Regurgitation (normal in budgerigars)					enlarged thyroid (iodine deficiency)
Protruding vent (female)				"egg-bound"	
Pale mucous membranes (mouth, inside eyelids)	internal bleeding (various)		various	ruptured, fatty liver	
Whitish swellings of toe joints		gout			
Swollen wing or leg joints	various				vitamin D and calcium deficiency
Drooping wing	nerve damage (various)	injury			
Wings held out from body				overheated	
Walking on hocks					vitamin D and calcium deficiency
Rubbery beak and legs (young birds)	enteritis (various)				vitamin D and calcium deficiency
Crusts around base of beak (canary)	canary pox				
Swelling of face and/or nodules of skin	pox				
Thickenings of scales of legs	scaly-leg mites				

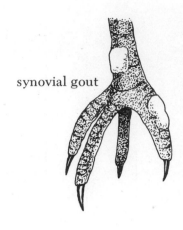

synovial gout

GOUT. This is probably due to a variety of causes. Some cases are associated with low intake of water, due to poor supply or ill-tasting water; still others are of unknown cause. Gout is manifested by urate crystal deposits in joint tissues (synovial gout) or in various body organs (visceral gout). Synovial gout impairs body movements. The deposits may be seen as whitish or yellowish swellings of the feet or of the leg. Visceral gout has no specific signs. Often it is not detected until the bird dies and is examined.

If an aviary has persistent gout problems, the water supply should be investigated. Make sure water is available to all birds and that the water is palatable. Birds with synovial gout may be helped by additional heat in cool climates. Consult your veterinarian about the use of allopurinol and other gout remedies.

CHRONIC DIARRHEA. If many birds are affected with diarrhea, there is generally an acute infectious disease present. Chronic diarrhea, in individual birds, is often due to pituitary gland tumors affecting kidney function; this bird drinks large quantities of water, and promptly excretes it through the kidneys. There is no known treatment for pituitary tumors.

reproduction and baby birds

It is important to remember that it is difficult to get wild birds to breed in captivity. It takes much effort and time in experimentation to make birds feel at home in their surroundings before they will respond by breeding. Many caged birds are wild-caught specimens and are unlikely to breed readily.

On the other hand, the more popular and common caged birds are really domesticated species, having been bred in captivity for many years (many hundreds of years in the case of the society finch). These birds include the canary, the society finch, the zebra finch, the gouldian finch, the budgerigar, and the cockatiel. The novice aviculturalist should begin with one of these species.

Breeding between species results in hybrids, which are usually sterile. This crossing of species is practiced by canary breeders, who cross the canary with other finches. The offspring are called "mules," and combine physical features of the two parent species.

No special food need be provided for baby birds; the parents will take care of feeding their young, though proper diet for the parents is especially important during the breeding season. If you find orphaned birds and want to try to care for them, they generally need a high-protein feed; hence the bugs and worms carried by the parents. Hamburger and liver with a mineral mix make a suitable diet. But be careful, baby birds may pick up bacterial infections from poorly kept foods.

Feeding a baby bird is a big job, and it would be difficult to handle more than one. Blend the food ingredients until they are combined in a homogeneous paste. Insert food material partway down the bird's esophagus, using a plastic eyedropper (check the dropper first for any cracks or jagged edges around the tip). Make sure you get it behind the bird's pharynx, behind the entrance to the trachea, to avoid suffocating the bird. Squeeze out a few drops at a time and rub your finger down the bird's neck to promote swallowing — the problem with newborn birds is that they don't know yet how to swallow. They must be fed every half hour.

CANARY

Sexing: during breeding season, adult males may be distinguished by the vent protruding outward and downward. At other times of the year sexing is very uncertain.
Breeding season: late winter and early spring.
Nest: a strawberry basket, or the wire cup of a wire food strainer, with burlap ravelings, cloth scraps, shredded paper, and similar materials as nesting materials.

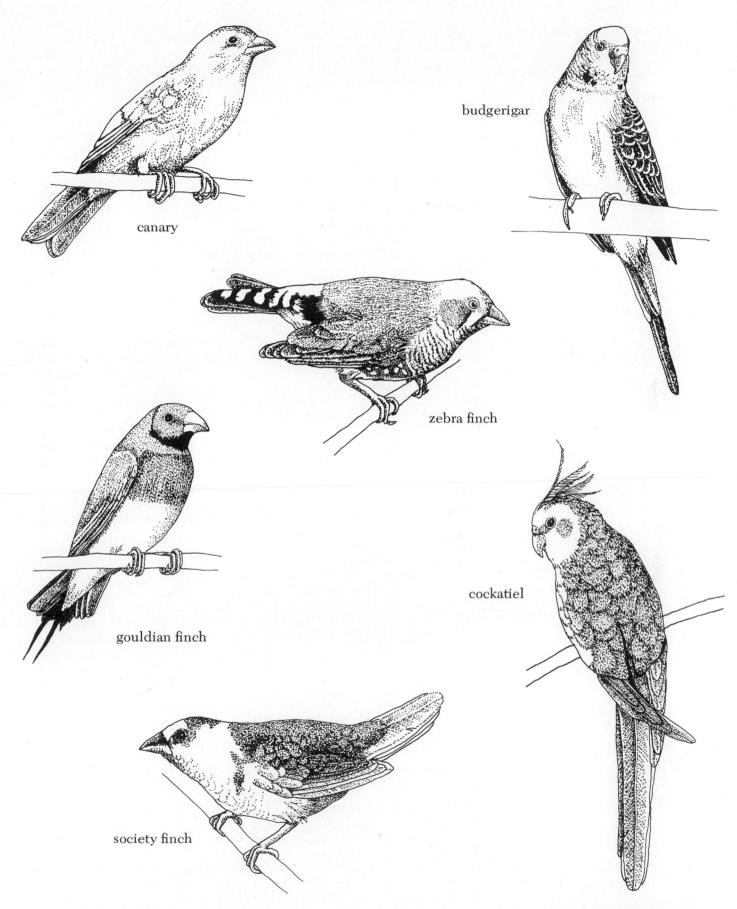

canary

budgerigar

zebra finch

gouldian finch

cockatiel

society finch

Clutch size (clutch is the number of eggs per brood): four to five.
Incubation time: about thirteen days.
Safe number of broods per season: three.
Which sex broods: female.

FINCHES   *Nest:* a 5-inch cube box (half of the front open), or a similar size basket as a nest, and burlap ravelings, cloth scraps, shredded paper, and similar materials as nesting materials.

SOCIETY FINCH. *Sexing:* sexes generally indistinguishable. Male bows to female during breeding.
Breeding season: will breed all year.
Clutch size: four to eight.
Incubation time: about fourteen days.
Safe number of broods per year: three to four.
Which sex broods: both.
Important note: the society finch has well-developed brooding and nurturing instincts. It is used to incubate the eggs and raise the young of other finches.

ZEBRA FINCH. *Sexing:* males (adult) are brightly colored with an orange cheek spot, with penciled markings of the upper breast (hence "zebra").
Breeding season: will breed all year.
Clutch size: four to seven.
Incubation time: fourteen days.
Safe number of broods per year: three to four.
Which sex broods: female.
Important note: zebra finches are very fond of nest making and will often make a nest, deposit eggs, and then make another nest on top of the first and deposit a second clutch. This may continue until there are five or more layers.

GOULDIAN FINCH. *Sexing:* male has much more vivid colors than the female.
Breeding season: late fall and early winter.
Clutch size: usually six.
Incubation time: about thirteen days.
Safe number of broods per season: three.
Which sex broods: both.
Important note: female gouldians are more prone to become egg-bound in cold weather. A heater in the aviary helps prevent this.

BUDGERIGAR   *Sexing:* the budgerigar is perhaps the easiest of all birds to sex. Adult males have a deep blue cere (a waxy swelling at the base of the upper bill). Adult females have a wrinkled brown cere. Birds lacking in sexual development (both sexes) may have a smooth, faintly blue cere.
Breeding season: will breed year-round; best in spring.
Nest: a box 6 inches square by 10 inches high. A rounded cup is made in the bottom, about ½ inch deep to 3 inches in diameter. The rounding serves to bring the eggs under the nesting hen. These nests are available at pet shops.
Clutch size: six.
Incubation time: eighteen days.
Safe number of broods per year: three to four.
Which sex broods: female. (No nest is built; use round-bottomed cup or tea strainer.)
Important note: in community cages, make sure that there are no unmated females. They are likely to cause trouble, destroying nests and eggs and fighting. Unmated males are not a problem.

COCKATIEL *Sexing:* males have bright yellow in face; bright orange patch on cheek; underside of tail is dark slate color (female has yellow streaks in tail).
Breeding season: October.
Nest: a 12-by-24-inch box, 12 inches high, with a 3-inch front hole. Most breeders use a concave bottom, similar to that used for budgies. Commercially manufactured nests are not as easy to find for cockatiels as for budgies.
Clutch size: six.
Incubation time: twenty days.
Safe number of broods per season: three.
Which sex broods: both.

further readings

American Cage Bird Magazine, 3449 N. Western Ave., Chicago, Illinois, 60618.

BERTIN, L. *The Larousse Encyclopedia of Animal Life* (English ed., rev. from the 1949 French ed.). New York, McGraw-Hill, 1967.

CLEAR, V. *Common Cagebirds in America.* Indianapolis, Bobbs-Merrill, 1966.

DAVIS, J. W.; ANDERSON, R. C.; KARSTAD, L.; AND TRAINER, D. O. *Infectious and Parasitic Diseases of Wild Birds.* Ames, Iowa, Iowa State University Press, 1971.

HONDERS, J. ed. *The World of Birds.* New York, Peebles Press International, 1975.

PETRAK, M. L. *Diseases of Cage and Aviary Birds.* Philadelphia, Lea & Febiger, 1969.

ROOTS, C. *Softbilled Birds.* New York, Arco, 1970.

SPARKS, J. *Bird Behavior.* New York, Grosset and Dunlap, 1970.

WETMORE, A. *Water, Prey, and Game Birds of North America.* Washington, D.C., National Geographic Society, 1965.

WETMORE, A., ed. *Song and Garden Birds of North America.* Washington, D.C., National Geographic Society, 1964.

Small rodents

STEPHEN M. SCHUCHMAN, D.V.M.

Despite the general aversion to their close relatives, there are several rodents, including certain rats and house mice, enjoying a vogue as household pets — and household pets they are, quite literally. Rodents should not be taken outdoors because they are likely to scamper away and get lost. Guinea pigs are an exception to this rule. The most popular rodents at present are gerbils, hamsters, albino mice and rats, and guinea pigs. While having some similarities, each species has its own special merits as a pet.

GERBILS

The Mongolian gerbil (*Meriones unguiculatus*), the common field mouse of eastern Asia, was first introduced to this country in 1954, to be used in medical research. In little more than a decade, its handsome appearance and gentle personality had won it many fans in the general public. Overall, the gerbil grows to about 8 inches, half of which is sleek, furry tail. An animal this size weighs around 3 ounces.

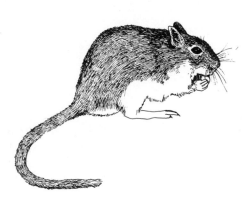

The gerbil's back is a rusty brown, with dark guard hairs over a dense gray undercoat. The underside is cream or light gray. The head is broad and proportionately shorter than that of a rat, with long expressive whiskers and large dark eyes. The long tail, small forefeet, and much longer hind legs give the gerbil something of the appearance of a pocket-size kangaroo, especially when it stands up to look around. But its coloring, size, curiosity, and sudden, swift movements are more reminiscent of chipmunks and ground squirrels.

Gerbils are easily tamed and, while they do not like to be cuddled, seem to enjoy being handled. Normally they do not bite, but attempts to grasp a gerbil may well earn the perpetrator a nip.

Gerbils are monogamous, choosing their own mates and remaining together as a couple for life, which may be as long as four years. In their native, desert habitat, they live in colonies, each family digging its own burrow. Living as they do far from water sources, their bodies are highly efficient at using what they can get — and this is a factor in one of their virtues as house pets: they are virtually odorless. The reason is that their urine, with its small amount of liquid, is highly concentrated and gives off little odor.

Because they are social animals, gerbils seem happiest in mated pairs rather than alone. They are usually nonaggressive toward one another and toward humans, and make quiet pets. Their most active period is during the daytime, when they will be busy burrowing and scratching. Before deciding to purchase gerbils, you should check your state laws. Gerbils are illegal in California.

HAMSTERS

The Syrian golden hamster (*Mesocricetus auratus*), which abounds in its Mideastern homeland, was practically unknown in the West until the early

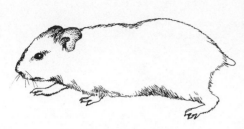

thirties, when a few were introduced to England. The roly-poly, short-tailed little animal, with its short legs, quickly caught on as a pet and shortly thereafter crossed the Atlantic. The hamster's back is brown, flecked with yellow, and the underside a creamy gray. At full growth, they reach around 4½ inches and weigh approximately 4½ ounces. The usual life span is from two to two and a half years, with occasional animals reaching a ripe old three.

Compared to gerbils, hamsters are pugnacious creatures and far more likely to take offense — and to let you know about it with a swift bite. They are also far less sociable and, when they are kept together, fights are not uncommon. The smaller male is anything but chivalrous toward his mates. Yes, mates, for hamsters are not, like the gerbil, monogamous. Usually they are bred in threes, one male to two females, and form no permanent bonds.

Hamsters are extremely clean and, in Asia, are sometimes eaten. These nocturnal animals live in burrows and are notorious hoarders. Even though they have an adequate food supply, pets will often store part of their meal in their cheek pouches to be stashed away in the nest just in case a rainy day *does* show up.

MICE   Albino mice are merely a pure strain of the common house mouse (*Mus musculus*). By virtue of their ancestry, they can be said to be man's oldest rodent companion, though until modern times the association was not one our species chose.

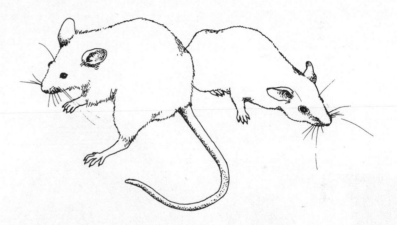

Mice, while they may tolerate humans in the sense of losing their fear, are animals that should be handled with care, for they will not hesitate to bite if startled. Their biggest drawback as pets is their odor. Mice urinate a more watery and less concentrated urine than gerbils do. These factors add to the stronger odor that is found with caged mice.

Mice are nocturnal. They can be kept in groups and will divide off into family pairs, each building its own nest. The average adult mouse weighs approximately 1 ounce. The normal life span is about three years.

RATS   Albino rats are a strain of the brown or Norway rat (*Rattus norvegicus*) commonly used in laboratory research work. Like the house mouse, the brown rat is of Asiatic origin, first appearing in Europe in the eighteenth century. By 1775, it had reached America. Again, while these animals are normally gentle, the possibility of a bite should be taken seriously. If the rats are to be handled at all, they should be handled frequently until they have become quite tame.

Cage odor is much less a problem with rats than with mice. In virtually every other respect, with allowances for size, what applies to keeping mice is equally good for rats.

Their life span is approximately three years and their weight, ¾ pound to over 1 pound.

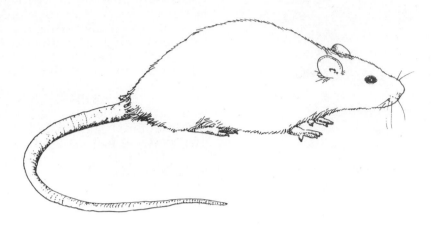

GUINEA PIGS   Guinea pigs are a beautiful example of just how confused we humans can become when we assign names to things. While there may well be guinea pigs in Guinea, they will have been taken there by man, and they are not even closely related to the pig family. Their orignial home was on the slopes of the Andes mountains of South America, where they were first domesticated by the Indians as a food animal. The original stock, the Brazilian or Peruvian cavy (*Cavia aperea*), still exists there in the wild state. The domestic guinea pigs (*Cavia porcellus*) have been selectively bred to produce a number of varieties, distinguished from one another primarily by the color and texture of their fur.

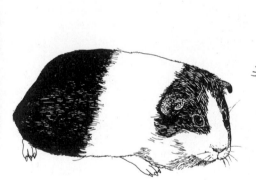

English guinea pig

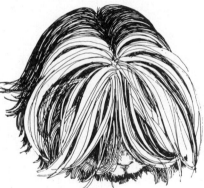

Peruvian guinea pig

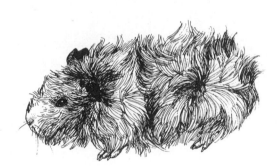

Abyssinian guinea pig

To compound the naming problem even further, the short-haired English guinea pig is much closer to the original stock than the long-haired Peruvian guinea pig, or angora. Both these are popular breeds, as is the Abyssinian guinea pig, another longhair — though the coat is considerably shorter than the angora's — with hair that grows in swirling cowlicks.

Despite these differences, guinea pigs have in common stocky, rounded bodies on which there are neither noticeable necks nor tails. They grow to a length of between 8 and 12 inches and may weigh in excess of 2 pounds. Guinea pigs are capable of giving a bite, with their large rodent incisors, but they rarely do. While males will fight, females get along quite amiably, even nursing one another's babies. As many as six females may be kept with a single male for breeding purposes. Normally, the guinea pig will live from

	KEEP IN PAIRS	RESPONSIVE TO OWNER	CAGE ODOR PROBLEM	BITING	OVER-BREEDING PROBLEM	LIFE SPAN	FREQUENCY OF CAGE CLEANING
Mouse	yes	very little	yes	may nip or bite	yes	3 years	every 2–3 days
Rat	yes	good	less than mice	rarely bite once they are used to people	yes	3 years	once every 3 days
Hamster	may fight unless kept separate	fair	not usually	may nip or bite	not usually	2–2½ years; sometimes 3 years	once every 5–7 days
Guinea pig	yes	good	not usually	very rarely nip, least likely to bite	not usually	4–5 years	once every 5–7 days
Gerbil	yes, pairs mate for life	good	no, very little odor	not usually	sometimes	4 years	once every 7–10 days

four to five years, though some have been reported to have survived as long as ten. Guinea pigs are clean pets and are not usually carriers of communicable disease.

preventive medicine

While in many ways less bother than larger species, small mammals actually impose an even greater responsibility on the pet owner, because they are totally dependent. If you forget to put out food for your dog or cat, the animal won't hesitate to remind you, but a rodent in a cage has very few ways to do so. So, while they are usually thought of as children's pets, adult supervision is essential to their welfare. It is up to the parent to make sure they regularly receive fresh food and bedding, get the gentle handling they require, and to watch for indications of poor health.

CAGES   The starting point in caring for your pet is to make sure the animal has a proper environment. Choosing the proper cage will both enhance your enjoyment of the animal and be an important factor in its health. Small rodents do quite well either in aquariums made for fish or in plastic rodent cages, which are available in pet stores. It is essential to have a well-secured and ventilated cover.

While plastic cages seem to have many advantages, bear in mind that they do crack if handled frequently, and some discolor when cleaned over a period of time. Because of its porosity wood cannot be easily disinfected; and if you use a wooden box, remember that all rodents are gnawers. Screening — using mesh hardware cloth — should cover all the inside wooden surface.

Mice should have a minimum floor space of 8 by 10 inches and the cage should be at least 6 inches high. Cages for rats should, of course, be somewhat larger. The floor space should be about 10 by 12 inches and the height around 10 inches. Commercial cages are available for both mice and rats. Extensive testing has established that rats have an extremely low tolerance

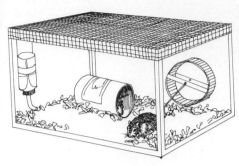

for overcrowding. For gerbils, cages should be at least 10 by 14, with a height of 8 inches. Hamsters' cages should have a floor area of no less than 10 by 12 inches and be at least 10 inches high. Cages for guinea pigs need a floor surface of 30 by 36 inches and a height of 18 inches.

The floor of the cage should be covered with some form of absorbent litter. Substances commonly used include dried rice hulls, wood shavings (preferably not colored), or dried corncob pieces. Because of the strong urine odor problem with mice, you might very well prefer to use some commercially available cat litter. Even so, to prevent odor buildup, this should be changed at least every other day. For the other species, at least once a week should be adequate.

There must be some place in the cage where the animals can hide, completely out of sight. Bedding material should be placed in the cage for their use. Materials include burlap, which the animal will shred, dried grass, hay, and shredded paper. These should be changed every two to ten days, depending on the animal (see chart, page 221). If the animal eats its bedding or nesting material, switch to another type.

In cleaning the cage, mild disinfectants such as a diluted Chlorox or ammonia solution may be used safely. They should be rinsed off well with water as an added precaution.

Regardless of the type of cage, it is a good idea to have an exercise wheel. A dripless watering bottle is absolutely necessary — even for gerbils, despite the fact that they are desert dwellers; many people have the mistaken idea that they will get all the water they need in their diet. Free access to water should be available to all animals.

HANDLING   There are three basic methods you can use to safely and securely handle your pet. For animals accustomed to people and for people accustomed to small rodents, gently using a cupped hand works satisfactorily. But if the animal is unaccustomed to being handled, proceed with caution. With some animals, especially if they are jumpy, you may want to do all your handling on the floor. Most small rodents, if they are frightened, will run off the edge of a table and injure themselves.

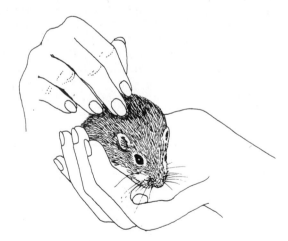

When getting the animal out of the cage, it is important to move slowly rather than chasing the pet around and increasing its fear. If possible, when dealing with pets unaccustomed to handling, remove the exercise wheels and close off escape routes first. With animals showing a tendency to bite, such as untrained hamsters, it is wise to use a pair of canvas gardening gloves until they begin to become tame.

If restraint is needed, there are two good techniques for handling:

TOWEL METHOD. This is especially useful for aggressive or frightened pets.

Place a small unfolded towel, thick enough to withstand the animal's teeth, in the hand you will use to hold it. With the toweled hand, grasp the rodent behind its head gently but securely. The body can be supported either in the palm of the hand holding it or by the other hand. With mice and rats it is easiest to start by using the free hand to gently lift the animal by its tail and place it on top of the cage. Once the rodent is on a surface where it can get traction, it will start walking forward. Keep holding the tail and simultaneously, with the toweled hand, grab the mouse or rat. This should not be attempted with gerbils since tail injury can occur; and it is impractical with short-tailed species.

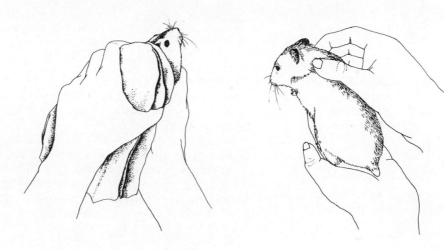

HAND METHOD. This is essentially the same process, but without the towel. When the rodent has been grasped by the nape of the neck, support the body in the palm of the hand holding it or by the other hand.

QUARANTINE

It is wise to isolate incoming pets for two to three weeks in a separate room of the house before allowing them to come into contact with your other pet rodents. Always feed, clean, and handle the new animals last, after you have cared for the others. Wash your hands and change your clothes before you come in contact with your original pets.

TEMPERATURE

Because these animals come from different habitats, each has a temperature range which is best for its health. There should be a thermometer mounted on the cage so that it can easily be checked. Optimum temperatures are:

Gerbils: 65–75°F.
Hamsters: 65–80°F.
Mice and rats: 70–80°F.
Guinea pigs: 65–75°F.

If nesting material is adequate, gerbils can stand temperatures as low as 50°F. Guinea pigs, on the other hand, are not usually subjected to temperatures below 65°F. without the risk of pneumonia or other respiratory problems unless they are slowly acclimated to the lower temperature.

HUMIDITY

For mice, rats, guinea pigs, and hamsters, a relative humidity of around 50 percent is optimal. Gerbils like slightly drier air, but 50 percent humidity will be fine for them too.

SENSITIVITY TO SUNLIGHT Burrowing animals, even those active during the day, take shelter when the sun becomes too intense. With the smaller rodents, especially, it is vitally important that their cages not be kept where they will be hit by direct sunlight. Their small body size has a larger relative surface area than larger rodents have, so they heat up faster, and the result can be fatal within minutes. It is equally important that cages not be placed where they are exposed to drafts — which might lower temperatures suddenly.

LETTING OUT OF CAGE Mice, because they are harder to tame, should be kept in their cages. The other rodents, however, can be let out for periods of play, so long as care is taken to prevent their getting outdoors and escaping. It is wisest to keep them on the floor, rather than risk a fall off a table or shelf.

CATCHING ESCAPED RODENTS If frightened, or sometimes prompted simply by curiosity, your pet might pull a disappearing act. The important thing to remember is that the animal must, in time, return to find food. The worst mistake would be to start rushing around pursuing it. This will only generate fear and make retrieval more difficult. If the cage is placed on the floor, the pet usually will return to it voluntarily if it sees no signs of danger. If it is under a piece of furniture and cannot be reached, try luring it out with a favorite treat such as a sunflower seed, sitting beside it, and remaining still until it comes within reach. Then pick it up as you ordinarily would, moving slowly and giving it the opportunity to climb onto your hand.

FEEDING All these species are mainly herbivores, though in the wild state hamsters may be omnivorous. The following diet for each of these species is geared to its nutritional needs:

GERBILS. Commercial mouse or rat chow, with the lowest fat content possible, makes a good basic food; it should be supplemented with seeds (sunflower, pumpkin, watermelon, or birdseed). This diet can be varied with grains such as corn, wheat, rice, oats, rye, or chicken scratch. Fruits and vegetables should be offered, but only in small quantities, and leftovers should be removed daily. A gerbil consumes around ½ ounce (10 to 15 grams) a day.

HAMSTERS. Commercial rat, mouse, or hamster chow supplemented with kale, cabbage (both better sources of nutrients than lettuce), apples (with their peels), and milk (for protein). Mealworms, crickets, and grasshoppers are fine sources of protein. Small pieces of cooked meat and liver will also be accepted, but leftovers must be removed at the end of the day. A hamster will eat less than ½ ounce daily (7 to 12 grams).

MICE AND RATS. Commercial mouse and rat chows will provide the basic needs, but can be supplemented, in small quantities, with fruits such as apples, raw carrots, potatoes, and other vegetables. Grains and wild birdseed will also be eaten. A mouse's average consumption is less than ⅐ ounce (2.5 to 4 grams) a day. Rats will normally eat around ten times this amount, a little over an ounce daily (20 to 40 grams).

GUINEA PIGS. Commercial guinea pig chow, supplemented with good quality hay, kale, cabbage, fruits, and carrots. The essential thing to remember is that guinea pigs cannot synthesize vitamin C themselves and it must be included in their diet. Commercial guinea pig chow should contain it — because the vitamin deteriorates, the pellets should be dated; this date must be checked. Nevertheless, fruits high in vitamin C should be provided. Ascorbic acid (vitamin C) tablets may also be added to the water at a concentration of 50 milligrams to 8 ounces of water. This solution should be made up fresh daily and placed, preferably, in a glass watering bottle. Cod-liver oil can also be added to the food to improve the animal's coat. In the summer, grasses, dandelions, plantains, and clover will be well received. A guinea pig will consume in excess of an ounce (30 to 35 grams) of food daily. Guinea pigs can also be given salt blocks.

Fresh food and water should always be available — even the gerbil will consume some water each day. Water bottles should be emptied and refilled daily and checked to make sure they're not leaking. Checking the bedding beneath the spout will give you a clue that leakage is occurring.

GROOMING

All of these species are extremely clean in their habits, grooming themselves and each other as a matter of habit and a major activity. Unless something is spilled on them that is either dangerous or beyond their capacity to handle, bathing should be avoided. Not only is it not necessary — by keeping their cages clean, you assure yourself of (with the exception of the mouse) an odor-free pet — but it could be dangerous to their health. Only the long-haired guinea pigs need any human assistance in normal circumstances. For brushing tangles out of their coats, a toothbrush is excellent.

TRAINING

With these small species, the only real training necessary is actually taming, winning their trust by handling them properly and frequently enough for them to become accustomed to the experience. The essential is to convey your own confidence by remaining calm, moving with slow deliberation, and speaking in a low voice. Allow the animal to climb onto your hand, offering it food in your palm. If, when you try to raise the hand when the pet is sitting on it, the pet seems fearful — let it go. In time it will become used to the experience, and to you. So far as tricks are concerned, the pet will provide those itself out of its store of instinctive behavior. Give them things they can climb into and out of — such as the paper tubes on which paper towels are rolled — or ladders they can climb up. Their natural curiosity will do the rest. And if you reward them with special treats, they will quickly learn that out-of-the-cage time means playtime.

the home clinic

STOCKING A MEDICINE CABINET

Only the most minor first aid can be handled in the home, but it might be useful to have a few basic items on hand that could help prevent minor problems from becoming major. These are:

mild antiseptic, such as tamed iodine or a 3 percent solution of hydrogen peroxide

flea powder or spray, certified to be safe on cats or hamsters

"SICK CAGE"

If you are keeping more than one animal, it might be a wise precaution to have an "isolation ward" to which an animal showing possible signs of trouble might be moved until the problem either clears up or is diagnosed by your veterinarian. Animals showing symptoms of colds should always be removed from the group to another room.

ADMINISTERING MEDICINE

To apply medication to the animal's exterior or to examine it for injury, use the towel or hand methods described above in restraining the pet.

first aid Minor scratches and bites received in fights should be treated with a mild antiseptic, such as hydrogen peroxide, to destroy bacteria and prevent infection.

GENERAL PURPOSE EXAMINATION If your pet appears to be either injured or in poor health, the most important thing you can do for it as owner is to spot signs of trouble early. Treatment with patent medicines may be useless at best, and could actually worsen a condition. Any problem that persists for more than twenty-four hours should be brought to the attention of your veterinarian. But only your alert eye can spot the early warning signs. The following outline will serve as a guide in judging both animals you already have and those you may be considering buying.

1. Skin and hair
   a. General condition: is it well groomed or scruffy in appearance?
   b. Any signs of scratching, small scabs on the skin?
   c. Any hair loss on face or body?
   d. Any pustules, boils, abscesses, or lumps (firm masses) anywhere on the animal?
2. Front feet, hind feet, and tail
   a. Sores on feet, toes, foot pads, or tail.
   b. Loss of pink color of tail of mice.
   c. Presence of ingrown toenails (especially guinea pigs).
3. Ears
   a. Crusty accumulation in ear canals (sometimes guinea pigs).
   b. Shaking head or scratching at ears.
4. Movement
   a. Reluctance to move.
   b. Weakness of all limbs.
   c. Dragging hind limbs (hamsters).
   d. Favors a particular side when lying down.
5. Central nervous system (brain and spinal cord)
   a. Loss of coordination; walks as if drunk.
   b. Walks in small circles.
   c. Head tilted to one side.
   d. Quick movement of eyes from side to side (constantly).
   e. Convulsion (seizure or fit) can occur in gerbils when excited or overhandled; animals recover quickly, back to normal after seizure.
6. Respiratory system
   a. Listen for sneezing sounds.
   b. Look for red-tinged nasal discharge or reddish blood-tinged staining around nostrils in rats, mice, and hamsters.
   c. Does breathing appear labored?
7. Gastrointestinal system
   a. Check for signs of slobbering (saliva staining around mouth), seen in guinea pigs. This can be the result of malformed teeth (incisors or molars).
   b. Examine anus and surrounding areas for signs of diarrhea or abnormal swelling or protrusion of rectum.
   c. Check consistency of droppings. It is normal for guinea pigs to eat their own stools. Periodically have stool specimens checked by a veterinarian to detect the presence of internal parasites.
8. Urinary tract and genital tract
   a. Observe and measure amount of water consumed in twenty-four hours. Make sure the bottle is not dripping. Use water bottles as opposed to dishes of water.
   b. Observe urine. Gerbils produce very little watery urine; their urine is quite concentrated.

c. Determine the correct sex of your animal (see page 232).
d. Female hamsters may show a very obvious cream-colored vaginal discharge; this is usually normal.
9. Eyes
a. Look for any signs of crusty or purulent eye discharge (especially in guinea pigs). This can be evidence of infection even though it appears mild.

NORMAL WEIGHTS FOR YOUNG AND MATURE ANIMALS (GRAMS)*

	AT BIRTH	FULL GROWN	
Gerbil	3.0	(F)	75
		(M)	85
Hamster	2.0	(F)	120
		(M)	108
Mouse	1.5	(F)	30
		(M)	30
Rat	5.5	(F)	300
		(M)	500
Guinea pig	100.0	(F)	850
		(M)	1,000

*1 gram = .035 ounce

If growth rates seem abnormal or there are obvious signs of illness you should ask yourself whether the cause lies in the care the animal is receiving or in a disease process. The former you are capable of handling; the latter is a problem for your veterinarian to help solve. The following checklist is designed to give you an organized approach in order to analyze the nature of your pet's problem.

PROBLEM CHECKLIST

1. Species _____
2. Sex _____
3. Age of animal _____
4. Weight of animal before problem and now _____
5. What type of diet is fed and by whom? _____
6. How is the water dispensed and by whom? _____
7. What is the room temperature — daytime?____ nighttime?_____
8. What is the cage temperature? _____
9. Where is the cage kept? _____
10. What is the humidity of the cage? _____
11. What type of cage is the animal kept in (wood, plaster, painted wood, or metal)? _____
12. How often is the cage cleaned? _____
13. What type of litter is used? _____
14. Are there other animals in the room or in the cage? _____
15. Among other animals in the house, what age group are you having problems with? _____
16. What do you think is the major problem? _____
17. What signs of illness is the animal showing? _____
18. How long has the problem been going on? _____
19. If the animal is a female, has she had a litter? Is she kept with a male? _____
20. Have you given any medication to the animal? _____

21. Have any new animals been brought into the household? When? _____

22. Do you or any other member of your household come in contact with other small mammals outside your home (in school, at friends', or at work)? _____

23. Have there been any major changes in the household (painting, exterminating, or moving animals from one room to another)? _____

external parasites

Lice, fleas, and mites are all possibilities when your pet constantly scratches or bites its fur. The treatment for all three is the same: a dusting powder that is safe for use on cats or hamsters. If, while the animal is restrained, you can examine the fur and find either fleas themselves or "flea dust," the tiny pepperlike residue they leave in their wake, its cage should be emptied and sprayed with the dusting powder before new material is put in, and the animal should be sprayed or powdered.

internal parasites and disease

The similarity between the symptoms of some internal parasites and bacterial or viral infections makes it impossible to deal with these conditions apart from other possible causes.

Any sign of poor health should be an immediate signal to observe the animal carefully and separate it from others of the same species. Supplying the veterinarian with an accurate case history to aid in diagnosis is important. Keep the sick animal clean and warm and supply fresh food and water in the meantime.

ASSISTING YOUR VETERINARIAN. Diagnosis is essentially a job of detection in which the veterinarian needs all the clues possible to arrive at a correct diagnosis. Ideally, you should start accumulating information before anything goes wrong.

Small mammals have few means of communicating what they feel, but their bodies are constantly giving us data, if we can read them, on the state of their health. To properly evaluate them, you should keep some simple records. Record-keeping is the best way of detecting health problems.

One of the most important pieces of information you should gather deals with your pet's weight. Once matured, the animal should maintain its weight. Immature animals should show a steady increase in weight. A failure to do so or a loss of weight in a nonhibernating adult probably indicates a problem. (Of the animals discussed, only hamsters hibernate. In captivity, this will not occur if their environment is kept at the recommended temperature.) A weight scale marked in grams (available for measuring food in small portions) should be used for weighing small pets such as mice, hamsters, and gerbils. A scale marked in ounces and pounds can be used for guinea pigs.

Growth weights can be taken every other day for very young animals, while adults can be weighed weekly.

The list of diseases below will allow you, depending on the type of animal you own, to relate the findings on your checklist to possible causes — both in terms of the care the animal is receiving and infectious conditions known in the species.

GERBILS

RESPIRATORY SYSTEM. Sneezing and labored breathing could be caused by viral, bacterial, or fungal infections. They can show up in animals of all ages and usually follow stress. To arrive at a definitive diagnosis, your veterinarian may rely on physical examination, cultures, and radiography. Antibiotics are usually used in treatment. Chances of recovery depend on the individual case.

EYES. In older animals, conjunctivitis (pinkeye)* and swollen eyes may occur. Treatment such as mild ophthalmic ointment may be dispensed by your veterinarian.

DIGESTIVE TRACT. Mild diarrhea can be due to a number of causes. There is the possibility that it may be a result of diet, or parasitism. Unwashed greens, intestinal parasites (most unlikely in gerbils), protozoan or salmonella infection can be a cause (this is not the usual type of salmonella that infects humans).

SKIN AND COAT. Scanty or patchy hair growth in unweaned young is not uncommon. No cause is known for this condition but hair will grow in as the animal gets older.

Nose and jaw inflamed and ulcerated — while dermatological problems cannot be ruled out, these symptoms are usually traceable to mechanical abrasion. The cage should be checked and any sources of irritation removed.

Bare spots on base of tail of mature animals usually indicate that they are fighting as a result of overcrowding. Correcting this condition will automatically bring the fights to an end.

NERVOUS SYSTEM. Some younger animals are especially prone to seizures when they are being handled. The body becomes rigid and the legs stiffen and tremble. As the animal gets older, the seizures become less frequent. The cause is believed to be a form of catalepsy.

HAMSTERS

EYES. Runny eyes, sneezing, nasal discharge, and a tendency to huddle may be due to either bacterial or viral infection. Young animals are particularly susceptible. Deaths are not frequent. Treatment relies on antibiotics.

DIGESTIVE TRACT. Mild diarrhea in mature animals that appear otherwise healthy is often an indication of a protozoan infection. Your veterinarian will probably prescribe a high-protein diet if a microscopic examination of the stool proves negative. Deaths are infrequent.

Diarrhea-stained anus, lethargy, difficulty in breathing, and protrusion of the colon through the anus (intussusception and prolapse of colon) are the classical symptoms of a disease called "wet tail." The exact cause is unknown, but factors believed to be influential are a possible infectious agent, viral and/or bacterial, improper caging, overcrowding, and lack of fresh water. Improved care, antibiotics, and even surgery are used in treatment, but fatalities are high.

SKIN AND COAT. Loss of hair, especially around the face, is probably an indication of mites. Itching is not a major problem. A special safe ointment prescribed by your veterinarian may correct this problem.

NERVOUS SYSTEM. Partial paralysis, inability to lift the head, and abnormal crawling can occur in mature hamsters. Degenerative nervous and muscle diseases can cause these symptoms. Nutritional problems also can mimic these signs. Administering vitamin D may be effective, although recovery rate is poor.

MICE AND RATS

RESPIRATORY SYSTEM. Sneezing, labored breathing, a runny nose at which the animal paws, unkempt coat, and a general appearance of poor health — these make up the clinical picture describing a number of diseases in mice and rats. They may be controlled with antibiotics, but can recur and become long-term problems.

* Not contagious to humans.

DIGESTIVE SYSTEM. Mustard-colored stains around the tail of a nursing mouse or rat and running stools are indications of a common and highly fatal disease. Prime attention should be given to preventing its transmission by placing filter caps over the top of the cage.

Mild diarrhea in an otherwise healthy adult mouse or rat is a common symptom that may be due to protozoan infection, usually treated with a diet of apples, cabbage, and ground beef and the administration of antibiotics.

SKIN AND COAT. Scratching around the head and ears, abrasions, scabs, and bald spots are indicative of mites, which are common in mice. Insecticide strips (dichlorvos or pest strips) and powder are usually effective in combating them.

Sores around the ears and on the ear tips in mature animals are usually the result of fighting among the males. Simple observation will confirm this and they can be separated.

NERVOUS SYSTEM. A tilted head and a tendency to go in circles may be suggestive of a bacterial infection of the inner ear, sometimes associated with an upper respiratory infection. Antibiotics are used in treatment.

GUINEA PIGS

LYMPH AND RESPIRATORY SYSTEMS. "Lumps," a disease named for the swollen lymph glands on animals that appear otherwise healthy and active, is usually a streptococcal infection. Often the lymph nodes will discharge pus and must be drained. The animal must be separated from other guinea pigs and may be given antibiotics — but cautiously. Oral antibiotics, especially penicillin, given to guinea pigs may cause sudden death by killing off good bacteria.

Difficulty breathing, a ruffled coat, runny nose, dried mucus on the inside of the foreleg, and itching conjunctivitis are among the symptoms of a number of bacterial infections, the most common being a streptococcal infection. Your veterinarian can isolate the specific cause with a culture and use antibiotics in treatment, but fatalities are high.

DIGESTIVE SYSTEM. Difficulty chewing or moving the mouth, slobbering when eating, and overlong molars can be the results of malocclusion. Your veterinarian may attempt to solve the problem temporarily by cutting and filing the teeth.

Blood-tinged diarrhea may be indicative of protozoan parasites. In young animals it is sometimes fatal. Your veterinarian may prescribe medication along with supportive care.

Poor weight gain, a rough coat, low resistance to disease, a tendency to huddle, and reluctance to move about are some symptoms that may occur with a vitamin C deficiency. Your veterinarian will check over the diet the animal is receiving and may increase its intake of ascorbic acid through injections, or by supplements in the water and food, as well as adding such items as kale, cabbage, citrus fruits, and orange juice to the diet.

SKIN AND COAT. Generalized bald spots or patchiness without itching is usually associated with a stress situation. No specific cause is known and if other dermatological causes are ruled out, treatment usually consists of a diet of hay, cabbage, or kale.

Scaly, patchy skin lesions and broken hair shafts with itching can be symptoms of a fungal infection. Since ringworm fungus may be the cause, the animal should be handled with disposable gloves, for this condition is communicable. Griseofulvin is used in treatment but cautiously, because of the possibility of a reaction to Penicillium cultures, from which it is derived.

Sores on the hocks or soles of the feet and abscesses are usually the result of infections resulting from the abrasions of a wire cage floor. The animal should be put on a softer surface and the affected areas treated daily with medicated dressings.

mothers and young

Closely related as they may be, the small rodents and guinea pigs vary quite widely both in the frequency with which they have litters and in the number born. While the guinea pig bears from two to three litters annually, with between one and four in each, the prolific mouse is producing twice as many litters of four to ten young. Rats may have as many as seven litters annually, averaging eight to ten births each but ranging as high as fourteen. It has been estimated that, under ideal conditions, one pair of rats could have as many as twenty million descendants in only three years. Gerbil litters contain one to twelve and hamsters eight to ten young.

Survival among the small rodents, targets for so many predators, both afoot and airborne, depends on speed of reproduction and these animals waste little time getting about it.

Only six weeks after her birth, the female hamster is ready to mate, outstripping even the mouse by at least two weeks. Rats reach breeding age at three months. Gerbils come of age between ten (males) and twelve (females) weeks and guinea pigs, while capable of conceiving at one month, are best not mated until they are a half year old.

Mating the animals is a fairly simple procedure: with mice and rats no more than putting males and females together in the cage is needed. They then form their family units and construct the nests in which they will raise their litters. With the gerbils, there is much more a question of self-determination. Putting a pair of opposite sexes together may accomplish nothing if they fail to take to each other. It is far wiser to try putting several of each sex in a cage, letting them pair off, and then isolating each couple while they go about building a family.

The fact that hamsters are not so particular does not mean that all will automatically go well once they have been introduced. Quite often, rather than turning to the pressing business of mating, the two will apparently find each other not only uninteresting but enemies at first sight. This does not mean that they will not later get together successfully. The battlers should be separated for a couple of days and a second female put in with the male. Breeders sometimes arrange mass matings, a number of males and twice as many females being placed in one cage. When all the females have been mated, they are removed and placed in breeding cages to bear and rear their young.

The harem system of mating can also be used with guinea pigs. A single male may be used with as many as six females.

PREGNANCY

Female hamsters have an incredibly brief gestation period, giving birth a mere 16 days after mating. Mice gestate for 20 days, rats take 21 to 23 days, gerbils 24, and guinea pigs 68. A further factor in the quick rate of reproduction among these animals is the rapidity with which they mate again. Within one day after delivering a litter, the female guinea pig is willing to accept a male again. The gerbil will mate while nursing, gestating one litter while bringing an earlier one to weaning.

The rodents, in general, require little special attention during pregnancy — though as she nears term, you might wish to give your female guinea pig a diet supplement of bread that has been soaked in milk, fresh or diluted condensed. Actually, the wisest course is to leave the prospective mother, of whatever species, alone as completely as is possible. Nervous mother hamsters often abort or kill their young. Try not to disturb a hamster's nest for nine days after the young are born.

NESTS

Mice, rats, and gerbils will construct their own nests, given the materials, in which the litters will be born and reared; hamsters and guinea pigs, though, may be provided with nesting boxes. Each hamster can have a box, approximately 6 by 6 by 6 inches; place some of the nesting material within it and the rest anywhere in the cage. There should be an opening for the mother to

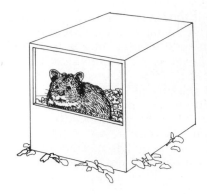

enter and leave. The guinea pig's nest should be just large enough for her and her litter to be comfortable. Nesting boxes should be placed so that they will be exposed to neither drafts nor dampness.

Because of the possibility that under stress the mother might destroy her young, every effort should be made to assure her total privacy until she cares to venture out of the nest herself. Aside from this, rodents are excellent mothers and, experts in their role, should be left to it without human interference. Most rodent fathers — except hamsters — will either help to care for or not interfere with the young; male hamsters can become aggressive, though, and should be kept in a separate cage. The young should have as little contact with humans as possible, until they have reached a point of maturity where they leave the nest themselves.

LACTATION   Weaning takes place in an amazingly short time, in comparison with most mammals. Young mice are completely converted to an adult diet in only 21 days, gerbils at about the same time, and hamsters in 25 days. Guinea pigs and rats nurse their young until they are three weeks old, though guinea pigs can be weaned earlier.

SEPARATING   To prevent overcrowding, indiscriminate breeding, and the combativeness of males as they reach sexual maturity, the young animals should be removed from the cage and either sold, given away, or established in new colonies when they have been weaned.

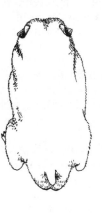
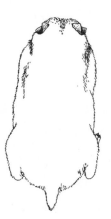

male hamster   female hamster

SEXING   Determining the sex of rodents is not difficult if you know what to look for. In males, a penis can be protruded from the prepuce, and testicles can be felt either in a scrotal sac or under the skin in the groin area. Males have only two external openings in the groin: the anus, and a urethral opening at the tip of the penis. Females have three: anus, vagina, and a urethral opening at the tip of a small papillalike structure (or a small urethral protruberance). An additional way to judge the sex of hamsters is to view them from above: those with rounded rumps are female and those with pointed sterns are male.

further readings

ROBINSON, D. G., JR. *How to Raise and Train Gerbils.* Neptune, New Jersey, TFH Publications, 1967.

VILLIARD, P. *Raising Small Animals for Fun and Profit.* New York, Winchester Press, 1973.

Rabbits

LESTER E. FISHER, D.V.M.

Gentle, unexcitable animals, domestic rabbits make marvelous pets for families with children. Equally important, their care is relatively simple compared to the majority of other animals. Given a dry, clean shelter for their protection and a sufficient diet of vegetable matter, these hardy pets will survive for as long as ten years.

Our wild, native species are altogether another matter, however. While related, their ancestry is quite different. Jackrabbits are actually hares — unlike rabbits, young hares are born with fur and open eyes. The cottontails, too — while rabbitlike — are not true rabbits. The problem lies in the temperaments: these are wild animals, whether they are raised in captivity or not. They are easily frightened: any loud, sudden noise or a well-intentioned visit by the friendliest family dog may bring on a panic — in which they injure themselves, leaping frantically at the sides of their cages in futile attempts to escape — or even a total collapse. They would be bound to prove an enormous disappointment for a child who wants a pet. They could actually be a danger: they defend themselves by kicking and biting, and a panic-stricken jackrabbit or cottontail can inflict painful injuries on a youngster. Cute as they may be, then, those tiny baby bunnies you come across in the country are far better off left in their native habitat.

selecting rabbits

Fortunately, man has succeeded in breeding this excitability out of the domestic rabbit. Nonetheless, in selecting a young rabbit, any sign of a disposition to use teeth or claws should be grounds for rejection.

The other bases for picking a pet from the order Lagomorpha (rabbits and their relatives are not rodents) are largely a matter of size and appearance but the choices are surprisingly varied. More than sixty-five breeds and color varieties are officially recognized in America, all descendants of the European wild rabbits. Among the most popular breeds available in this country are:

BELGIAN "HARE." This is an active, elegant, and hardy animal. Unlike the majority of domestic rabbits, it assumes the upright position so familiar from illustrations in children's books. Despite the name, this is actually a rabbit, evidently descended from the wild Belgian land rabbit. There are three accepted color variations — red, tan, and chestnut — with hazel eyes surrounded by white circles. A medium-sized rabbit, an adult's optimum weight is around 8 pounds.

ANGORA. This rabbit was originally bred for its fur, and the name is indicative of the result. As an owner, bear in mind that the price you pay for this animal's spectacular appearance is in the extra brushing and combing its long, silky coat requires. Four basic colors are available — white, fawn, blue,

Flemish giant

Belgian hare

Himalayan rabbit

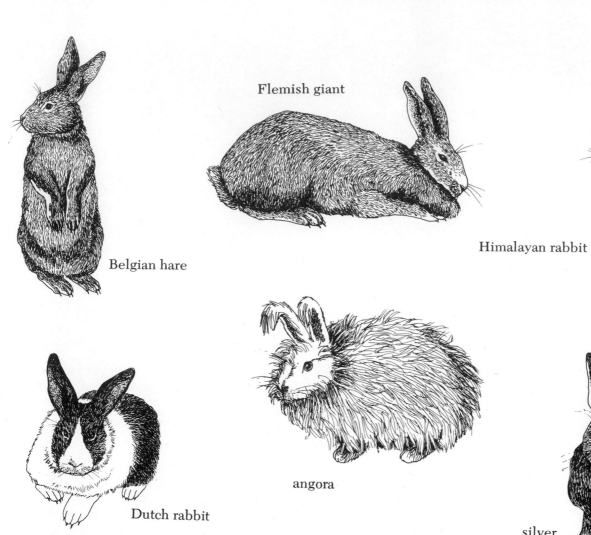

angora

Dutch rabbit

silver

Polish rabbit

harlequin rabbit

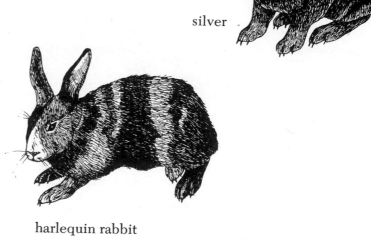

English spot

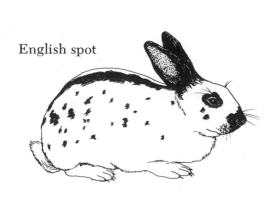

New Zealand rabbit

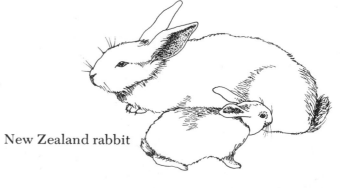

and black. There are two breeds of angoras, the English and the French. The ideal weight for the smaller English breed ranges from 6 to 7 pounds, while the larger French will top 8 pounds.

POLISH. This rabbit is the handsome little favorite of the magician. As a performer, the Polish is familiar as a pink-eyed white albino, but there are also chocolate and black varieties with blue eyes. The fur is short, thick, and glossy. These charming, cheerful little rabbits weigh, ideally, around 2½ pounds.

DUTCH. These rabbits are far and away the most popular with breeders, because they are both prolific and excellent mothers. The greater part of the animal's body may be yellow-gold, chocolate, blue, tortoise, or steel gray, and there is a symmetrical white band that extends over the shoulders, down under the neck, and over the forelegs and hind legs. Ideally, these animals weigh between 3½ and 5½ pounds.

FLEMISH GIANT. This rabbit justly deserves its name, for some bucks weigh up to 22 pounds, though 13 pounds is considered the ideal. These are the largest rabbits raised at present. Their colors are steel gray, white, blue, sand, fawn, or black.

ENGLISH SPOT. This exotically marked animal, has short, sleek fur with a white undercoat and markings of black, blue, chocolate, gray, tortoise, and lilac. The lighter, contrasting spots include butterfly wings on the lower jaw, eye circles, cheek spots, and markings on the ear, spine, and sides. No two of the breed are identical. These rabbits range up to 8 pounds.

SILVER. The silvers get their name from the ticking of light-colored guard hairs against backgrounds that may be gray, fawn, black, or chocolate. The silver gray, the commonest color variation, is actually a mixture of black and white on the animal's head, ears, feet, and tail. The basic color of the silver fawn is a deep, bright orange. In buying, bear in mind that the silvering is not visible in the young rabbits, but will appear by their sixth month. As adults, their weight will range from 4 to 7 pounds.

HIMALAYAN. This rabbit has velvety, colored markings on the nose, ears, feet, and tail that contrast with the short, soft, white hair of the body. Only jet-black markings are available in the United States, but European breeders have come up with blue and brown variations. The markings are not present at birth; they show up on the nose no earlier than the third week and on the legs and tail in the fourth week. The later they appear, the stronger they will be. There is a price the owner pays for the animal's dramatic appearance: Himalayans are heat-sensitive and if kept in bright sunlight will lose their coloring. On the other hand, keeping them in a cold place will not only restore but intensify the contrast.

NEW ZEALAND. This large rabbit is bred in red, black, and white color variations. This densely furred rabbit is a favorite in laboratories because of its rapid growth. It reaches weights between 9 and 12 pounds, which is about par for the breeds that follow.

HARLEQUIN OR JAPANESE. This is the most spectacular of the domestic rabbits in its color patterns. The basic colors are combinations of black and yellow or black and gold. The latter is preferred in the United States. There are ideally at least four vertical stripes of alternating colors on the animal's sides. The head is black on one side and colored on the other, but the ears reverse the pattern: the black ear is on the colored side of the head, and vice versa. Also, one foreleg should be black, the other colored, with the hind legs taking the opposite pattern of the forelegs. The fur is medium long with a dense undercoat and a fine, even ticking of guard hairs.

Other popular breeds include the champagne d'argent, or champagne silver rabbit, which is white with a silver or blue undercoat; the American, in blue or white; the American chinchilla, blue, chocolate, tortoise, gray, steel gray, or black and white; and the tans, on which the basic black, blue, chocolate, or lilac pales to a lighter color on the flanks and belly.

DETERMINING THE SEX   If you're picking only a single rabbit as a pet, sex is of little importance; if you plan on keeping more than one, it is a factor that must be considered. By the time they reach three months, the males and females should be separated, to prevent both indiscriminate breeding and fights between the males over the females. In general, the only pair of rabbits that are practical to keep in a single cage are two females.

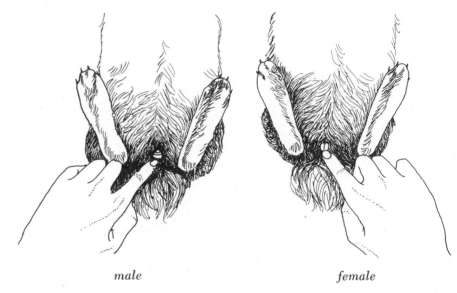

male   *female*

MUCOUS MEMBRANE

Determining the sex of young rabbits before weaning is both pointless and a job that requires an expert. At two weeks, however, it's a relatively simple matter. Gentle pressure with the finger just to the rear of the urogenital opening will expose the mucous membrane. In the male the shape will be circular, and in the female, a slit, which extends almost to the anus.

Wild rabbits are largely nocturnal in their habits, but this does not mean that domestics are dormant during the day and therefore useless as pets for young children (as are many nocturnal animals that seek refuge in order to sleep). They may simply be less active. They pick up in the evening, however, and are quite busy before it is time for youngsters to go to bed.

preventive medicine

For an animal with many natural enemies in the wild, the instinctive emphasis is on protection. With your assistance, your rabbit will do a good job of avoiding both injury and disease. And it must, for when things go seriously wrong, the tendency is in favor of a high rate of fatalities. Often, by the time symptoms of illness become apparent, it is already too late. Also, the light bone structure of animals like rabbits that rely on speed seriously increases the likelihood of fractures. The key to good health and long life, therefore, is to give your rabbit what it needs.

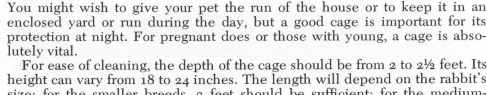

CAGE You might wish to give your pet the run of the house or to keep it in an enclosed yard or run during the day, but a good cage is important for its protection at night. For pregnant does or those with young, a cage is absolutely vital.

For ease of cleaning, the depth of the cage should be from 2 to 2½ feet. Its height can vary from 18 to 24 inches. The length will depend on the rabbit's size: for the smaller breeds, 3 feet should be sufficient; for the medium-sized, 4 feet; yet with an active breed such as the Belgian hare you might allow even more space. Larger breeds require a minimum length of 5 feet, but for the big Flemish giants a full 6 feet is desirable. As a general rule, allow a square foot of floor space for each pound of body weight at maturity.

Proper cage size is more than a matter of giving the animal enough room to exercise, so that its growth won't be stunted. In a cage with a solid floor, the danger of disease is seriously increased if the pet is unable to get away from the corner of the cage where its wastes are deposited.

With solid-floored cages, a straw, hay, or sawdust bed is also needed; and it should be changed at least every second day to keep it dry. Hay and straw, however, are impractical for a long-haired breed such as the angora because they might get tangled in the pet's coat. A wire-bottomed cage is usually a far better bet, from the standpoint of both the animal's health and the owner's convenience. The floor should be made of 12-gauge welded wire and can either rest on a sawdust-filled tray, from which it can be lifted, or be suspended over an easily cleaned, removable tray. All types of cages should be cleaned at least every other day. This will prevent the buildup of any obnoxious odors. For dryness, the floor of the cage should be at least 9 inches above the ground. For the owner, it is even better to raise it to 30 inches, a more convenient working height.

The wire used on the side of the cage should be at least 14-gauge. The frame can be either metal or wood — 5-inch boards will ensure strength. To make it easy to get the rabbit in and out of the cage, or a nest if you're breeding your pets, a door should be provided at least 20 inches wide. For a doe that has been bred, you may wish to attach a second hutch with a hinged door that can be opened up to double the space when she has a litter.

If the cage is kept indoors, it should not be placed directly against the wall. A gap of at least 9½ inches should be left, for sufficient ventilation. However, since rabbits are highly resistant to cold and it actually improves their coats, it is quite practical to keep the cage outdoors all year round if you wish. With a wire-bottomed cage, there is no chance of the floor becoming flooded. A roof is a necessity in an outdoor cage to protect the pet not only from snow and rain but from direct sunlight in the summer, for rabbits are quite sensitive to heat. Part of the cage can be left open to sunlight. In colder climates, it is important to make the sides and back of the cage solid to provide protection from the wind. For additional protection, give the rabbit a nest box (see page 245).

OUTDOOR FREEDOM The removable wire-bottomed cage that rests on a stand is ideal if you wish to give your rabbit a chance to nibble at fresh grass on the lawn to supplement its diet. It should be regularly moved around the yard to avoid overgrazing.

If you allow your pet out of the cage in a fenced yard, remember that rabbits are expert diggers. Unless your fence has been buried to a depth of at least two feet under the soil, the rabbit must constantly be watched to prevent its escaping.

No matter how close an eye you keep on it, the rabbit should not be allowed out on an unenclosed lawn. You'll be providing an irresistible temptation for the neighborhood dogs, and sudden death can strike before you're even aware of the danger. The very lack of excitability that suits the domestic rabbit so well to the role of pet was gained by breeding out the alertness that serves to protect its wild relatives.

INDOOR FREEDOM Giving a rabbit the run of the house is not the unsanitary proposition it might seem on first thought. These animals are quite clean by nature and at least as easily housebroken as cats. Instinctively, your pet will pick a special corner as its bathroom. A low box placed there and filled with kitty litter will prevent odors if it is regularly cleaned. Put newspapers under it to protect the floor. You may need to place young rabbits in the box a few times to help them learn. A word of caution before you give your rabbit the run of the house: do not simply ignore it because it seems harmless. Left to their own devices, rabbits are quite capable of finding trouble. Among other things, they like to chew on the insulation surrounding electrical wiring, a good means of getting electrocuted.

On the subject of sanitation, it might be well to mention one habit of rabbits that some people unreasonably find offensive: coprophagy or pseudorumination. Many rabbits will eat their own pellets as they emerge from the anus, though only the soft ones that have passed through the digestive tract a single time. This is a perfectly natural trait, comparable to cud-chewing in cows, and is an important means of obtaining vitamin B complex. Fortunately, rabbits seem to have an instinctive modesty and usually do this only during the night and in the early morning.

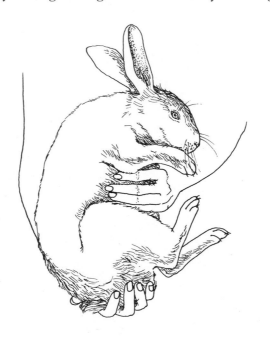

HANDLING AND HOLDING Obviously, in the process of getting your rabbit in and out of its cage it is going to receive a great deal of handling. This is all to the good and will make it a better pet as it gets accustomed to you, so long as it is done *properly*. There is a widespread and dangerous misunderstanding about how rabbits should be picked up. Despite all you may have heard, rabbits were not given ears to serve as handles. *They should never be picked up by the ears.* Besides causing the rabbit pain, it will break the cartilage in the ears and cause them to droop unattractively.

To lift a rabbit, place one hand under its rump to support its weight. The other hand should be used to prevent its struggling. One method is to place your hand under the animal's abdomen, beneath its front legs; or you could grasp the loose skin between its shoulder blades; or lightly grip the ears close to the head, the forefinger between them with the thumb and second finger each serving to contain an ear. Carry the animal against your chest facing you with a hand under it for support. If you hold it gently but firmly, the animal will feel secure and will rapidly become accustomed to human handling.

TOENAILS Despite their obvious advantages, wire-bottomed cages do tend to create at least one problem. Lack of contact with a solid surface eliminates the friction that would normally serve to wear down the rabbit's toenails. This can be dangerous if the rabbit kicks, and sharp nails should be regularly trimmed to within ¼ inch of the quick. Either side-cutting pliers or toenail clippers can be used. If the toenail is held toward a light the quick will be easily visible.

COAT As do most thickly furred animals, rabbits shed seasonally. Regular brushing, particularly as the weather warms or if the animal is kept indoors, will not only keep loose hairs to a minimum but will also improve the condition of the rabbit's coat and skin.

FEEDING Giving your rabbit a proper diet, never a serious problem, has been made even simpler today by prepared foods that contain all the essential nutritional elements. Many of these food pellets also include Aureomycin to help prevent infection. A proper green pellet for rabbits should contain hay, but if you are unable to obtain a product that does, supplement the prepared food with clover hay or alfalfa without the stems. Do not buy pellets in large quantities. Their nutritional value rapidly diminishes in storage; therefore, they should be used promptly.

Since rabbits will regulate themselves in eating, you should always have food available in the cage.

While the pellets will give your pet its normal requirements for protein and grains, it is good to vary its diet occasionally for added assurance that all nutritional needs are satisfied. Oats, wheat, barley, bran, wheat germ, ground corn, and dry bread will supply the rabbit's grain needs. Proteinaceous foods it should receive include soybeans, peanuts, and linseed. Changes in diet should be made gradually in order to avoid upsetting the animal's digestive system. For the same reason, when buying a rabbit you should make sure to find out what its diet has been and continue it before making any changes.

FRESH VEGETABLES AND FRUITS. Particularly in hot weather, give your rabbit fresh foods that have a high water content twice a week. These include carrots, potatoes, apples, lettuce, dandelions, and plantain. In addition, the cage should always contain a piece of salt brick where the animal can easily reach it. This is available at both pet and feed stores.

WATER. A constant supply of fresh, clean water is also essential. Hamster bottles are fine for this pupose because they eliminate spillage. The bottle should be checked daily. Patented feeders are available for use with the food pellets too, but homemade containers for both food and water serve just as well. An easily cleaned heavy crock that cannot be turned over is excellent for watering. Glazed earthenware bowls with in-turned lips to prevent spilling are also satisfactory. If a tin can is used, it should be anchored to the corners of the cage. A convenient feeding arrangement is a built-in food trough with a screen bottom (rabbits dislike dusty food) that can be filled through a hopper from outside the cage.

the home clinic
STOCKING A MEDICINE CABINET

rectal thermometer
small, sharp scissors
cotton balls
cotton ear swabs
hydrogen peroxide, 20 percent solution
antiseptic dusting powder

HOW TO TAKE TEMPERATURE

For the most part, the health of a rabbit can be described as an all-or-nothing proposition. They are cautious animals and do not tend to be subject to the minor illnesses common among more active species, such as dogs and cats. Their diet virtually eliminates the possibility of their consuming poisons — if a rabbit did consume posion, death would be a virtual certainty.

Challenges for the home diagnostician are quite limited. Neither pulse nor heartbeat are important indicators for any of the common complaints. Temperature, however, can serve as a danger sign for some of the diseases that will be discussed.

The normal temperature of a domestic rabbit is 102.5°F. (plus or minus 1°). This can be measured easily with a rectal thermometer. Holding the rabbit firmly but gently on a table, insert the lubricated (with Vaseline — or, if there's no Vaseline, salad oil will do) thermometer in the anus to approximately 1 inch. This should not disturb the animal or cause struggling. After two or three minutes, extract the thermometer and read the temperature.

MEDICATION

The forms of internal medication used to treat common conditions in rabbits eliminate the necessity of administering pills or force-feeding. They are given in such a manner that the rabbit will consume them as part of its normal diet.

optional operations

While both spaying female and castrating male rabbits are possible means of controlling fertility, the desirability of doing so is questionable in normal circumstances. Adult males and females should be kept separated and be brought together solely for the purpose of breeding. As it is totally impractical to allow these pets the freedom given dogs and cats, the possibility of an unplanned conception is virtually nonexistent.

first aid

EMERGENCIES

Again, the nature of the animal, for better or for worse, severely limits the possibilities of an owner's assisting a pet rabbit in an emergency that would qualify as acute. If the rabbit has been seriously injured, the chances of recovery are usually negligible. The obligation of the humane owner in such a case is to provide the rabbit with as quick and painless a death as possible by taking it to a veterinarian, who will probably inject an overdose of an anesthetic.

WOUNDS AND BITES

Again, degree is the prime determinant in what can and should be done. In the case of the minor scratches and bites that result from the battles between males, treatment is designed primarily to prevent the possibility of secondary infections. If these are allowed to develop, the effects can be serious enough to cause death.

Trim away the fur around the wound so that it will not become matted, then cleanse it with diluted hydrogen peroxide — equal parts water and hydrogen peroxide. Apply antiseptic dusting powder. Do not bandage.

BONE INJURIES

In a light-boned animal such as the rabbit, simple "greenstick" fractures are most unlikely. Any force powerful enough to break a bone will almost invariably result in a compound fracture with the bone badly shattered; there is limited hope of restoring the animal to a normal condition.

Nonetheless, you will undoubtedly want to take your pet to a veterinarian to determine the seriousness of the injury. The rabbit may be in a state of collapse after a severe trauma; you should apply a temporary splint to avoid accidentally moving the injured limb. Simply lay a short stick alongside the injured limb and bind them together with bandages wrapped firmly but not so tightly as to interfere with circulation. The bandages should be of uniform tightness along the splint to minimize swelling.

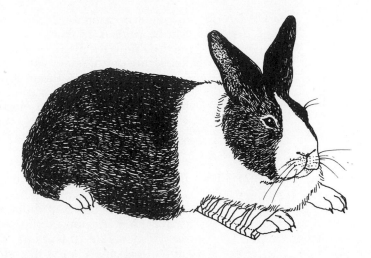

HEAT STROKE   Heat stroke in rabbits is a not uncommon type of emergency in which your prompt help could be of enormous importance. This is usually a result of hot, humid weather and poorly ventilated cages. Rabbits suffering from the effects will lie on their sides, breathing rapidly. A rabbit in this condition should immediately be immersed in a bucket of lukewarm water, up to its head, in order to lower its body temperature. To avoid the problem, bring your rabbit's cage indoors in such weather. A wire-bottomed cage outdoors can be sprinkled with water from the hose.

INTENSE COLD   If, by some accident, your animal is exposed to intense cold or a high wind outdoors in an improperly protected cage, bring it into a normally warm room.

POISONOUS PLANTS   Although your rabbit may not come into contact with the plants that are poisonous and sometimes fatal, or eat them if it does, you should be aware of and watch out for these: blue and scarlet pimpernel, anemone, aconite, hemlock, belladonna, meadow saffron, foxglove, mustard, poppy, primula, buttercup, and Saint-John's-wort. Also, parsley and chervil may harm a mother's milk.

parasites
COCCIDIOSIS   Rabbits are subject to several types of internal parasites. Coccidiosis, important to those who raise rabbits commercially for meat or fur, is rare among pets because the opportunities for its spread are limited. Nevertheless, there is a possibility a newly purchased pet may be infested.

Coccidiosis occurs in two forms: in the liver and in the intestines. If the liver is attacked by these protozoan parasites, the symptoms are diarrhea, difficult breathing, and a rough coat. Young rabbits, which are especially susceptible, will fail to gain weight at a normal rate. This infection must be diagnosed by a veterinarian but you will administer the medicine prescribed by mixing it into the animal's food and water. At the same time, sanitary arrangements must be intensified to make doubly sure the pet's cage is kept dry and clean.

Intestinal coccidiosis can show up in rabbits no matter how well cared for they might be. The symptoms include failure to grow, difficult breathing, as well as a potbelly. Diagnosis should be left to a veterinarian, who will prescribe the proper medicine.

TAPEWORMS Tapeworm infection is far more likely in pet rabbits than coccidiosis, for this can be picked up from the family dog or cat. Check the appropriate sections in this book for symptoms and treatment of other animals in the house, and keep dogs and cats away from the rabbit's food, water, cage, or any items regularly used with them. With the exception of cysts, or warbles, under the skin — surgically removable — the symptoms of tapeworms in rabbits are far less obvious than in dogs and cats. But should the other animals be infested, your veterinarian should examine the rabbit as well, to prevent the establishment of a cycle in which the animals pass the parasites back and forth.

EAR MITES Rabbits are bothered by two types of mites. The most common are ear mites, and the symptoms are easily recognized. The animal will shake its head, flap its ears, and scratch at them with its hind legs. These tiny insects are more than mere annoyances: they weaken the rabbit's health and make it susceptible to secondary infections. Thick brown crusts accumulate in the ears and must be cleaned out with cotton soaked in hydrogen peroxide diluted to half strength with water. While the veterinarian will do this initially at the time the diagnosis is made, there must be follow-up and you will be expected to do this job at the time you administer the medicine, which is swabbed into the ear. The rabbit's cage must also be cleaned and disinfected.

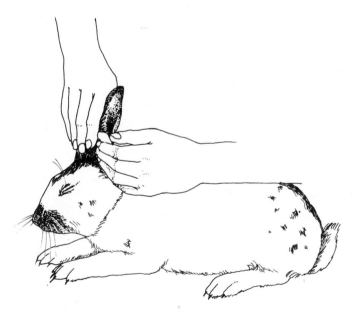

MANGE MITES Mange mites are far less common but a great deal more serious than ear mites, for the treatment is much more difficult. Commercial breeders will automatically destroy all but the most valuable animals who pick up these parasites. The symptoms are constant scratching and loss of hair on the chin, nose, head, and around the eyes and the bases of the ears. This condition is transmissible to humans, as well as to other pets, and should be brought to a veterinarian's attention immediately for diagnosis and treatment. Wash your hands after handling the animal.

TULAREMIA Tularemia, or rabbit fever, is most unlikely in a pet rabbit, and deserves discussion only because some potential owners may have heard of it and become alarmed at the possibility. This can be contracted by humans and is potentially fatal but is fortunately rare. The problem is that the symptoms are extremely difficult to detect in rabbits. The only clear symptom would be a sudden and inexplicable death, for the onset of tularemia is sometimes rapid and virulent in animals. Should this happen, the dead pet must be taken to a veterinarian for autopsy. If evidence of infection is discovered, any humans who have been in contact with the animal should see a physician immediately.

disease

While they pose a problem to the commercial breeder, infectious diseases are relatively uncommon among pet rabbits. The primary cause of troubles for pets is, probably, the owner's negligence. A newly purchased animal, however, might already be infected.

VACCINATIONS

Certain vaccinations are available and this is an important preventive measure to be taken after the rabbit is twenty-five days old. Following the nature of the diseases, these vaccinations are seasonal: enterotoxemia in the spring; myxomatosis in the summer; pasteurellosis in the fall; and mucoid enteritis in the winter.

SYMPTOMS OF DISEASE

The general signs of illness in a rabbit include listlessness, rubbing of its eyes or nose, labored breathing or shortness of breath, sneezing, and coughing. Watch for abscesses or sores on its head or body; swollen or discharging eyes or nose; drooping or swollen ears; loss, thinning, or matting of hair; discharge from or inflammation of the sex organs; or an abnormal temperature. Since many of these symptoms are indicative of more than one disease, read through the symptoms listed after each to identify which matches best your animal's condition.

MYXOMATOSIS

This viral infection is limited to coastal Oregon and California. Outbreaks occur every eight to ten years in the months between May and August, as it is spread by mosquitoes. A vaccine is available to immunize animals.

Symptoms include conjunctivitis (inflamed eyes) and a milky discharge from the eyes; swollen eyelids, nose, lips, and ears; drooping ears; swollen, inflamed anus; nasal discharge; labored breathing; and high fever.

Little can be done for an animal that has contracted myxomatosis, and fatalities are very high.

RABBIT POX

The mortality rate is high. Smallpox vaccine will give rabbits an immunity to this viral disease.

Symptoms include fever, discharge from nose and eyes, and skin rash.

PASTEURELLOSIS

Pregnant does are particularly susceptible to this bacterial disease. Infected wounds on males that have been fighting are often fatal within forty-eight hours. Antibiotics can be effective, but the prognosis is generally poor. The rabbit's cage, bowls, and other equipment must be disinfected before they are used again.

Symptoms include snuffles, sneezes, and coughs with a thin, puslike discharge from the nostrils; and the fur on the inside forelegs will be matted from wiping the nose. Abscessed wounds from fights, inflammation of the sex organs with a thick, yellow-gray discharge of pus from the vagina or penis, and sores or chancres on the penis are also symptoms.

PNEUMONIA
This frequently occurs as a secondary infection in rabbits which have pasteurellosis. Drafty, damp, poorly cleaned cages and a lack of good bedding are often to blame. The rabbit is often dead within four days. Antibiotics, however, can be quite effective in fighting pneumonia.

Symptoms include high fever (104°F.), shortness of breath, diarrhea, and listlessness.

PSEUDOTUBERCULOSIS
Humans can contract this disease and it is standard practice to kill rather than attempt to treat rabbits that have contracted it.

Symptoms include listlessness, thinness, shortness of breath, and difficulty breathing.

CONJUNCTIVITIS (WEEPY EYE)
The most frequent victims are mature males and young rabbits. The disease is relatively easily treated with antibiotic eye ointments, however.

Symptoms include inflamed eyes, eye discharge, and rubbing of eyes.

VENT DISEASE
This venereal disease of rabbits is quite similar to syphilis but cannot be transmitted to humans. Like syphilis, it can be effectively treated with penicillin administered subcutaneously.

Symptoms include sores or chancres on the sex organs, which may be covered with heavy scabs. Sores may also appear on the lips and eyelids.

HUTCH BURN
The symptoms are similar to vent disease, with which this infection is often confused. The cause, however, is totally different: owner neglect. Hutch burn is a result of the animal's having been exposed to urine in a cage that has been allowed to remain dirty and wet. Once it has occured, penicillin ointment should be applied to the lesions.

MUCOID ENTERITIS
Antibiotics are sometimes effective in treating this often fatal disease. Its cause is unknown.

Symptoms include subnormal temperature, listlessness, diarrhea, and difficulty breathing. The coat will be rough, the ears will droop, and the eyes will appear squinty.

RINGWORM
This highly contagious fungus disease can be spread both to humans and to other pets. It does yield to treatment, though the process is long and bothersome. After diagnosis, using either an ultraviolet lamp to examine the lesions or a microscope for cultures, the veterinarian will prescribe oral medication, ointments, and special shampoos. Return visits will be required.

Symptoms include loss or thinning of fur. Circular patches of skin will be reddened and covered with flaky, white, dry material.

WET DEWLAP
This disease is found in breeds characterized by double chins, loose rolls of skin under their necks called dewlaps. If the dewlap becomes soaked when the animal drinks from its bowl, inflammation of the skin results. Water bottles prevent this problem.

Symptoms include loss of hair under the neck and reddened skin.

SORE HOCKS
Bacteria on wet, dirty floors may infect minor sores or scrapes on the rabbit's hock, the leg just above the foot. Sulfonamide powder and pencillin injections are effective treatments.

does and bunnies Many parents find rabbits useful in teaching young children their first lessons in the nature of reproduction. Problems are rare, and most does make excellent mothers. For this purpose, you would probably be wisest to buy a doe who has already conceived.

But if you already have a doe and wish to breed her, this too is a relatively simple matter. Sexual maturity in the smaller breeds arrives at around five months, in the medium-sized around seven months, and among the giants between nine and twelve months.

MATING There is no regular estrus cycle in rabbits. Does are receptive to males as much as 75 percent of the time, and ovulation is stimulated by mating. The only real way to determine whether a doe is interested is by making the attempt.

Breeding should always take place in the male's cage. If you put him in with the doe, he is far too likely to be distracted by the strange setting and spend his time exploring. If the doe is receptive, the animals will mate within five minutes. If not, remove the doe and try again later. Does are sometimes selective, however, and if there is another male handy it is possible she might respond to him.

PREGNANCY Normal gestation is thirty-one to thirty-two days. By the seventeenth day, it is possible to determine whether the doe is pregnant: holding her by the ears and skin between her shoulders with your right hand, carefully feel her abdomen with your left; if she has conceived, you will easily detect the marble-shaped fetuses. False pregnancies do take place and if your test reveals nothing, the doe can be mated again on the eighteenth day after the first attempt.

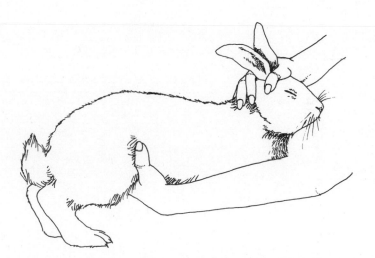

NEST BOX. The first essential is a nest box. Any wooden box about 12 inches high and wide and 20 inches long will serve for small or medium-sized rabbits. To prevent crowding, giants need somewhat larger quarters, so long as they are small enough to ensure warmth. Old apple boxes or nail kegs make excellent nests.

The bottom of the entrance, placed at one end, should be 6 inches above the floor of the nest, to keep the young rabbits in while allowing the mother freedom of movement. If the bunnies get out too soon, the doe will abandon them. A removable or hinged top will be convenient for cleaning and for inspecting the litter when it has arrived. Drill several large holes in the bottom of the floor for ventilation and drainage.

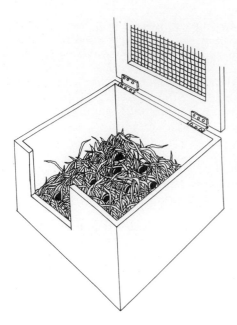

The box should be half filled with straw or wood shavings and cleaned once a week. Several days before the litter is due to arrive, it should be given fresh bedding. Around three to four days before she gives birth, the doe will make her own nest, lining it with fur she pulls from her breast. At this time she should be disturbed as little as is possible.

ISOLATION. When she goes into labor, the doe will retreat into her nest box, and she should be left alone for two to three days before any attempt is made to inspect the litter. If she is worried during this period, it could well cause her to eat her young. When you do check, remove her from the cage. If any of the young are dead or deformed, they should be disposed of immediately.

BUNNIES. The size of litters varies but will normally range from six to ten. The bunnies are born hairless and do not open their eyes until the ninth day after birth. By three weeks, they are old enough to get over the door and come out of the nest. If you have provided a second cage, this is the point at which it should be opened up to allow them extra space to roam.

While it is possible to wean the young rabbits as early as the fourth week, it is advisable to leave them with the mother until they are two months old, when she will take care of weaning herself. While she is nursing, the mother's diet can be supplemented with fresh leafy greens. When the young begin to feed themselves, they may receive rabbit food.

As mentioned earlier (see page 236), by the time the young rabbits are three months old they should be segregated by sex.

further readings   FAIVRE, M. I. *How to Raise Rabbits for Fun and Profit*. Chicago, Nelson-Hall, 1973.
NAETHER, C. A. *The Book of the Domestic Rabbit*. New York, David McKay, 1967.

Squirrels and chipmunks

LESTER E. FISHER, D.V.M.

Although charming pets for some people, squirrels are not for everyone. No matter how early they are acquired, they remain essentially wild animals whose instincts, throughout their lives, keep them in a perpetual state of alert to potential danger. They are far from the ideal pet for children. A squirrel will never tolerate hugging, rarely petting. Simple holding is a threat, because it restricts the animal's ability to flee in an instant. If squeezed inadvertently even the smallest, shyest, most gentle squirrels will automatically retaliate with a bite that can pierce a finger, nail and all.

The squirrel will do little to accommodate to you. You either keep it in an adequate cage — or you decide to accommodate to it, in order to really get to know the animal. The owner who allows these animals outside their cages in the home must be prepared to pay a price in chewed, scratched furniture — and drapes, which are by the squirrel's definition its territory. Housebreaking, except in the most literal sense of breaking a house, is impossible.

While a squirrel might obviously enjoy playing *on* people as if they were trees, it takes no delight in playing *with* them. This kind of sport will not endear the owner to guests wearing nylon hose, and bare legs simply mean the squirrel must, and will, find something else to dig its claws into as it charges upward.

And yet, with the varied habits and personalities of the different species, you might well find an animal ideally suited to your particular life-style. Take the working couple, for example. Wouldn't a nocturnal animal such as a lovely, gentle flying squirrel make an ideal pet? It sleeps all day while they are at their respective jobs. When they return home, it is ready and eager to get out and soar gracefully from room to room. And it is affectionate, delighting in climbing into pockets where it can curl up into a soft fur ball.

If acquired while very young, some squirrels adapt well to captivity. They are by nature hardy and the care they require presents no great difficulties. Disease is rare, and they are both cautious and nimble enough to avoid accidents.

different species

There are far too many species of squirrel in the United States alone to attempt to cover here. Briefly, we'll look at the most widespread and numerous of these, those most likely and best suited to become pets. This will show something of the diversity of personalities and illustrate what should be done to keep the different types of squirrel in good health. Different as their behavior might be, the care needed by one species of tree squirrel is the same as that needed by another. The chipmunk is distinguished in many ways from the true ground squirrels, yet the kind of treatment that is best for it will be equally good for other ground dwellers. The two species of flying squirrels have identical needs that must be satisfied if they are to remain healthy and happy.

GRAY SQUIRRELS   As they make the rounds of park benches, sitting up without the slightest sign of shame to ask for a handout, these most familiar of our native tree squirrels prove just how misleading it can be to try to categorize animals. A large part of their lives is spent on the ground, both looking for food and finding places to bury the surplus of the moment for the lean times ahead. The tree is there for nesting, rearing the young, and as a retreat in danger. The earth is for activities certainly no less important.

No squirrel has adapted better to man's invasion of its environment than the eastern gray, the dominant species within the genus Sciurus, animals with greater or lesser physical differences but basically similar in their personalities and habits. The prime reason for their success in living side-by-side with man is personality. Among tree squirrels, the grays are comparatively easygoing types, not so quickly given to panic but quite ready to put up a defense if pushed too far. Some, in fact, actually become aggressive, suddenly launching unprovoked attacks on humans. Though they grow to no more than 18 inches in length, half of which is bushy tail, an attack by an animal with razor-sharp teeth in a jaw powerful enough to open the shells of black walnuts is nothing to be shrugged off lightly.

The likelihood of such physical attacks is minimized if you get a gray young enough. They often prove to be very much one-person pets and very infrequently attack their owners. Interestingly, some assaults reported to take place in parks are believed by certain naturalists to be characteristic of pets that have been abandoned, rather than animals that grew up wild.

It was the impressive tail, incidentally, that gave this genus its name. *Sciurus*, Latin for "squirrel," had its own roots in Greek: *skia* (shadow) and *oura* (tail), or shade-tail, because the animal holds his brush up as though it were an umbrella.

In appearance, the gray is a handsome animal with his dark salt-and-pepper to tweed brown to black back and light gray undersurface. The interesting shadings result from the fact that each guard hair is made up of bands of different colors. The western gray, whose range picks up in the Dakotas and extends to the Pacific Coast, is distinguishable from its eastern relatives only by its larger size, ranging up to 22 inches in length.

FOX SQUIRRELS   A shyer member of the genus, the fox squirrel, has retreated from large parts of the heavily inhabited Northeast. Oddly, however, fox squirrels have been successfully introduced to parks in cities. Largest of the tree squirrels, the fox reaches a full 2 feet. This heavily built animal comes in a number of striking color variations — gray, buff, or black with white ears and tail. Like the eastern gray, its range ends in the Dakotas to the west. While the gray prefers low timberlands, the fox squirrel is found in country with alternating groves and open land.

But color variation is common in this genus. Melanistic (black) gray squirrels occur frequently, and albinos have even become dominant in some isolated communities. Among the most dramatic of the species are the Albert's and kaibab squirrels found in the Rocky Mountains, with bobcat tufts of long hair tipping their ears, reddish backs, and white or off-white tails.

RED SQUIRRELS   These, the smallest of the native tree squirrels, belong to the genus Tamiasciurus. Very obviously, the red considers size of little importance. Pugnacious creatures, they haven't the slightest hesitation in attacking larger grays indiscreet enough to invade their territory, and invariably put the intruder to flight. These chases rarely if ever lead to actual combat, however. If the gray is trapped on the end of a branch, the red will keep its distance, content to scold. While human interlopers need not fear actual physical assault, they too receive ample attention when they enter the range of these watchdogs of the forest. The stream of insults that follows has earned the red such names as chatterbox, barking squirrel, and boomer.

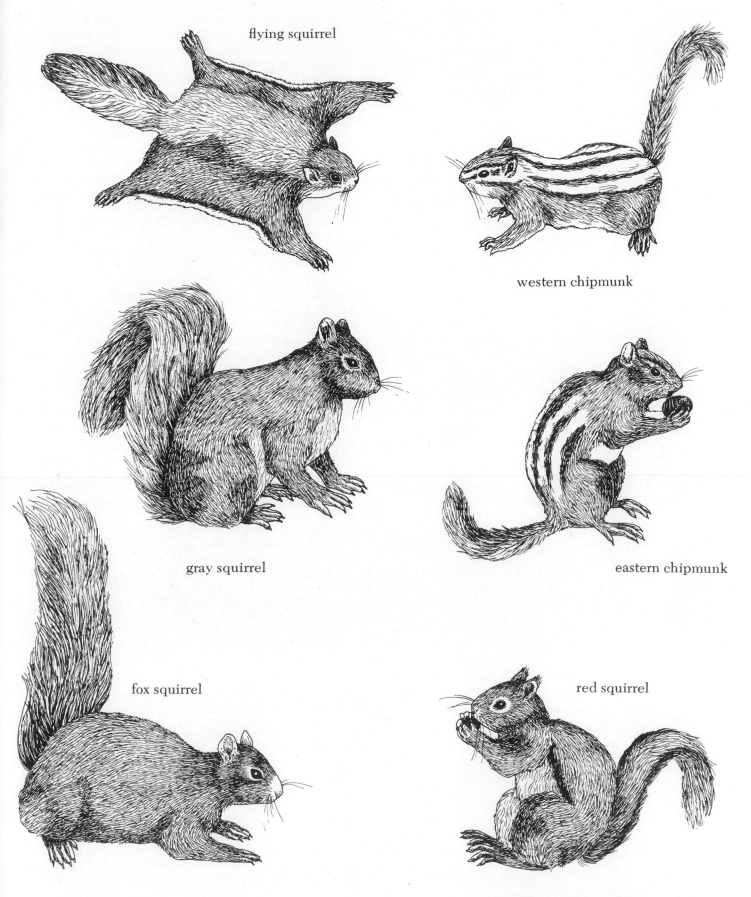

flying squirrel

western chipmunk

gray squirrel

eastern chipmunk

fox squirrel

red squirrel

Eastern reds range up to 14 inches in length, 5 inches of which is tail, and weigh no more than 11 ounces. The somewhat smaller Douglas red squirrel, or chickaree, of the West, is distinguished primarily by color. The general appearance is a rusty red with a gray vest.

These animals are far more excitable than the gray squirrels and are therefore not so easily adaptable to the role of pet. In captivity, tree squirrels have lived up to twelve years.

CHIPMUNKS   Chipmunks, the most widespread of our native ground squirrels, have at times made gentle, hardy pets. There are two groups of these handsome little animals: the eastern chipmunk (*Tamias striatus*), which ranges from the Atlantic Coast to the Dakotas; and the western, or least, chipmunk (genus Eutamias) with a range extending from the Great Lakes to southern Alaska. There are around sixteen species of the latter, distributed through most of the western states.

The basic colors of the eastern chipmunk are a rusty or brownish red on the back and light gray to white undersurface. The back is marked with five dark brown to black stripes, extending to the base of the tail. These alternate with two gray and two white stripes. The eye is offset with a dark stripe, outlined above and below by buff stripes. While it has a proportionately long tail, the chipmunk's lacks the bushiness of tree squirrels'. Eastern chipmunks grow to between 8 and 12 inches.

The western chipmunk tends to be smaller, rarely reaching 9 inches, and is more slender. Its color is more grayish than that of the eastern species. The stripes, while they maintain the same pattern of alternating dark and light, are thinner and more closely placed.

Chipmunks are more easily tamed than tree squirrels. Members of the western species are less shy and adapt more readily to life in captivity. As pets, chipmunks have lived as long as seven years.

FLYING SQUIRRELS   Flying squirrels, of the genus Glaucomys, are the most interesting and, with their large, soft eyes, possibly the most attractive of our native squirrels. Furthermore, despite the drawback of their being noctural, some of these gentle, sociable animals make excellent pets.

These animals do not actually fly despite their name, but glide from branch to branch or to the ground, covering distances as great as 125 feet. This is made possible not by wings, as in the case of the bat, but by expansible, furred membranes that run from the wrists of the forelegs to the hind feet and then to the base of the tail. When the squirrel leaps into space, it extends its legs, drawing the membranes taut and giving them the surface area necessary to soar. The flattened, featherlike tail is used for guidance. As the squirrel nears a tree trunk it wants to land on, it swoops upward at the last instant, making contact with all four feet. In the forest, you can hear the thumps as they land.

There are two native species, the northern flying squirrel — which ranges in the East from Labrador as far south as Georgia, and in the West from Alaska down to southern California — and the southern — which overlaps its cousin's range southward and eastward from Minnesota.

The larger northern flying squirrel grows up to 14½ inches in length, and weighs up to 6½ ounces. The southern does not exceed 10¼ inches and weighs no more than 4 ounces. The tail is almost half the animal's length. The undersurface of both species is a gray to cream white. While the upper surface of the northern flying squirrel is a soft, dark gray, that of the southern may range to a reddish brown. Pet flying squirrels have been known to live up to eight years.

Although the northern chipmunks retreat to their burrows for the winter, none of the squirrel family truly hibernates. In captivity, with a continuing supply of food, these animals should remain active throughout the year.

preventive medicine

FINDING A PET

None of these animals breed readily in captivity, so there is no true commercial supply. The prospective owner, therefore, must either rely on luck — such as finding a foundling or knowing someone whose animals have successfully mated — or secure a rarely available tame adult. The latter are to be approached with caution. Obviously, they are former pets and there is automatically the question of why they were given up. In the case of a red, inclined to be very much a one-person pet, it would be almost impossible to fit it into a new home.

Ideally, you should look for a squirrel no older than six weeks. Red squirrels are born in May and June, eastern grays around the end of January and in mid-June, western grays in the late winter or early spring, flying squirrels in late March and early April, and chipmunks usually in April.

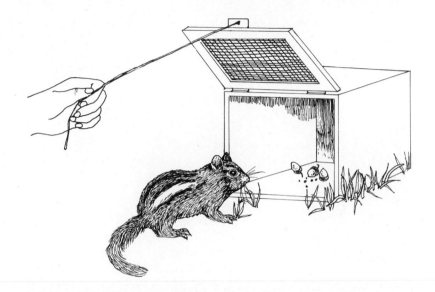

For securing chipmunks, traps are one method and the most suitable are the box variety. These are simply made with a drop door, which is triggered remotely by a string once the animal has been lured in. Precise age is not so crucial a factor, though youth is desirable and it would be best to trap your pet during its first days of exploration outside the nest. Grass seeds, berries, or acorns can serve as bait. Patience is a necessity.

The bait should be placed at the far end of the cage so that there is no possibility of the animal's being hit by the door as it descends. Regardless of species, any new animal that shows a tendency to bite should be promptly returned to the place from which it was taken.

HOUSING

Until the baby becomes active and shows that it is ready to begin inspecting its new home, housing is primarily a matter of protecting it from chills. Any small, strong, dry box will serve adequately if it is lined with clean, soft cloth such as flannel, or dry grass. Change regularly for cleanliness.

When it does start getting around, you can purchase a cage suitable for an adult squirrel at a pet store. If you plan to build your own, remember that these are gnawing animals; unless you plan on giving the squirrel the freedom of the house, you must be prepared for escape attempts. These can be forestalled by covering the wooden supports with wire or metal. Use 14-gauge welded wire for the sides and top. The bottom may be cut from heavy plywood and given sides that rise to 18 inches.

Squirrels need sufficient space in which to move around and to exercise. For a tree squirrel, a cage 6 feet long by 4 feet high by 3 feet wide would not be excessive. In it, place a tree limb large enough to extend from floor to ceiling and anchor it firmly at top and bottom. Chipmunks can have proportionately smaller cages and do not need a limb to climb on. An exercise wheel, however, is extremely important.

The floor of the cage can be covered with wood shavings, leaf mold, or soil to a depth of at least 1 foot. The covering should be changed at least twice a year. If leaf mold or earth are used, they should be dampened but not soaked whenever they become dry. This serves to prevent parasites. The cage should be kept where it will get sunlight in the morning.

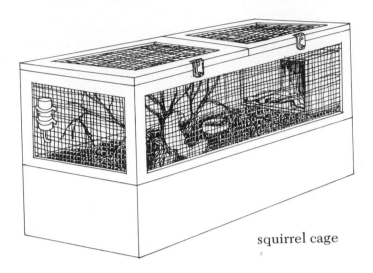

squirrel cage

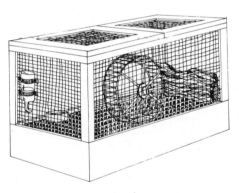

chipmunk cage

Facilities and materials for a nest must be provided. For tree and flying squirrels, the nest can be a wooden box with adequate space for the animal or animals to sleep comfortably. This must be raised off the cage floor, either on a shelf or bracketed to the side of the cage. One end should be open. A hollow log makes an ideal nest for a chipmunk.

The animal will construct its nest from the materials you put in the cage. These can vary, including coarse shavings, shredded paper, kapok, grass, and soft hay. Because it catches on the squirrel's claws, no form of floss should be used.

If your squirrel or squirrels are regularly allowed the run of the house, cages need not be so large. A large, ceiling-high limb with sturdy branches should be firmly mounted in one corner to give tree squirrels a place to climb and scamper. Cages for tree squirrels and chipmunks should be left open during the day and provided with entrances that make it easy for the animal to scamper in and out at will for food and water when it is let out.

While tree squirrels and chipmunks can be kept permanently caged, there would be no point in keeping flying squirrels if this were your intention. The animal could live nothing remotely resembling a normal life.

Tree squirrels are territorial and it is rare that one will accept others either in its cage or in the same house unless they are litter mates. Chipmunks, while they live individually, are much more tolerant of others of their kind, and several can usually be kept together. Flying squirrels, on the other hand, are sociable creatures who normally share their nests in the wild and are actually happier in a group.

GROOMING   A pet that cannot be held is hardly likely to be cooperative in any attempts at grooming. Fortunately, squirrels are conscientious about grooming themselves, and no efforts are needed.

Despite the discomfort they might cause when the squirrel decides that you are a walking tree, its claws should never be trimmed. These are essential to the animal's activities and you would be endangering it by doing so.

In one respect you can aid your squirrel in its own personal grooming:

there should be items in the cage that make it possible to sharpen its teeth. Rock salt, which can be purchased at pet or food stores, is ideal, because it is also desirable from a dietary standpoint. Hard-shelled nuts are good for larger squirrels but of little use to chipmunks or flying squirrels, which do not regularly feed on them.

FEEDING Food should always be at hand, particularly for the rapidly growing younger animals. Squirrels and chipmunks regulate their own diets, according to need. The ideal staple diet, both nutritionally and from the standpoint of convenience and expense, is hamster pellets. These should be supplemented with fruits, including berries, apple or orange slices, and melon seeds and rinds.

Fresh greens, such as spinach or lettuce, are also necessary to the animal's diet. Any kind of seeds and grain will be welcome. Tree squirrels are especially fond of mushrooms and will take them either fresh or dried.

Occasionally, larger squirrels should be given a few nuts. For economy's sake, gather acorns from beneath the nearest oak rather than pay the inflated prices of luxury nuts. Hard-shelled nuts are actually of more value for tooth-sharpening than nutrition.

WATER. There should always be a supply of fresh, clean water in the cage. The best means of providing it is with a hamster bottle, which can be obtained at any pet store.

TRAINING In the strict sense of the word, squirrels cannot be trained. They can, however, learn things when there is a proper reward. For example, they will delight in investigating your pockets if you customarily carry a treat in them. The smaller chipmunks and flying squirrels will learn to eat sitting on your hand. Bear in mind, while attempting to train your squirrel in this fashion, that it will have no tolerance whatsoever for being teased. Holding a nut too firmly for the pet to take, or grasped in a fist, will earn a painful bite.

FLYING SQUIRRELS AND OPEN WATER In general, squirrels are extremely cautious creatures, alert to all possibilities of danger. Thus, there is little possibility of their causing injury to themselves. There is one strange exception, however. Though they are unable to swim, flying squirrels are extremely fond of water. Any open water in a home in which there are flying squirrels is an invitation to drowning.

illness and injury

Obviously, with an animal that cannot readily be held, there is little that the layman can do in the event of illness or injury. Even such routine examinations as taking temperature or checking for fleas require professional care. Serious traumas are almost inevitably the cause of death, for the animal's nervous system is incapable of handling the strain. Death from shock is swift and, fortunately, painless.

The best that can be done is to remain alert to symptoms of illness. These are:

Bald patches or severe loss of hair (this does not include spring shedding of the winter coat)

Sniffling or running nose

Running eyes

Diarrhea

Scratching

All of these should be signals to take the animal to a veterinarian. There is simply no sense in getting badly bitten attempting to diagnose and treat problems yourself. While we are on the subject of both biting and illness, it might be well to point out that though squirrels are subject to rabies, no case has ever been reported of a human contracting rabies from a squirrel bite.

Squirrels are incredibly hardy animals with a strong resistance to infections and, living in a home, the opportunities of their picking up any transmissible disease are extremely limited.

mating and babies

Mating squirrels is largely a matter of determining whether they are willing to share quarters and are of opposite sexes — then leaving it in their hands (or paws) from that point. Sexing is best done while the animal is still young enough to permit handling. Pressure from a gentle finger immediately in front of the anus will reveal either the bulbous head of the penis or the distinctive fore-and-aft slit of the vagina. Females are usually ready to breed by the end of their first year, though some flying squirrels do not do so until their second.

With sociable animals such as the chipmunks and flying squirrels, there is little difficulty in introducing the male to the female. With the tree squirrels, the situation is somewhat more tricky. The best way to get over this hurdle is to bring them together on neutral ground, in a cage unfamiliar to either. Any immediate hostility will be overcome by the desire to explore the new environment, and territorial defensiveness will not provoke attacks.

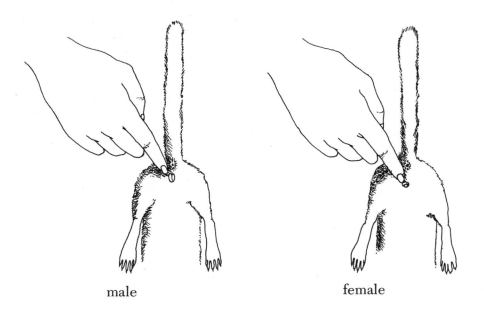

male   female

MATING   Mating seasons vary in number regionally and it is difficult to predict just what the pattern might be with squirrels reared inside households. Mating might take place in the spring, in the summer, or even in the winter. Litters usually consist of from two to five young, though there may be only one or as many as seven. At the indication of any hostility by the mother, the father should be removed from the cage.

BIRTH   Squirrels are excellent parents; if breeding is successful, the mother should simply be left alone. No human intervention is required at any time. When the young are born, they should not be interfered with until they emerge from the nest on their own initiative. The gestation period is approximately one and a half months, with some slight variation by species — though this is no greater a factor than individual differences.

HOUSING   No special nesting box is necessary if the babies are sharing the mother's nest, though if you suspect she is pregnant new nesting material should be placed in the cage. Nesting boxes for foundlings or babies removed from the nest are described on page 252.

FEEDING   There is no problem feeding the babies when the mother is tending them. She will care for them adequately without assistance until they are weaned.

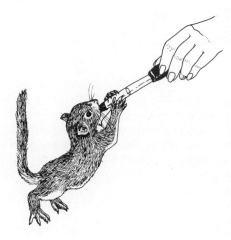

Foundlings and captured babies are another matter, of course. Age is the prime determinant in what they need. Very young squirrels must be fed every few hours — this time can gradually be lengthened.

Either a plastic eyedropper or a glass one, with the tip enclosed in a small piece of rubber tubing to protect it from young teeth, is excellently suited for giving the baby its milk. This can be either whole cow's milk or a mixture half of evaporated milk and half of water. It should be given at body temperature.

While vitamin drops or precooked baby foods, such as Pablum, may be added, baby squirrels should not be given a formula containing any sweetener, which can cause diarrhea. Immediately after feeding, any milk should be removed from the squirrel's fur with a warm, wet washrag to minimize the chances of diarrhea.

When the baby is able to feed itself, introduce bread soaked in milk, to supplement the bottle and to introduce it to more solid foods. This can be followed by soft fruits and vegetables until the squirrel gets its gnawing teeth, at which time a gradual transition may be made to the adult diet (see Feeding, page 252). By ten or eleven weeks, the squirrel should be completely weaned.

further readings   BARKALOW, F. S., JR., AND SHORTEN, M. *The World of the Gray Squirrel.* Philadelphia, J. B. Lippincott, 1973.

MacCLINTOCK, D. *Squirrels of North America.* New York, Van Nostrand Reinhold, 1970.

SNEDIGAR, R. *Our Small Native Animals.* New York, Dover Publications, 1963.

Chickens, ducks, and geese

W. J. MATHEY, V.M.D.

Almost any chicken, duck, or goose* will make a good pet if you get it early in its life.

CHICKENS The most numerous bird in the chicken world is the pheasant we call the chicken. All breeds of the chicken belong to one species.

Bantams are the ponies of the chicken world, about one-fourth the size of average larger breeds. There are bantam forms of all the standard breeds, as well as bantams with no standard counterpart. Their wide variety, their vigor, the small space needed for keeping them, and their smaller consumption of feed make them attractive as pets.

DUCKS While all the chicken breeds are variations of one zoological species, the ducks come from two subfamilies: Anatinae, the dabbling ducks (which feed by reaching down with their head and neck, often upending), and Cairininae, the perching ducks. Most of our domestic breeds are derived from the mallard, a dabbling duck. Although the mallard is also a game bird, it is kept as a pet by many people. If you breed or raise them in captivity, they should be banded and reported. Otherwise you might be accused of taking waterfowl out of season.

The muscovy, a perching duck, is favored in France, though there are many small farm flocks in Pennsylvania. "Muscovy" is apparently a mistaken derivation from the scientific name, *Cairina moschata*. It does not come from Russia, despite its name, but from Central and South America. Muscovies are as large as small breeds of geese (the male weighs 12 pounds, the female 7). They have unfeathered faces, covered with lumpy caruncles in the male.

In the same subfamily as the muscovy are two species with strikingly colored males: the mandarin, from Japan and Eastern Asia, and the similar wood duck, a North American bird. Both species nest in tree hollows, and live in freshwater ponds and streams. They are small birds, about two thirds the size of a mallard. The wood duck can stand cold much better than the mandarin.

GEESE The main breeds of geese in America come from four zoological species: the graylag goose of northern Europe, the Canada goose, the swan goose, and the Egyptian goose, which is really a duck.

* A note about swans. In general, swans can be treated similarly to geese — but one word of caution is needed. An owner or prospective owner should be aware that during the breeding season, when the swans are easily agitated, their great strength and size could create a serious hazard, especially to small children. A blow dealt by the wing, for instance, could be very dangerous.

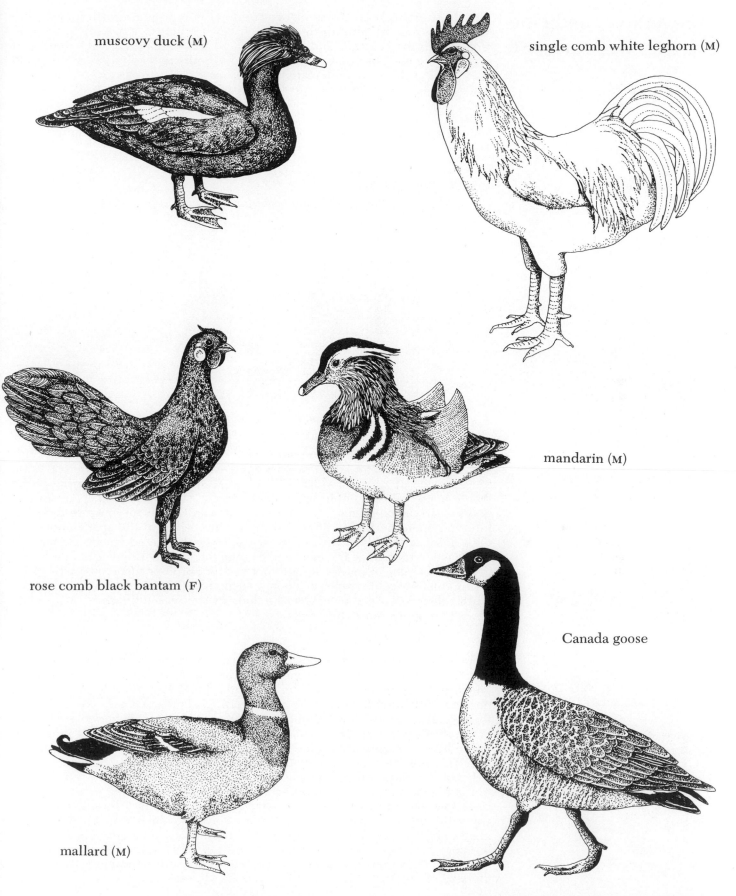

muscovy duck (M)

single comb white leghorn (M)

mandarin (M)

rose comb black bantam (F)

Canada goose

mallard (M)

preventive medicine

HOUSING

The best way to keep chickens or waterfowl is in a house with a cleanable floor. Birds can be kept all their lives in such a house, where they are protected from the weather and predators, and where they are safe from wild birds. With cleanable surfaces, you can control the spread of parasites — and openings can be screened against flying insects. Nests can be provided, so that clean table eggs are easy to secure. If you have only one bird, it can be kept in a wooden box, a small cask, or any waterproof container.

Birds need protection from the extremes of heat and cold, often more protection than just shelters will provide. See Temperature Requirements, page 259.

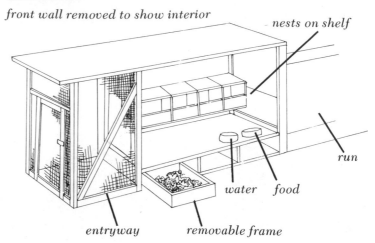

BIRDHOUSE

front wall removed to show interior

nests on shelf

run

water   *food*

entryway   *removable frame*

Ideally, a house for fowl should have a raised wire-mesh floor, through which droppings may fall. The wire mesh should be fastened to removable frames made of 2-by-4s, which will allow periodic thorough cleaning of the whole house. There should be an enclosed entryway, allowing space for two doors — and enough space so you can enter and close the outside door before you open the inside door. For laying hens, part of the space above the wire floor can be filled with nests equipped with hinged backs, so that you can reach in to remove the eggs and change the nest material as needed.

Leghorns need at least 1 square foot per bird of floor space on a wire floor; a 4-by-8-foot wire-floored space could easily have twenty-four hens. Birds on a litter floor require about twice the floor space. Such a house is dustier and tends to produce more dirty eggs.

RUNS

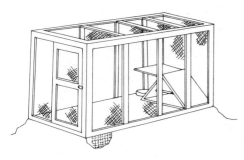

Although keeping birds in outdoor runs or letting them run free seems, at first thought, to be most beneficial for the birds, it is not. Diseases of all kinds multiply unless the area used for the birds is rotated to allow a long period of idleness; the eggs of certain worm parasites may survive in the soil for several years. Pet birds should run free only if there are no more than one or two birds per acre. If you plan to let your birds wander free around your grounds, it is important to remember that the droppings of all these birds are soft. Those of the goose, which eats much plant food, are the wettest.

If you are determined to have runs, make sure that the earth floor of the run is higher than the surrounding soil for good drainage. To protect against predators and prevent fly-aways, bury the wire fencing a foot or more and cover the top with wire netting. A wire floor is even better, for it tends to keep parasites away. Poultry fencing is available with more closely spaced horizontal wires at the bottom than at the top. This helps keep young birds from wandering off through the wire. Obviously, the wire mesh should suit the size of the bird you want it to fence in. Unfortunately, it is very difficult to protect against snakes, weasels, mink, and rats, which can squeeze through small openings.

SHELTER IN A RUN. If you are not providing a house, there should be a shelter to protect the birds against inclement weather, such as a small A-frame coop or an empty barrel, with a removable perch frame inside. The perches or roosts should be spaced at least 16 inches apart, and allow enough lateral room for the number and size of the birds using them — 3 or 4 inches for bantams, about 6 inches for leghorns, and 8 for heavy breeds. Feeders should be in a protected place, so that rain and snow do not wet the feed and the sun's rays do not destroy its nutrient value. Sheltered nests should be provided for egg-laying birds with straw or shavings in them, replaced as needed.

PONDS

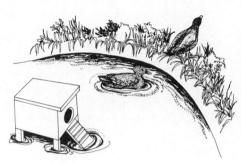

Ponds are not necessary for ducks and geese — except for ducks and geese kept in the colder parts of the United States, if they do not have housing and heat. As long as the pond water is not frozen, it will be warmer than the air, and the ducks or geese will dip their feet in the water to keep from freezing. Waterfowl seem to enjoy swimming, but shallow, stagnant ponds are a danger, especially in summertime. The botulism organism grows in organic material in the shallows, which is where waterfowl tend to feed. In deeper water or running water, where this is not a problem, various fish, turtles, and frogs feed on young ducks and geese. Ponds also attract migrant waterfowl, which may bring in infectious disease agents, such as the bacteria of fowl cholera or the virus of duck plague.

If you are determined to have a pond, build one without a shelving bank, so that there will be no shallows, or use coarse gravel in the shallows to avoid the mucky condition conducive to botulinus growth. A small container a few feet square can be used as a pond for several pet ducks, or you can build an elaborate swimming pool complete with vacuum cleaner and filter. The water should be changed often.

NUTRITION

Young chickens, ducks, and geese do well on turkey starter feed, which is higher in most vitamins than chicken starter, and nutritionally better than the corn they prefer. Breeder feed is a good idea during the breeder season. Grower feed costs less, and can be fed to adults the rest of the time. Supplemental green feed is a good idea — geese in particular are grazers and like to have a patch of fresh growing grass to cut for themselves. All three kinds of poultry like to feed on small invertebrates — worms and insects — and will also eat small frogs and other small vertebrates. A light-breed pullet before production starts will eat about .14 pounds of feed per day, as contrasted to a heavy-breed pullet's .32. Laying hens eat more: a light breed eats .27 pounds and a heavy breed .36. Bantams eat about a quarter the amount regular-sized fowl in the same breed do.

It is important to use only the best grain and to store it free of moisture, so that fungal toxins will not develop. Ducks are particularly susceptible to liver damage from even small amounts of these toxins. Always use a wooden floor or pallet for sacked feeds, and a metal, wooden, or plastic container for loose feed. Never store feed on the ground or on concrete floors. Examine the feed bins and containers for caking, a common sign of fungus growth. It is best to use feed within a week or so of manufacture, though refrigeration will preserve it longer.

TEMPERATURE
REQUIREMENTS

Birds need shelter from the heat of the sun if they are kept outside. If they are housed, they need fans and possibly air-cooling by fogging or roof sprinkling. Birds need more water in hot weather, since they evaporate it rapidly from their lungs in order to keep their body temperature down. They do best at temperatures between 50° and 65°F. At temperatures above 80°F., chickens are uncomfortable and egg production drops. At 100°F., many birds die of heat exhaustion, especially in areas where the nights are warm. Roofs should be painted white outside and black inside to help control heat and, ideally, should be insulated. An overheated bird pants rapidly, holding its wings away from its body — an extremely overheated bird becomes unconscious; often it can be saved if its head is cooled with water applied by sponging.

Chickens, ducks, and geese can survive in cold climates if given protection, though waterfowl can withstand colder temperatures. Single birds need more protection from the cold than do birds in groups. Chickens, in sufficient numbers, can keep a house warmed to about 50°F. Water temperature should be kept above 40°F., since birds do not like to drink very cold water. If the temperature falls below freezing, the water will freeze and the combs and wattles of the birds will be frost-nipped, turn black, and fall off. Waterfowl can survive the cold better if allowed access to ice-free water, for their feet are their cold-susceptible parts.

In cold weather, birds will eat more food. A chilled bird fluffs out its feathers to increase the layer of insulating air and sits down to protect its feet. A space heater or even containers of hot water can be used to build up the heat in the house.

GROOMING

Chickens do not like to be wet — they take dust baths. (If your chicken isn't allowed the run of the yard, and thus can't take dust baths, don't worry — the chicken will not suffer at all from the deprivation.) Ducks and geese bathe while swimming, ducking under and splashing water over themselves with their wings.

BIRD PSYCHOLOGY

Ducks and geese have a relationship with the first large moving thing they see at birth. Artificially hatched birds thus become attached to a human being and want to associate with people rather than with their own kind.

Chickens (and waterfowl) in a group have to adjust among themselves which one or ones will dominate — once this has been settled, life is smoother for all, except the lowest on the totem pole. Any new member of the group must fight for a place. This disturbance of the peck order is very stressful for the birds and may cause flare-ups of infectious disease.

During breeding season — which is all year long with chickens, and with many of the ducks — the males are aggressive. They fight with one another; they will endeavor to chase human beings away from their territory, and even a tiny bantam rooster will tackle a human being. Needless to say, poultry, especially muscovy ducks and the geese, are dangerous for small children. Females with a brood of young are also likely to be troublesome. The aggressiveness of the males in sexual activities may be damaging to the females if the flock consists of equal numbers of males and females. It is better, with chickens and ducks, to have ten or more females per male.

QUARANTINE

Newly acquired birds should be quarantined for a month or more before they join your other birds, for they may be carrying infectious agents. Prophylactic medication of both resident and new birds with one of the tetracycline antibiotics helps to reduce the chances of bacterial infections crossing from one group to the other. It should be remembered that the resident birds are possibly as much a source of infection to the new birds as vice versa.

Especially with chickens, for which many commercial vaccines are available for the various bacterial and viral diseases, preventive vaccination of both resident and new birds is advisable. Birds that have been to a show should be treated as though they were newcomers.

Blood tests are available for some of the more troublesome diseases that spread through the hatching egg from infected breeders. These are pullorum disease, *Mycoplasma gallisepticum* infection, and *Mycoplasma synoviae* infection. Your veterinarian can run these tests on your birds, or he may be able to teach you to do them yourself.

FLIGHT CONTROL   The chicken can make only short flights, whereas the wild ducks can fly long distances. Domestic ducks and geese often have been bred to be heavier and have lost much of their power of flight. Birds capable of flight, however, can leave your property even though you have 6-foot-high fences. There are a number of measures you can take to prevent this: brailing, wing clipping, day-old pinioning, adult pinioning, and tenotomy. Ask your veterinarian to demonstrate these.

BRAILING

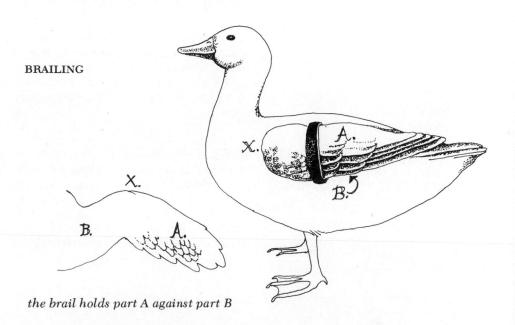

the brail holds part A against part B

BRAILING. This consists of putting a restraining strap or cord (the brail) on one wing to prevent it from being extended. This method has the advantages of being simple and of not irreversibly changing the bird. The disadvantages are that the brail may accidentally come off, allowing the bird to fly away, and that it should be moved every couple of weeks to the other wing to prevent atrophy of the brailed wing from disuse.

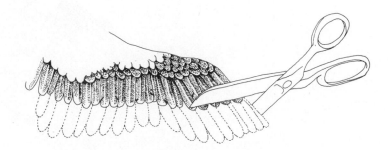

WING CLIPPING. In this procedure, the primary flight feathers of one wing are cut with sharp scissors or shears. Be sure to boil the scissors or shears

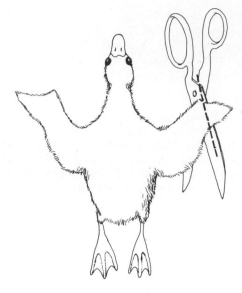

before clipping. Wing clipping disfigures the bird until the next molt, when the procedure must be repeated.

DAY-OLD PINIONING. In this procedure, the outer part of one wing — the part that corresponds to the human hand — is surgically removed from a newly hatched bird. Again, use boiled sharp scissors or shears and place the bird in a clean container. Bleeding is not a serious problem at this age, and the bird rapidly recovers from the operation. It is permanently disfigured, though, since the primary flight feathers are gone, and it can never develop the ability to fly.

ADULT PINIONING. This is an operation better left to your veterinarian. The fully grown wing has hard bones and a well-developed blood supply to cause problems in the removal of the outer segment.

TENOTOMY. This is another operation better left to a professional. It involves cutting out a section of the tendon passing over the "wrist" of one wing. This prevents the bird from extending the outer portion of the wing into flight position. It is an irreversible operation, which has the advantage of leaving the bird looking completely normal.

the home clinic
EXAMINATION OF THE BIRDS

Watch the birds in their pen without getting them excited. Look for droopy individuals, for dragging legs or wings, for blood on feathers or beaks. Listen carefully for unusual sounds: sneezing, coughing, or gurgling. Watch the birds at the feeders and waterers for unusual actions (sometimes something prevents them from eating and drinking). Look for feathers on the floor. Since small feathers are always being shed, their absence may mean they are being eaten — a sign of nutritional deficiency.

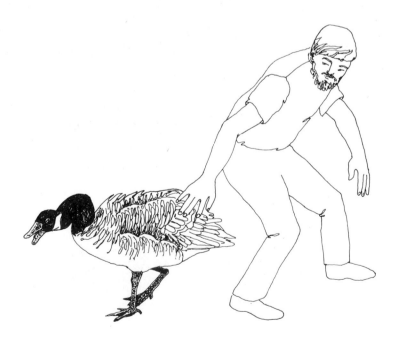

Next you may want to examine certain birds. One way to catch them by hand is to maneuver them into a corner. With large birds like muscovy ducks or geese, back up to them in the corner — wear thick clothing on your own posterior — and squat down on them, while reaching back to grasp them.

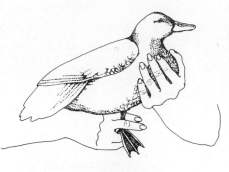

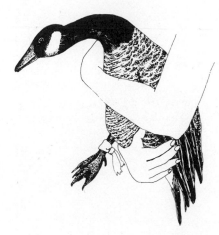

This prevents them from escaping by causing you to flinch and also prevents them from injuring your eyes.

The catching hook can also help — a long metal rod with a wooden handle; the hook end is bent into a tapered U shape. It is used to catch the bird by the leg and to draw it quickly toward you, so that you can grasp it before it frees itself. A pole net may also be used.

It is important to hold the bird properly to prevent it from struggling. Usually if you place the palm of one hand under the front of the bird's chest, catching its legs between your fingers so that the bird rests on your palm, it will not struggle. Of course, this is difficult or impossible to do with a large bird. These must be placed on a table and restrained with the help of an assistant. If you are alone, tie the legs together with a strip of cloth. It is often helpful to restrain the wings by wrapping the bird in a heavy towel or feed bag.

Use a bright light — a spotlight or a high-intensity light — to examine the bird. This allows you to detect changes caused by disease and to see small external parasites.

Handle your birds regularly so that you will be able to recognize changes from the normal. Look for changes in the appearance of the eyes: color of the irises, discharges, swellings of the lids or the area below the eye. Look at the nostrils for discharges. Listen to the bird's breathing. Look in its mouth: there may be color changes, ulcers, and the like. Look at the vent: there may be caking of feces and urates. Look at the feather coat. Look at the legs and feet. Feel the bird: run your fingers along its back, its breast muscle, its legs; feel its head. Gently try to bend the beak and the leg to see whether they feel weak.

ADMINISTERING MEDICINE

Many drugs for treating chickens are available directly mixed with feed at the feed mill. Far fewer drugs are available in this form for waterfowl — the clearance procedures with federal agencies are too expensive to the drug companies for the number of sales that might result.

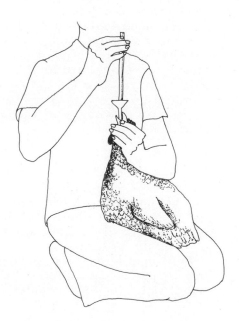

An alternate way to administer drugs to large numbers of birds is in their drinking water. Care should be taken when giving such potentially dangerous drugs as the sulfa drugs in this way during hot weather, when the bird

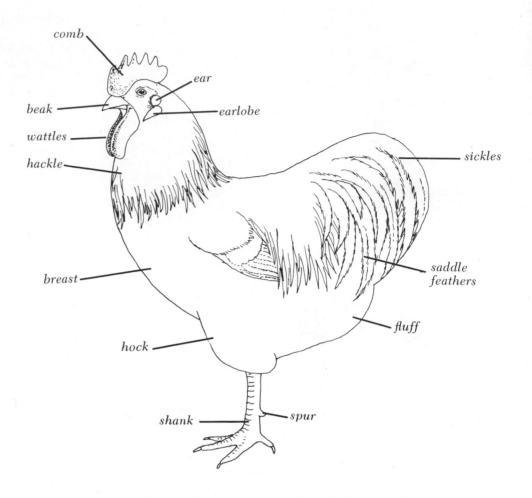

comb

ear

beak

earlobe

wattles

hackle

sickles

breast

saddle
feathers

fluff

hock

shank

spur

drinks more: the drug is then concentrated in the body and may cause trouble. Calculate a proper dose of the drug per bird, mix it in a given volume of water, and switch to unmedicated water when the drugged water is gone.

Individual birds may be given drugs by capsule (pushed back over the tongue), by esophageal tube (a piece of rubber or plastic tubing and a funnel), or by pill. Syringe and needle may be used to inject drugs by various routes.

For most diseases, your veterinarian will recommend drugs and methods of treatment.

HEAT AS THERAPY   Heat is a very valuable therapeutic agent, either applied to a group of birds en masse or given individually. Increasing the temperature of the building that houses birds sick with almost any problem will work wonders in reducing the length of illness and the number of deaths, and any drug will be more effective if the birds are warmer. An increase of 5 to 10 degrees may make all the difference.

Individual birds, such as ducks with swollen joints, may be given heat treatment. Soaking a swollen foot in hot salt water (as hot as your hand can stand) for ten to fifteen minutes four times a day often speeds recovery.

first aid   Injuries can be caused by many agents — other birds, mammals, snakes, human beings, objects in the surroundings. Penetrating wounds from beaks,

TRAUMA   claws, or teeth may lead to immediate death or to slow death from wound infection. Broken bones may cause lameness, inability to walk, fly, or swim, or the sudden deformity of a limb. See "Caged Birds," pages 203ff., for ways to treat these injuries.

FOREIGN BODIES   Birds are prone to swallowing all kinds of objects. Pieces of aluminum roof trimmings over 6 inches long and 2 inches wide have been removed from turkeys. It is common to find in a dead bird that roofing nails, needles, pins, and pieces of wire have pierced the wall of a gizzard. Waterfowl on ponds that are fished get hooks in them and are tangled in line. The rings from easy-open beverage cans can snare a beak, or be swallowed and damage the digestive tract.

Sometimes vicious human beings catch birds and put heavy rubber bands around their beaks or tongues, causing slow death from starvation. Or careful examination of a dead bird will reveal a bullet wound, inflicted by a modern Viking.

POISONS   FUNGAL TOXINS. Poisonings are fairly common in poultry. The most common is caused by fungal toxins formed in feed containing high moisture levels. Moisture, precipitating on the wall of a metal feed tank in an area with hot days and cool nights, is often the cause.

BOTULISM. Botulism is seen commonly in waterfowl. The bacterium, which forms a potent poison, grows in decaying animal and plant material in the shallows of lakes and ponds. The carcass of a dead chicken or duck may also contain much toxin, which can be picked up by maggots feeding on the carcass or can be absorbed by the earth under it. Signs of the poisoning are lack of control of the neck muscles (limber-neck) and the loss of feathers.

CHEMICALS. Poisoning by chemicals is also common, from careless use of drugs and insecticides. Always read carefully the labels of any products you use.

The treatment of poisoning depends on correct diagnosis and is best left to the veterinarian. Often all that can be done is careful nursing: protecting the bird from chilling, injury, and other hazards.

parasites   (See "Caged Birds," pages 207ff.) Control of arthropods is very important when any group of animals is kept together. Mite and louse populations can
ARTHROPOD PARASITES   build up to very sizable proportions if the birds are not regularly examined.

Bantams, in particular, are likely to have scaly-leg mites (see page 207), air sac mites (which are usually not pathogenic), and subcutaneous mites (which would be noticed only if a bird were dressed for the table, as whitish granules just under the skin). Ticks of all kinds can cause trouble in birds that are out in vegetation, and fleas can be very troublesome.

Birds ranging outside or kept in unscreened buildings are subject to attack by various winged bloodsucking insects. Waterfowl, particularly, may become infected with the blood protozoans by insects' bites. These are particularly bad near the Great Lakes, but can occur anywhere.

Read the label on any insecticide you use on your bird, especially if you sell eggs or meat. Call your local office of the Cooperative Agricultural Extension Service for advice.

ROUNDWORMS   There are numerous worms that affect poultry, especially birds that are out running on the ground.

Most of the nematodes, or roundworms, live in the digestive tract, but some live in the respiratory tract, under the skin, in the eye, and so on. The most likely to be noticed is probably the least important, the large roundworm *Ascaridia galli*, which causes trouble only if present in large numbers in birds under six weeks of age. It is a white worm several inches long, round in cross-section, and pointed at each end.

SMALLER ROUNDWORMS   The more dangerous roundworms are smaller and less likely to be seen. The threadworms, which are like pieces of fine thread, burrow into the mucous membrane of various parts of the digestive tract from the mouth to the vent and cause considerable irritation and death. The gizzard worm, in geese and ducks, burrows under the horny lining of the gizzard. The blood-red tetrameres worms are buried in the wall of the glandular stomach, looking like areas of hemorrhage. Another stomach worm, *Dispharynx nasuta*, may cause the formation of ulcers. A nematode parasite of the glandular stomach of ducks, *Eustrongylides ignotus*, bores through the wall and causes the formation of fleshy tubes. Young chickens on the ground are likely to be plagued by a nematode of the respiratory tract, the gapeworm *Syngamus tracheal*, which lives attached to the wall of the trachea and may cause asphyxiation. A similar worm affects geese and may cause 20 percent mortality. Birds in Gulf Coast states and Hawaii may have eyeworms. Their eyes become watery and they scratch at them.

ACANTHOCEPHALIDS   The acanthocephalids are the thorny-headed worms. They have a proboscis armed with heavy hooks by which they attach themselves to the wall of the intestine. The chicken is very seldom troubled with these, but the duck may die from one that causes a severe inflammation of the intestine.

TAPEWORMS   The cestodes, or tapeworms, are found in various parts of the intestine. Like many of the other worm parasites, they require intermediate hosts for transmission. A tapeworm egg has to be eaten by, say, a beetle, and develop to an infective stage within it, before it is dangerous to the chicken who eats the beetle. In general, there are waterfowl tapeworms and chicken tapeworms. Intermediate hosts vary — they can be slugs, snails, crayfish, water fleas, flies, earthworms, ants, grasshoppers, and others. Obviously the bird running on the ground is more likely to have tapeworms.

TREMATODES   The trematodes, or flukes, may be found in the eye, under the skin, in the respiratory tract, the digestive tract, the liver, the urinary system, the circulatory system, or the reproductive system. All require intermediate hosts, usually some sort of snail. Birds running free are the most likely to have flukes.

In general, diagnosis of the presence of worms in the living bird depends on finding the worm eggs in the droppings or finding larval stages in the blood. This requires a good microscope and experience. There are no specific signs different from those caused by other diseases.

diseases   Because more money is spent on research and diagnosis of chicken diseases than on pet bird diseases, there are many more infectious diseases of chickens known.

VIRAL   Some viral diseases can be recognized from signs, but most manifest themselves in the death of the bird. When vaccines are available, use them regularly — unless your birds are housed and protected from insects and other sources of trouble, and you live far away from other flocks of poultry.

Viral diseases are treated with nursing care. Keep the birds warm, give them plenty of clean water, and try to tempt their appetites with cooked grains (oatmeal, Wheatena, and so on).

LYMPHOID LEUKOSIS AND MAREK'S DISEASE. Two of the most important diseases of chickens are lymphoid leukosis and Marek's disease, both of which cause tumors. Though many commercial strains of chicken are free of lymphoid leukosis, which is transmitted through the hatching egg from an infected hen, the fowl kept by bird-fanciers are likely to be infected. Marek's disease is transmitted by infective feather-follicle debris inhaled by the bird at an early age. There is a vaccine available now to prevent this disease, which must be given at hatching time or shortly thereafter.

INFECTIOUS BRONCHITIS. Infectious bronchitis is a widespread viral disease of chickens. It causes respiratory disease and serious damage to the reproductive system. There are several vaccines effective in preventing it.

NEWCASTLE DISEASE. Newcastle disease is really a series of respiratory, reproductive, nervous, and digestive tract diseases, ranging from extremely mild to highly lethal, caused by a series of related viruses. Fortunately the viruses are enough alike so that vaccination with one (repeated several times) will protect against all.

AVIAN INFLUENZAS. This is also a series of diseases caused by a series of similar viruses. One of the very severe diseases is fowl plague, which much resembles the most severe of the Newcastle disease series in appearance and lethality. Unfortunately, there is no commercial vaccine available.

LARYNGOTRACHEITIS. This disease causes severe damage to the trachea and larynx, resulting in the coughing up of blood; a bird may die from blockage of the air passages — though some strains of this virus are manifested only by a mild inflammation of the eyes. Vaccines are available but some states do not allow their use, because the disease does not occur within their borders.

ENCEPHALOMYELITIS. Avian encephalomyelitis is transmitted through the hatching eggs laid by an infected hen, which usually shows no signs of sickness. In the flock, there may be a sudden drop and rise in egg production. The chicks hatched from the infected egg, and then their hatch mates, are afflicted with muscular tremors and paralysis, and surviving birds may develop cataracts a few weeks later. A vaccine is available.

Equine encephalomyelitis viruses are usually spread by insects or other arthropods, and one of these has caused deaths in Long Island ducklings. Little or nothing is known about the effectiveness of a vaccine made for use in horses.

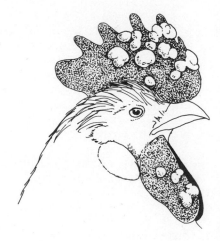

AVIAN POX. This is a group of diseases caused by a group of viruses, for which many vaccines are available. Chickens quite commonly have pox, especially in areas with high mosquito populations; waterfowl are less commonly affected. Lesions may be external, internal, or both. You may see small nodules on the comb and wattles or on the body. Sometimes they do not grow; other times, they form large tumorlike masses, eventually forming a scab to protect the virus.

INFECTIOUS BURSAL DISEASE. This disease damages the bursa of Fabricius, an organ involved in the development of the capacity to form antibodies, which exists only in young birds. The problem most commonly strikes at four to six weeks of age. The bursa first becomes swollen and then much smaller than normal. Affected birds are likely also to get miscellaneous bacterial infections.

ARTHRITIS, HEPATITIS, AND DUCK PLAGUE. Viral arthritis is often manifested as ruptured tendons of the leg. Apparently healthy birds are seen walking around on their hocks. The inflammation caused by the infection prevents the tendons that run down the back of the leg over the hock from sliding in their sheaths, and causes them to break.

Duck virus hepatitis is a disease of young ducks. It affects the liver and causes 50 to 100 percent mortality in ducklings under three weeks of age.

Duck plague (also called duck virus enteritis) has a firm foothold in the United States. It causes severe hemorrhages, particularly of the digestive tract, in all kinds of fowl, and particularly in the muscovy duck.

BACTERIAL

PULLORUM AND FOWL TYPHOID. Perhaps the most important bacterial disease of chickens is one that is almost nonexistent today in commercial poultry. This is pullorum disease, which now is found in small flocks and flocks containing birds of the less common breeds. Usually these originate from Kansas, Missouri, Iowa, or some other place where there are many small supply flocks for mail-order enterprises. In this disease chicks are stunted, chicks the same age are of uneven size, and many die. The area around the vent is pasted up with urates. Older birds may die suddenly. Pullorum disease, caused by *Salmonella pullorum,* and a very similar disease called fowl typhoid, almost wiped out the rapidly developing poultry industry in the early years of this century, until testing methods that can be done in the chicken house were developed. The infection is passed through the hatching egg from the infected hen. The chick from the infected egg may in turn infect the other chicks in contact with it.

PARATYPHOID. Paratyphoid infections result from contamination of feed or water with the salmonella bacteria. In the paratyphoid diseases as well as in pullorum typhoid, the intestine is most commonly affected, but no part of the body is safe. The signs are similar to those of pullorum.

A very common bacterial disease, much like that produced by the salmonella organism, is *E. coli* infection.

CORYZA. Infectious coryza is a bacterial infection of chickens, manifested by lacrimation, swelling of the sinuses below the eyes, an offensive odor, and a drop in egg production. This is more common in the South and in Mexico.

MYCOPLASMOSES. The mycoplasmoses of chickens can cause respiratory disease as well as joint troubles. To a large extent, they have been eliminated from commercial poultry by blood testing.

TUBERCULOSIS. In poultry, tuberculosis is still seen in small backyard flocks or hobby flocks that have birds of all ages, usually running on the ground. Young birds are most susceptible to infection but the disease takes a long time to develop. The signs are seen in older birds, which are shedding the bacteria in their droppings. These contaminate the soil for months or years, infecting young birds and perpetuating the disease. Birds affected with tuberculosis tend to get thin, although they continue to eat. The liver, spleen, and intestine usually have nodules of various sizes.

FOWL CHOLERA. This is an important problem in small backyard flocks of chickens and waterfowl. The disease may be quite mild, amounting to no more than a runny nose; or it can be devastating, killing most of a flock overnight. The bacterium may be carried by various mammals (dogs, cats, rodents, rabbits) or birds. Vaccines are available and are of value if vaccination is repeated frequently (every two or three months). Treatment is generally palliative, not curative.

Bacterial diseases are treated with drugs determined by the veterinarian. Again, nursing care is very important.

FUNGAL

In general, owners should consult a veterinarian before treating fowl. Symptoms of different diseases are often very similar — though the treatments of the diseases are quite different.

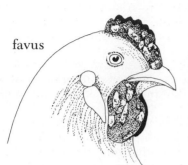

favus

ASPERGILLOSIS. This disease is most often seen as brooder pneumonia, a disease newly hatched chicks pick up in the hatchery. Often lesions are undetectable with the naked eye, and the birds sicken and die within a short space of time. Aspergillosis of older birds is more chronic in nature, and produces large lesions, which often have pockets of greenish fungi growing in them. Some birds will develop Aspergillus infection of the brain. Valuable birds may be treated with amphotericin (available from a veterinarian) if the disease is diagnosed early enough.

FAVUS, OR RINGWORM. Favus is a form of ringworm most common in the Asiatic breeds. It is usually seen as a whitish crusting of the comb and wattles. Athlete's foot ointments may be used on the lesions.

CANDIDIASIS, OR THRUSH. Candidiasis affects the digestive tract, often producing whitish coatings of the mouth, crop, or other parts. The disease is fostered by feeding honey or other substances containing simple sugars. Mycostatin (available from a veterinarian), although expensive, will control it, as will formic acid. Formic acid is a dangerous liquid, which should be used with caution. However, one can obtain it at a drugstore without a prescription. To use formic acid, dilute it to a 3 percent solution and spray it on the feed; wear goggles to protect your eyes.

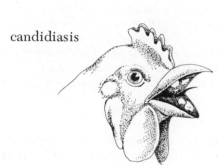

candidiasis

MYCOTOXICOSES. Mycotoxicoses are caused by poisonous substances produced by fungi in feedstuffs. Grains or mixed feeds with too high a moisture content allow the growth of the fungus, which in a certain temperature range will produce toxins. The temperature range that allows toxins to be produced is very broad — and moisture and other factors play a role. The problem is worse in the summer, but there are toxins that can develop at refrigerator temperature, too. Ducklings are most susceptible, responding with liver damage to doses that do not affect chickens. Mycotoxicoses have no really distinctive signs, though hemorrhages and death are common. If the condition is recognized, changing the feed, adding a vitamin supplement (a few drops of general baby vitamins each day), increasing the heat in the house, and similar supportive measures may help.

PROTOZOAN

There are many protozoan diseases of poultry. The most well known are the coccidioses.

COCCIDIOSES. These generally affect young growing birds. Intestinal species cause diarrhea, sometimes with bloody discharge. Kidney species cause weakness, diarrhea with whitish feces, grayish spots on the kidneys, and death.

HISTOMONIASIS OR BLACKHEAD. This disease is seen occasionally in chickens. They tend to have yellowish droppings and are very weak; the ceca and the liver are severely affected.

BLOOD PROTOZOANS. Various blood protozoans may be found in poultry, especially in ducks and geese. They are spread by biting insects. The signs are droopiness and death but diagnosis depends on microscopic examination of blood smears.

TRICHOMONIASIS. Trichomonads cause this disease, the signs of which are diarrhea, droopiness, and death. Diagnosis depends on microscopic examination.

TREATMENT. Protozoan diseases are treated with drugs determined by the veterinarian.

NUTRITIONAL There are a great number of nutritional diseases. One common cause is the feeding of mash mixed with whole grains, which dilute the nutrients in the mash. Since oxidation, which destroys vitamin A and vitamin E, is catalyzed by the minerals contained in a mixed feed, the feed should be purchased freshly mixed and stored for as short a time as possible. It keeps better if refrigerated.

Nutritional problems are most likely to be found in young growing birds, and in females in active egg production. Both need calcium and phosphorus for bone or eggshell formation, and vitamins of all kinds, for active body building or storage in the egg.

Bone weakness or deformity is probably the most commonly seen nutritional problem. The growing bird may develop rickets from lack of calcium and phosphorus. If it lacks certain of the B vitamins, its bones will have an abnormal growth pattern, resulting in deformities. The laying hen may put more calcium into eggshells than she takes in, and develop osteoporosis.

Skin problems are perhaps the next most common nutritional disease. These can be caused by deficiency of vitamin A, riboflavin, pantothenic acid, or nicotinic acid.

A diet deficient in vitamin E can result in a nervous disorder in chicks and changes in the gizzard and voluntary muscles in chickens and ducks.

Chickens and waterfowls may be affected with thyroid enlargement resulting from iodine deficiency in the feed.

METABOLIC GOUT. The most common metabolic disease seen in poultry is gout. Uric acid and urates, instead of being excreted by the kidneys, are precipitated in the joints, in the muscles, and in the serous cavities. The affected joints are swollen and white. Sometimes newly hatched chicks are afflicted with gout. Gout may be provoked by a shortage of drinking water — but little is really known about the cause in birds (or in human beings). The disease is usually

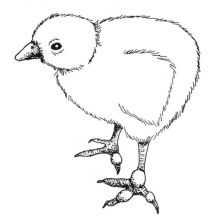

diagnosed only after death, but if it is discovered earlier, your veterinarian may prescribe allopurinol or another drug.

reproduction If chickens are being kept for their reproductive efforts — for the eggs they produce — it is cheaper to keep an all-hen flock. The roosters in a mated flock eat lots of feed; and it is better for the well-being of the hens, since roosters tend to rip their feathers and skin. For eating purposes, the unfertilized egg is nutritionally equal to the fertilized egg.

Sexing of baby chicks is a fine art. Chick-sexers, whose accuracy is higher than 90 percent, learn their trade by sexing hundreds of chicks, and then killing them to see if they were right. In some breeds there is a color difference between male and female chicks; or a difference in early feather development.

male duckling

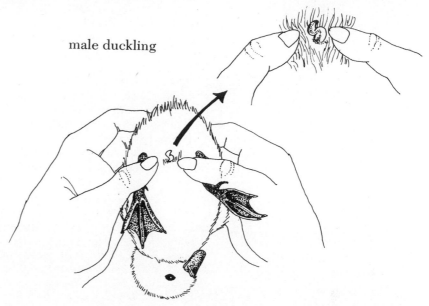

Waterfowl are easier to sex because males have what is called a penis, which can be seen as a pigtail-shaped little body when the cloacal lips are parted. Great care in the manipulation of the cloaca is advisable to avoid killing the baby duck or goose. It is best to wait until the birds are several weeks old. Another sex difference in ducks (not geese) is a one-sided bulbous enlargement of the syrinx in the male duckling, which can be felt by gently pushing the forefinger into the thoracic inlet.

In the sexually mature bird, the male chicken can usually be distinguished by his feathering. He has silky hackle feathers, long thin feathers covering the neck, and curled tail feathers. His head is more massive in appearance, and his appendages are bigger than those of the hen.

Some of the waterfowl have a sex difference in the adults. In addition, most male ducks have tail feathers curled up and forward, a more massive appearance, and a penis much larger than that of the immature bird. Some male ducks have a nuptial plumage, which appears during breeding season.

The adult female chicken or waterfowl has an oviduct opening into the cloaca on the left side. This may be seen as a small mound with a small depression in the center — the opening.

It is often very difficult to open the cloaca of waterfowl. It is helpful to use a human nasal speculum in immature birds, and a small vaginal speculum in mature birds, available from a druggist.

Chickens and many breeds of duck breed year-round; other ducks and all geese breed only in the spring.

orphan chicks and ducklings

The regrettable (and in some jurisdictions, criminal) practice of selling newly hatched chicks or ducklings as toys for children at Easter still exists. These poor animals are condemned to a short miserable life of chilling, semistarvation, and mishandling. Compared to the people who indulge in this torture, cockfight promoters and pit-bull fanciers are nature's noblemen.

In the hope of preventing some of this misery, I offer the following advice: the chick needs to be kept warm — 95°F. the first week, dropping 5° per week until 70° is reached in the sixth week. Heat may be furnished by a light bulb, a heating pad, or hot water containers.

Feed should be nutritionally balanced, with small particle size during the first two weeks. Corn is inadequate. Feed consumed by a single chick is very slight during the first weeks — about 0.15 pound for the first week, 0.25 pound the second week, finally reaching about 1 pound per week when the chick is an adult. (These figures are for light breeds; bantams should have less and heavy breeds, more.) Feed should be kept in sealed plastic bags in the freezer. Remove enough for a few days each time. This will help prevent the chemical deterioration resulting from the mineral components' catalysis of fats and vitamins.

Clean fresh water should be available at all times. The chick would use perhaps ½ ounce the first day, increasing to about 4 ounces a day by six weeks (more in hot weather).

To make clean-up easy, the chick should be in a wire-floored cage, with several layers of newspaper covering the droppings pan. Remember that an adult bird produces a ¼ pound or so of droppings per day.

further readings

THE AMERICAN POULTRY ASSOCIATION. *The American Standard of Perfection*. Atlanta, Georgia, The American Poultry Association, 1953.

AUSTIN, O. L., JR. *Birds of the World*. New York, Golden Press, 1961.

EWING, W. R. *Poultry Nutrition*, 5th ed. rev. Pasadena, California, Ray Ewing, 1963.

HOFSTAD, M. S., ed. *Diseases of Poultry*, 6th ed. Ames, Iowa, Iowa State University Press, 1972.

HYDE, D. O., ed. *Raising Wild Ducks in Captivity*. New York, E. P. Dutton, 1974.

NORTH, M. O. *Commercial Chicken Production Manual*. Westport, Conn., AVI Publishing, 1972.

ROMANOFF, A. L., AND ROMANOFF, A. J. *The Avian Egg*. New York, John Wiley, 1949.

SIEGMUND, O. H., ed. *The Merck Veterinary Manual*, 4th ed. Rahway, New Jersey, Merck, 1973.

TAYLOR, L. W., ed. *Fertility and Hatchability of Chicken and Turkey Eggs*. New York, John Wiley, 1949.

UNIVERSITIES FEDERATION FOR ANIMAL WELFARE. *Handbook on the Care and Management of Laboratory Animals*, 4th ed. Baltimore, Williams & Wilkins, 1972.

Sources, Conversion Table, and About the Authors

SOURCES OF EQUIPMENT, FOODS, AND MEDICINE

Most of the equipment, foods, and medicines mentioned in the text can be found at pet stores, aquarium supply stores, feed stores, drugstores, hardware stores, or suppliers of scientific equipment. In some cases you will have to get them from your veterinarian, whom you also should consult if you are unsure about brands. For chickens, ducks, and geese, you may want to contact the Agricultural Extension Service of the U.S. Department of Agriculture in your state. Many poultry supplies can be ordered through the Sears, Roebuck, Montgomery Ward, and Nasco Company farm catalogs.

METRIC CONVERSION TABLE

APPROXIMATE COMMON EQUIVALENTS

1 inch	=	2.5 centimeters
1 foot	=	.3 meter
1 ounce	=	28.0 grams
1 pound	=	.45 kilograms
1 quart	=	1.0 liter

$$\tfrac{5}{9}\,(°F-32) = °C$$

ABOUT THE AUTHORS

Dr. Paul G. Cavanagh received his B.S. and his D.V.M. from the University of Minnesota. He interned and completed a two-year medical residency program at the Animal Medical Center in New York City where he is currently Associate Staff. His special interests are nephrology, endocrinology, immunology, and basset hounds.

Dr. Lester E. Fisher received his D.V.M. from Iowa State University in 1943, was Attending Veterinarian at the Lincoln Park Zoo in Chicago, Illinois, from 1947 to 1962, and since 1962 has been Director of the zoo. He is Associate Professor of Biology at De Paul University and Adjunct Professor of Zoology at the University of Illinois. He has been Associate Editor of the *British Small Animal Journal* and the *Small Animal Clinician*.

Dr. Fredric L. Frye received his B.A. and his D.V.M. from the University of California, Davis, where he is now Clinical Professor of Medicine. He was Chief of Staff at the Berkeley Dog and Cat Hospital until he joined the research staff of the Donner Laboratory, University of California, Berkeley, and the United States Public Health Service Hospital, San Francisco. Dr. Frye is the author of *Husbandry, Medicine and Surgery in Captive Reptiles*, on the editorial board of the *Journal of Herpetology,* and a guest editor of *Current Veterinary Therapy.*

Dr. Jean Holzworth, a veterinarian who specializes in cats, is a member of the clinical staff of the Angell Memorial Animal Hospital in Boston, Massachusetts. She is a graduate of Bryn Mawr College and received her D.V.M. from the New York State College of Veterinary Medicine at Cornell University. She has contributed frequently to veterinary journals and has lectured to many veterinary and laymen's groups on diseases of cats.

Dr. Jay D. Hyman is a veterinarian with a specialty in marine animal medicine. He graduated from Cornell College and received his D.V.M. from the New York State College of Veterinary Medicine at Cornell University. Dr. Hyman is a past President of the Metropolitan Veterinary Medical Practitioners Society and is President of the International Association for Aquatic Animal Medicine. From 1968 to 1975 he was Consulting Veterinarian to the New York Aquarium and he is now a consultant to the United States Department of Commerce.

Dr. W. J. Mathey received his B.S. from the University of Notre Dame, his V.M.D. from the University of Pennsylvania, and his Ph.D. from the University of California. He was an army veterinarian in World War II, a biological researcher, and is now doing teaching and research at the Department of Veterinary Science at Louisiana State University, where he supervises the avian disease diagnostic laboratory. His own pets have included falcons, hawks, parrots, canaries, crows, ducks, and pheasants.

Dr. Stephen M. Schuchman is the owner and director of Boulevard Pet Hospital in Castro Valley, California. He graduated from Cornell University and received his D.V.M. from the New York State College of Veterinary Medicine at Cornell University. He belongs to numerous professional associations, including the American Association of Zoo veterinarians, and has written on the care and management of rodents and rabbits for *Current Veterinary Therapy.*

Roger Caras is a Vice President of the Humane Society of the United States and the author of numerous books on animals, the two most recent of which are *The Roger Caras Pet Book* and *Skunk for a Day.* Mr. Caras is also a commentator on CBS radio ("Pets and Wildlife") and Animal Correspondent for ABC Television News. He lives on Long Island with a family which includes six dogs (Yorkshire terrier, golden retriever, Siberian husky, English bulldog, random-bred shepherd, bloodhound), one horse, one pony, a number of cats, three ducks, one to two hundred fish, and various short-term pets.

Dr. Michael W. Fox holds a veterinary degree and doctorate degrees in animal behavior/ethology and medicine, both from London University, and has been Associate Professor of Psychology at Washington University and Associate Director of the St. Louis Zoo. He is now Director of the Institute for Animal Problems of the Humane Society of the United States. Dr. Fox writes the monthly column "Understanding Your Pet" for *McCall's* magazine and the syndicated newspaper column "Ask your Vet." He is the author of *Understanding Your Dog, Understanding Your Cat,* and *Between Animal and Man.* His scholarly studies of animal behavior have won wide acclaim in the scientific community.

Index

abrasions in reptiles, 171
abscesses in reptiles, 176
Abyssinians. *See* cats
acanthocephalids. *See* thorny-headed worms
acne in cats, 103
Afghan hounds. *See* dogs
aggressiveness: in caged birds, 194, 196; in chickens, ducks, and geese, 260; in fish, 142, 143, 144, 145, 150; in hamsters, 219, 232; in multipet family, 5
air-sac mites in chickens, ducks, and geese, 265
Albert's squirrel. *See* squirrels, fox
algae in fish tank, 144, 148, 151
allergies: in cats, 102, 108–109; in dogs, 47, 54
alligator lizards. *See* reptiles (lizards)
alligators. *See* reptiles
American rabbits. *See* rabbits
amphibians: acquiring, 181–182; advantages of, as pets, 178; aquariums for, 182–183; bleeding in, 185; breeding, 186; cannibalism in, 182, 185, 186; dehydration in, 186; diseases and disorders of, 185–186; eggs of, 181, 182, 186; feeding, 184–185, 185–186; first aid for, 185; handling and holding, 181–182; housing, 182–184, 185; life spans of, 178; light requirements of, 183–184; metamorphosis in, 178–181; parasites in, 186; quarantining, 182, 186; regeneration in, 185; sexing, 186; species of, 178; starvation in, 185–186; symptoms of illness in, general, 185; temperature requirements of, 183; terrariums for, 182; thermal shock in, 185; water requirements of, 183, 186
CAECILIANS: appearance and size of, 178; feeding, 185
FROGS: appearance and size of, 178; cannibalism in, 182; development of, 181; diseases and disorders of, 186; feeding, 184; handling and holding, 181; shedding of skin of, 183; temperature requirements of, 183; terrariums for, 182
SALAMANDERS: appearance and size of, 178; cannibalism in, 182; development of, 181; diseases and disorders of, 186; feeding, 184–185; handling and holding, 181–182; shedding of skin of, 183; temperature requirements of, 183; terrariums for, 182
TOADS: appearance and size of, 178; diseases and disorders of, 184; feeding, 184; housing, 182

anacondas. *See* reptiles (snakes)
anal glands (sacs): in cats, 111, 121; in dogs, 56
anchor worms in fish, 156
anemia in cats, 83, 101–102, 115
anemone fish. *See* fish, marine
angelfish. *See* fish, marine
angelfish scalare. *See* fish, freshwater
angora rabbits. *See* rabbits
aquariums: for amphibians, 182–183; for reptiles, 164; as rodent cages, 221
FOR FISH: freshwater, 146–150; marine, 150–151; second, for breeding or quarantining, 141, 142, 153
argulus (fish louse), 156
arthritis: in cats, 122; in chickens, ducks, and geese, 267
arthropod parasites: in caged birds, 207; in chickens, ducks, and geese, 265
artificial respiration: for cats and skunks, 82–83; for dogs, 32
ascarids. *See* roundworms
aspergillosis: in caged birds, 210; in chickens, 269
asthma: in cats, 83, 108–109; in dogs, 54
aviaries for caged birds, 196, 197
axolotls. *See* amphibians (salamanders)

bacterial diseases. *See* diseases and disorders
balanoposthitis in dogs, 57
bandages: for caged birds, 203; for cats and skunks, 86–87; for dogs, 33–34; *see also* splints
bantams. *See* chickens
barbs. *See* fish, freshwater
bathing: of amphibians, 183; of caged birds, 197; of cats, 74; of dogs, 23–24; of rodents, 225; of skunks, 129; *see also* shampoos
beak, care of, in caged birds, 195–196, 202
bedding: for dogs, 22; for rabbit cages, 237, 246; for rodent cages, 222
beds: for cats, 69; for skunks, 127
Belgian hares. *See* rabbits
bettas. *See* fish, freshwater
birds, caged: advantages of, as pets, 191; aggressiveness in, 194; attachments of, to humans, 194; bandaging, 203; beak, care of, 195–196; bleeding in, 195, 205; blood tests on, 201; breeding, 214–217; breeds of, 193; budgerigars, 196, 197, 198, 211, 214, 216; cages and aviaries for, 196–197; canaries, 197, 206, 209, 214–216; chilling of, 197; claws, care of, 196; cockatiels, 194,

214, 217; diseases and disorders of, 206, 209–214; dispositions of, 193; environmental hazards to, 197–198, 206–207; examination of, 201–202; feather coat of, 195; feeding, 193, 198, 211, 214; finches, 196, 197, 214, 216; first aid for, 203–207; foreign bodies in, 205–206; handling and holding, 201; heat exhaustion in, 197; heat therapy for, 203; injuries of, 203–205, 206; Java sparrows, 194; life spans of, 191; lovebirds, 194; medication, administering to, 202–203; medication, preventive, 198–201; nests for, 214–217; obesity in, 211; observing, 201; parasites in, 207–208; parrots, 197, 209; peck order of, 194; poisoning in, 206–207; psittacines, 195–196, 201, 207, 209; psychology of, 194; quarantining, 198; regulations governing, federal, 194; restraint of, protective, 201; sexes and species, mixing, 196; sexing, 214–217; sizes of, 193; songbirds, 194; splints for, 203–205; starvation in, 211; symptoms of disease in, general, 212–213; talking, 194, 196; temperature requirements of, 197; vaccination of, 201; water requirements of, 198; young, care of, 214
birds, wild: breeding, 214; care of, 194–195; and oil spills, 207; passeriformes, 191; psittaciformes, 191; regulations governing, federal, 194
birth control: in cats, 75–76; in dogs, 26, 60; in rabbits, 240; in skunks, 131
birth defects and abnormalities in cats, 67, 68, 120–121
bites and bite wounds: in cats and skunks, 87; in dogs, 38; in rabbits, 240
blackhead in chickens, 269
black spot in fish, 156
bleeding
EXTERNAL: in amphibians, 185; in caged birds, 195, 196, 205; in cats, 86; in dogs, 33–34; in reptiles, 175
INTERNAL: in caged birds, 205; in cats and skunks, 85; in dogs, 34–35
blind cave fish. *See* fish, freshwater
blind characin. *See* fish, freshwater
blood diseases and disorders of cats, 83, 114–116
boa constrictors. *See* reptiles (snakes)
bone diseases. *See* skeletal diseases and disorders
bones: for cats, 72, 107; for dogs, 22, 23, 42, 53
bones, broken. *See* fractures

box tortoises. *See* reptiles (tortoises)
brailing of chickens, ducks, and geese, 261
breathing. *See* respiratory rate
breeding: of amphibians, 186; of caged
    birds, 214–217; of cats, 116–119; of
    chickens, ducks, and geese, 270, 271; of
    dogs, 60–64; of fish, 139–140, 141–142,
    143, 144; of rabbits, 245–246; of reptiles,
    177; of rodents, 221, 231–232; of skunks,
    134; of squirrels and chipmunks, 254–255
bronchiectasis in dogs, 54
bronchitis: in cats, 108–109; in chickens,
    267; in dogs, 54
brushing: of cats, 72, 121; of dogs, 24; of
    guinea pigs, 225; of rabbits, 239; of
    skunks, 129
bucket collar. *See* collars, Elizabethan
budgerigars. *See* birds, caged
bullfrogs. *See* amphibians (frogs)
Burmese. *See* cats
burns: in cats and skunks, 89; in dogs, 37,
    41; in reptiles, 171–172
bursal disease, infectious, in chickens,
    ducks, and geese, 267
butterfly fish. *See* fish, marine

caecilians. *See* amphibians
cages: for birds, 196–197, 198, 207; for
    rabbits, 237, 241, 242, 246; for reptiles,
    164–166, 167, 171; for rodents, 221–222,
    225; for skunks, 128; for squirrels and
    chipmunks, 251–252
caimans. *See* reptiles
Canada goose. *See* geese
canaries. *See* birds, caged
cancer: in cats, 106, 108, 109, 115, 122; in
    dogs, 49, 54
candidiasis. *See* thrush
canker. *See* trichomoniasis
cannibalism: in amphibians, 182, 185, 186;
    in reptiles, 171
cardiovascular system. *See* heart disease
carrier for cats, 80
castration: in cats, 76; in dogs, 26; in rabbits,
    240; in skunks, 131
cataracts in dogs, 50
catching: caged birds, 201; chickens, ducks,
    and geese, 262–263; escaped rodents, 224
catfish. *See* fish, freshwater
catnip, 70
cats: Abyssinians, 68, 117; acquiring, 66–67;
    advantages of, as pets, 66; artificial res-
    piration for, 82–83; bandaging, 86–87;
    bathing, 74; beds for, 69; birth defects and
    abnormalities of, 67, 68, 73, 120–121; bite
    wounds in, 87; breeding, 116–119; breeds
    of, 67–68; Burmese, 68; burns in, 89;
    carrier for, 80; castration of, 76; claws of,
    trimming, 72–73; collars and harnesses for,
    81; convulsions in, 84; declawing, 76–77;
    devocalization of, 77; diseases and dis-
    orders of, 68–69, 74–75, 83, 84, 99–116;
    diseases of, transmissable to humans, 68–
    69; ears, care of, 73–74; embolisms in, 83;
    environmental hazards to, 93; euthanasia
    in, 121–122; eyes of, cleaning, 74; feeding,
    70–72, 80; first aid for, 82–93; foreign
    objects in, 91–92; frostbite in, 90; fur balls
    in, 109; grooming, 72; hand feeding, 80;
    handling and holding, 81–82; heartbeat,
    checking, 77; heart massage for, 82; heat
    cycles in, 75; heat stroke in, 89–90;
    Himalayans, 68; housebreaking, 69–70;

injuries of, 85–88; insect bites in, 90–91;
    life span of, 68, 121; longhairs, 67; Manx,
    68; medication, administering to, 79–80;
    medicine cabinet for, 77; mismating of, 76;
    in multipet family, 5, 7–8; old age in, 121–
    123; taking outdoors, 69; paralysis in, 83;
    parasites in, 93–99; Persians, 68, 74, 75,
    105, 116; play and toys for, 70; poisoning
    in, 40, 85, 92–93; pulse, checking, 77;
    punishing, 70; restraints for, protective,
    80–82; shock in, 84; shorthairs, 67;
    Siamese, 67, 70, 75, 77, 104, 117;
    snakebites in, 90–91; spaying of, 75–76;
    splints for, 88–89; spraying of urine in, 76,
    113; stretchers for, 88; temperature of,
    taking, 77; training, 69–70; urinate,
    inability to, 84; vaccination of, 74–75, 100;
    young, care of, 66, 119–120
cestodes. *See* tapeworms
chameleons. *See* reptiles (lizards)
chelonians. *See* reptiles: terrapins; tortoises;
    turtles
chickaree. *See* squirrels, red
chickens: advantages of, as pets, 256;
    aggressiveness in, 260; attachments of, to
    humans, 6; bantams, 256, 259, 263, 265,
    272; blood tests on, 261; breeding, 271;
    breeds of, 256; catching, 262–263; diseases
    and disorders of, 266–270; examining, 263;
    feeding, 259, 260, 271–272; first aid for,
    264; flight control in, 261–262; foreign
    bodies in, 265; grooming, 260; handling
    and holding, 263; heat exhaustion in, 260;
    heat therapy for, 264; housing, 258, 259,
    260; injuries of, 264; leghorns, 258, 259;
    medication, administering to, 263–264;
    medication of, preventive, 260; observing,
    262; parasites in, 265–266; peck order of,
    260; poisoning in, 265; quarantining, 260;
    restraint of, protective, 263; runs for,
    outdoor, 258–259; sexes, balance between,
    in flock, 260, 270; sexing, 270, 271;
    temperature requirements of, 259–260,
    264, 271; vaccination of, 260; water
    requirements of, 259, 260, 271; young,
    care of, 271–272
chipmunks. *See* squirrels
cholera, fowl: in caged birds, 201; in
    chickens, ducks, and geese, 268
circulatory emergencies in cats, 83
civets. *See* skunks
clawed frogs. *See* amphibians (frogs)
claws, trimming: of caged birds, 196; of cats,
    72–73, 121; of skunks, 129; *see also* nails
clown fish. *See* fish, marine
collars: for cats, 81; for dogs, 21–22
    ELIZABETHAN: for cats, 81; for dogs, 32
    FLEA: for cats, 97, 98; for dogs, 45
coccidiosis: in caged birds, 210, 211; in cats,
    95; in chickens, ducks, and geese, 269; in
    rabbits, 241–242
cockatiels. *See* birds, caged
cocker spaniels. *See* dogs
cold and wind, protection from: for caged
    birds, 197; for dogs, 22; for rabbits, 241;
    for reptiles, 164; for rodents, 224
colds: in cats, 100; in rabbits, 225; in skunks,
    133; *see also* respiratory diseases and
    disorders
columnaris in fish, 155
combing of cats, 72
conjunctivitis: in cats, 105; in dogs, 50; in
    gerbils, 229, 229n; in rabbits, 244

constipation: in cats, 110, 122; in dogs, 55; in
    hamsters, 229; in reptiles, 175
convulsions: in cats and skunks, 84; in dogs,
    36–37; in gerbils, 226, 229
coprophagy: in dogs, 55; in guinea pigs, 226;
    in rabbits, 238
coral fish. *See* fish, marine
coral fish disease, 155
corneal ulcers in dogs, 50
coryza: in cats, 100; in chickens, 268
cottontails. *See* rabbits, wild
cotton wool mouth in fish, 155
coughs in dogs, 53–54
crocodiles. *See* reptiles
crocodilians. *See* reptiles: alligators;
    caimans; crocodiles; gavials
cuttlefish bone for caged birds, 198, 211
cystitis: in cats, 112; in dogs, 56–57, 59
cysts in rabbits, 242

dachshunds. *See* dogs
Dalmatians. *See* dogs
damsels. *See* fish, marine
dandruff in dogs, 48
danios. *See* fish, freshwater
de-barking of dogs, 27
declawing of cats, 76–77
deficiency diseases. *See* diseases and
    disorders
dehydration: in amphibians, 186; in reptiles,
    173–174
dermatitis: in cats, 102; in dogs, 47, 57
dermatoses in cats, 104
de-scenting of skunks, 126–127, 130
devocalization of cats, 77
dewclaw removal in dogs, 26–27
diabetes: in cats, 110, 122; in dogs, 35
diarrhea: in caged birds, 214; in cats, 110; in
    dogs, 55; in gerbils, 229; in guinea pigs,
    230; in hamsters, 229; in mice, 230; in rats,
    230; in skunks, 134
diet. *See* feeding; water requirements
dietary deficiencies. *See* vitamin and
    mineral deficiencies and supplements
digestive diseases and disorders: in caged
    birds, 198, 209, 210; in cats, 109–111; in
    chickens, ducks, and geese, 267, 268, 269;
    in dogs, 54–56; in gerbils, 229; in guinea
    pigs, 230; in hamsters, 229; in mice and
    rats, 230; *see also* parasites
disciplining. *See* training
discus. *See* fish, freshwater
diseases and disorders: of amphibians, 185–
    186; of caged birds, 201–202, 209–214; of
    chickens, ducks, and geese, 263, 266–270;
    of fish, 153–157; of rabbits, 243–244; of
    reptiles, 173–177; of rodents, 226–227,
    228–230; of skunks, 133–134; of squirrels
    and chipmunks, 253–254; *see also* parasitic
    infections and infestations; vaccination
    OF CATS, 68–69, 99–116, 122; of the blood,
    114–116; digestive, 109–111; of the ears,
    106; of the heart, 114; of the mouth and
    teeth, 107–108; in old age, 122;
    panleukopenia, 99–100; reproductive,
    113–114; respiratory, 108; skeletal, 109; of
    the skin, 102–104; transmissible to
    humans, 68–69; urinary, 111–113
    OF DOGS, 20, 46–60; digestive, 54–56; of
    the ears, 51–52; of the eyes, 49–51;
    genitourinary, 56–59; of the heart, 59–60;
    of the mouth and throat, 52–53; of the
    nose, 42, 52; respiratory, 53–54; skeletal,

54; of the skin, 47–49; transmissible to humans, 20
dislocations: in cats and skunks, 88; in dogs, 38
distemper: in dogs, 21, 25, 60; in skunks, 133
distemper, cat. *See* panleukopenia
dobermans. *See* dogs
dogs: acquiring, 19–20; advantages of, as pets, 17, 20; Afghan hounds, 18, 36; artificial respiration for, 32; bandaging, 33–34; bathing, 23–24; bite wounds in, 38; bleeding in, 33–35; bones for, 42; breeding, 60–62; breeds of, 17–19; brushing, 24; burns in, 37, 41; castration of, 26; cocker spaniels, 48; collars for, 21–22, 32; convulsions in, 36–37; coprophagy in, 55; dachshunds, 18, 35, 48; Dalmatians, 42; de-barking, 27; dewclaw removal in, 26–27; disciplining, 20; diseases and disorders of, 20, 35, 46–60; diseases of, transmissible to humans, 20; dobermans, 18; ears, care of and problems with, 24, 51–52; electrical shock in, 41; environmental hazards to, 22; euthanasia in, 65; examining for injuries, 32–35; exercise for, 22; eyes, problems with, 41–42, 49–51; feeding, 23, 30, 62–63; first aid for, 30–42; foreign bodies in, 41, 42; frostbite in, 22, 37; German shepherds, 19, 48; grooming, 23–24; hand feeding, 30; heartbeat, checking, 29, 32; heart massage for, 32–33; heat cycles in, 60; heat stroke in, 22, 37; housebreaking, 21; housing, 22–23; injuries in, 33–35, 37–39, 41–42; insect bites in, 39; leash training of, 21–22; life span of, 64; medication, administering to, 29–30, 51, 52; medicine kit for, 27; mouth and throat problems in, 52–53; in multipet family, 5, 7, 8, 23; nails of, trimming, 24; nose problems in, 42, 52; obesity in, 56; old age in, 64–65; taking outdoors, 21, 22; paralysis in, 35–36; parasites in, 42–46; personalities of, 18; poisoning in, 39–41; Pomeranians, 53; poodles, 24, 35, 38, 50, 51, 53; pulse, checking, 29; purebreds, 18–19; respiration of, checking, 29, 32; restraint of, protective, 30–32; Saint Bernards, 47; schnauzers, 24, 48; shock in, 35; skin problems in, 41, 47–49; smoke inhalation in, 41; snakebites in, 39; splints for, 30, 38; stretchers for, 32, 35; temperature of, taking, 29; training, 20–22; tourniquet for, 33, 39; tumors in, 49, 53, 54, 57–59; unconsciousness in, 35; urinate, inability to, 42; vaccination of, 21, 25–26; Yorkies, 38; young, care of, 62–63, 64
Douglas red squirrels. *See* squirrels, red
dressings. *See* bandages
dry eye in dogs, 50
ducks: aggressiveness in, 260; attachments of, to humans, 6, 260; breeding, 271; breeds of, 256; catching, 262–263; diseases and disorders of, 266–270; examining, 263; feeding, 259, 260; first aid for, 264; flight control in, 261–262; foreign bodies in, 265; grooming, 260; handling and holding, 263; heat exhaustion in, 260; heat therapy for, 264; housing, 258, 259, 260; injuries of, 264; mallards, 256; mandarin, 256; medication, administering to, 263–264; medication of, preventive, 260; muscovy, 256, 262–263, 268; observing, 262; parasites in, 265–266; peck order of, 260;

poisoning in, 265; ponds for, 259; quarantining, 260; restraint of, protective, 263; runs for, outdoor, 258–259; sexes, balance between, in flock, 260; sexing, 271; temperature requirements of, 259–260, 264; vaccination of, 260; water requirements of, 259, 260; wood, 256
Dutch rabbits. *See* rabbits
dystocia in dogs, 61–62

ear diseases and disorders: in cats, 73–74, 91, 106; in dogs, 51–52; in rodents, 226
ear mites: in cats, 73; in dogs, 46; in rabbits, 242
ears, cleaning: in cats, 73; in dogs, 24; in skunks, 129
eclampsia in dogs, 63
egg-laying fish. *See* fish, freshwater
eggs: of amphibians, 181, 182, 186; of chickens, 270; of fish, 141; of reptiles, 159, 177
Egyptian geese. *See* geese
Egyptian mouth breeder. *See* fish, freshwater
Elizabethan collar. *See* collars
embolisms in cats, 83, 114
emphysema in dogs, 54
encephalomyelitis, avian, 267
English spot rabbits. *See* rabbits
enteritis: duck virus, 268; mucoid, in rabbits, 243, 244
enteritis, infectious. *See* panleukopenia
enterotoxemia in rabbits, 243
environment, natural, importance of preserving for reptiles, 162
environmental hazards: to caged birds, 197–198, 206–207; to cats, 92–93; to dogs, 22, 40–41; to rabbits, 241; to flying squirrels, 253
eosinophilic granuloma in cats, 102
epilepsy in dogs, 36, 37
epiphora: in cats, 105; in dogs, 50
euthanasia: in amphibians, 185; in cats, 122–123; in dogs, 65; in fish, 153; in rabbits, 240
examination, for symptoms of disease: of caged birds, 201–202; of chickens, ducks, and geese, 262, 263; of rodents, 226–227
exercise wheel: for rodents, 222; for squirrels and chipmunks, 252
eye diseases and disorders: in caged birds, 205; in cats, 91, 104–106; in dogs, 49–51; in gerbils, 229; in hamsters, 229; in rodents, 227
eye injuries: of cats, 85; of dogs, 41–42; of reptiles, 172
eyes, cleaning in cats, 74, 105–106
eyeworms: in cats, 95; in chickens, ducks, and geese, 266

fasting in reptiles, 167
favus. *See* ringworm
feathers: bleeding from, in caged birds, 195; eating of, in chickens, ducks, and geese, 262
feeders: for caged birds, 196, 197; for chickens, ducks, and geese, 259; for rabbits, 239
feeding: of amphibians, 184–185, 185–186; of caged birds, 193, 198, 206, 211, 214; of chickens, ducks, and geese, 259, 260, 270, 271–272; of cats, 70–72, 100, 117, 118, 120, 122; of dogs, 23, 56, 62–63, 64; of fish, 140,

141, 143, 144, 150, 151; of guinea pigs, 224–225, 231; of rabbits, 239, 246; of reptiles, 167–171, 173–174, 177; of rodents, 224–225; of skunks, 128–129, 135; of snakes, 161, 167–168; of squirrels and chipmunks, 252–253, 254–255; *see also* hand feeding; water requirements
filtration systems: of amphibian aquariums, 182–183; of fish tanks, 147–148; in reptile pools, 164
finches. *See* birds, caged
fin rot in fish, 155
first aid: for amphibians, 185; for caged birds, 203–207; for cats, 82–93; for chickens, ducks, and geese, 264–265; for dogs, 30–42; for fish, 151–153; for rabbits, 240–241; for reptiles, 171–172; for rodents, 226–228; for skunks, 131, 82–93; for squirrels and chipmunks, 253–254
fish: advantages of, as pets, 139; destroying of diseased or injured, 153; diseases and disorders of, 153–157; first aid for, 151–153; handling and holding, 149, 150, 153; light requirements of, 146, 148; in multipet family, 8; overcrowding of, 150; overheating of, 148, 154; parasites in, 153; quarantining, 153, 156; species of, 139–145; symptoms of disease in, general, 153–154; tropical, 139–144; wounds of, treating, 153
FRESHWATER, 139–144, 155; acquiring, 149; aggressiveness in, 142, 143, 144, 150; angelfish, 143, 150; appearance and size of, 140, 141, 142, 143, 144; aquariums for, preparing, 146–150; barbs, 142; bettas, 142; blind cave fish, 142; blind characin, 142; breeding, 139–140, 141, 143, 144; catfish, 144; discus, 143, 150; danios, 142; egg-laying, 141–144; Egyptian mouth breeders, 143; feeding, 140, 141, 143, 144, 150, 151; gouramis, 142–143; guppies, 140, 141; hatchetfish, 142; Jack Dempseys, 144; labyrinths, 142–143; life spans of, 141, 143, 144; live-bearing, 139–141; loaches, 144; mollies, 140, 141, 151; oscars, 144; piranhas, 143–144; platys, 140–141; scavengers, 144; Siamese fighting fish, 142; species, segregation of, 143, 144; sucker fish, 144; swordtails, 141; tank size requirements of, 143, 150; temperature requirements of, 141, 142, 143, 144, 146, 148, 156; tetras, 142, 150; tigers, 142; zebra fish, 142
MARINE, 144–145, 154; acquiring, 149, 151; aggressiveness in, 145, 150; anemone fish, 145; angelfish, 145; appearance and size of, 144, 145; aquariums for, preparing, 147–148, 150–151; butterfly fish, 145; clown fish, 145; coral fish, 154; damsels, 144–145; feeding, 150, 151; species, segregation of, 145; tank size requirements of, 150; temperature requirements of, 146, 150, 156; trigger fish, 145
fits. *See* convulsions
flatulence: in cats, 110; in dogs, 56
fleas: in caged birds, 208; in cats, 97–98; in chickens, ducks, and geese, 265; in dogs, 45; in rodents, 228; in skunks, 132
Flemish giants. *See* rabbits
flies and maggots: in cats, 99; in dogs, 46; in reptiles, 172–173
flight control of chickens, ducks, and geese, 261–262

sea snakes. *See* reptiles (snakes)
seborrhea in dogs, 48
seizures. *See* convulsions
septicemia, bacterial hemorrhagic, in fish, 155
sexes, segregation of: in chickens, 270; in rabbits, 236; in rodents, 232; in squirrels and chipmunks, 254
sexing: of amphibians, 186; of caged birds, 214, 216, 217; of cats, 120; of chickens, ducks, and geese, 270–271; of rabbits, 236; of rodents, 232; of skunks, 131; of squirrels and chipmunks, 254
sexual maturity: in cats, 75, 76; in dogs, 60; effects of, on multipet family, 7; in rabbits, 245; in rodents, 231; in squirrels and chipmunks, 254
shampoos: for cats, 74, 102, 103; for dogs, 23–24, 45, 46, 48; for skunks, 129, 132
shock: in cats and skunks, 84; in dogs, 35
  ELECTRICAL in dogs, 41
  THERMAL in amphibians, 185
Siamese. *See* cats
Siamese fighting fish. *See* fish, freshwater
skeletal diseases and disorders: in amphibians, 186; in cats, 109, 122; in dogs, 54
skin diseases and disorders: in caged birds, 202, 211; in cats, 91–92, 92–93, 102–104; in chickens, ducks, and geese, 270; in dogs, 41, 47–49; in gerbils, 226, 229; in guinea pigs, 226, 230; in hamsters, 226, 229; in mice and rats, 226, 230
skin, shedding of: in frogs, 183; in reptiles, 172; in salamanders, 183
skunks: acquiring, 135; advantages of, as pets, 124, 126–127; artificial respiration for, 82–83; bandaging, 86–87; bathing, 129; bite wounds in, 87; breeding, 134; brushing, 129; burns in, 89; castration of, 131; civets, 125; claws of, trimming, 129; convulsions in, 84; de-scenting in, 126–127, 130; disciplining, 127; diseases and disorders of, 132–134; ears of, cleaning, 129; escaped, 131, 133; feeding, 128–129, 135; first aid for, 82–93, 131; frostbite in, 90; grooming, 129; handling and holding, 127–128; heartbeat of, checking, 77; heat stroke in, 89–90; hibernation in, 126, 128; hog-nosed, 125; hooded, 125; housebreaking, 126, 127; housing, 127, 128, 135; injuries in, 88–89; leash training, 126, 130; medication, administering, 79–80; medicine cabinet for, 77; in multipet family, 127, 131; nocturnal habits of, 126, 130; paralysis in, 83; parasites in, 131–133; poisoning in, 40, 85, 92–93; rabies in, 124, 126, 133; rectal prolapse in, 131; regulations concerning, 126; restraints for, protective, 80–82; runs for, outdoor, 128; sexing, 131; shock in, 84; spaying of, 131; species of, 124–125; spotted, 125; spray of, 127; striped, 124–125, 125–126; symptoms of disease in, general, 133–134; temperature of, taking, 77; training, 127–128, 129–130; vaccination of, 133; water requirements of, 129; young, care of, 127, 135
smoke inhalation in dogs, 41
snakebites: in cats, 90–91; in dogs, 39
snakes. *See* reptiles
socialization in multipet family, 5–6
songbirds. *See* birds, caged

sore hocks in rabbits, 244
spaying (ovariohysterectomy): in cats, 75–76; in dogs, 26; in rabbits, 240; in skunks, 131
splints: for caged birds, chickens, ducks, and geese, 203–205; for cats, 88–89; for dogs, 30, 38; for rabbits, 240–241
spotted skunks. *See* skunks
sprains in cats, 88
spraying of urine in cats, 76, 113
squirrels: acquiring, 251; advantages of, as pets, 247; breeding, 254; claws, care of, 252–253; diseases and disorders of, 253–254; feeding, 252–253, 255; first aid for, 254; grooming, 253; groups, keeping in, 252; housebreaking, 247; housing, 251–252; injuries in, 254; nesting boxes for, 252; outside the cage, 247, 252; rabies in, 254; sexing, 254; species of, 247–250; symptoms of illness in, general, 253–254; training, 253; water requirements of, 253; young, care of, 255
  CHIPMUNKS (ground), 247; acquiring, 251; advantages of, as pets, 250; appearance and size of, 250; breeding, 254; cages for, 251–252, 254; feeding, 253; life spans of, 250; nests for, 252; training, 253
  FLYING: acquiring, 251; advantages of, as pets, 250; appearance and size of, 250; breeding, 254; cages for, 252; feeding, 253; life spans of, 250; nests for, 252; training, 253; and open water, 253
  FOX (tree): appearance and size of, 248; breeding, 254; cages for, 251, 252; feeding, 253; nests for, 252
  GRAY (tree): acquiring, 251; advantages of, as pets, 248; appearance and size of, 248; breeding, 254; cages for, 251, 252, 254; feeding, 253; nests for, 253
  RED (tree): 248–250; acquiring, 251; advantages of, as pets, 250; appearance and size of, 250; breeding, 254; cages for, 251, 252; feeding, 253; life spans of, 250; nests for, 252
starvation: in amphibians, 185–186; in caged birds, 211; in reptiles, 173–174
steatitis in reptiles, 176
stomach worms in chickens, ducks, and geese, 266
stomatitis: in cats, 107, 108; in dogs, 53; in reptiles, 176–177
stretcher: for cats, 88; for dogs, 32, 35
striped skunks. *See* skunks
stud tail in cats, 103
subcutaneous mites in chickens, ducks, and geese, 265
sucker fish. *See* fish, freshwater
surgery, optional: in cats, 75–77; in chickens, ducks, and geese, 261–262; in dogs, 26–27; in rabbits, 240; in skunks, 130–131
swan geese. *See* geese
swans, 256n
swordtails. *See* fish, freshwater
symptoms of disease, general: in amphibians, 185; in caged birds, 201–202, 212–213; in chickens, ducks, and geese, 263; in cats, 99; in fish, 153–154; in rabbits, 243; in rodents, 226–227; in skunks, 133–134; in squirrels and chipmunks, 253

tail, problems with in cats, 85, 104
tail rot in fish, 155
taming. *See* training

tanks for fish. *See* aquariums
tapeworms (cestodes): in caged birds, 208; in cats, 93–94; in chickens, ducks, and geese, 266; in dogs, 43; in rabbits, 242; in skunks, 132
tearing, heavy. *See* epiphora
teeth. *See* mouth and throat
tegus. *See* reptiles (lizards)
temperature, taking: of cats and skunks, 77–79; of dogs, 29; of rabbits, 240
temperature requirements: of amphibians, 183; of caged birds, 197; of chickens, ducks, and geese, 259–260, 264, 271; of fish, 140, 141, 142, 143, 144, 146, 148, 150, 156; of rabbits, 237; of reptiles, 159, 165, 166, 167; of rodents, 223
tenotomy in chickens, ducks, and geese, 262
terrapins. *See* reptiles
terrariums: for amphibians, 182; for reptiles, 164
tetrameres worms in chickens, ducks, and geese, 266
tetras. *See* fish, freshwater
thorny-headed worms (acanthocephalids): in caged birds, 208; in chickens, ducks, and geese, 266
threadworms in chickens, ducks, and geese, 266
throat. *See* mouth and throat
thrush: in caged birds, 210; in chickens, ducks, and geese, 269
tick paralysis: in cats, 98; in dogs, 36
ticks: in caged birds, 207; in cats, 98; in chickens, ducks, and geese, 265; in dogs, 36, 45–46; in reptiles, 172; in skunks, 132
tigers. *See* fish, freshwater
toads. *See* amphibians
tonsillitis in dogs, 53
tortoises. *See* reptiles
tourniquet: for cats, 90–91; for dogs, 33, 39
toxoplasmosis in cats, 95–97
tracheas, collapsed, in dogs, 53–54
tracheobronchitis (kennel cough) in dogs, 53
training: of cats, 69–70; of dogs, 20–22; of rodents, 225; of skunks, 127–128, 129–130; of squirrels and chipmunks, 253
trauma. *See* injuries; wounds
tree frogs. *See* amphibians (frogs)
tree squirrels. *See* squirrels: fox; gray; red
trematodes. *See* flukes
trench mouth: in cats, 108; in dogs, 53
trichinosis in cats, 94
trichomoniasis: in caged birds, 210; in chickens, ducks, and geese, 269
tricks. *See* training
trigger fish. *See* fish, marine
trout chow for amphibians, 185
tuataras. *See* reptiles
tuberculosis: in caged birds, 209; in chickens, ducks, and geese, 268
tuleremia in rabbits, 241–242
tumors: in caged birds, 211, 212–213; in cats, 103–104, 108, 109, 115, 122; in dogs, 49, 53, 54, 57–59
turtles. *See* reptiles
typhoid, cat. *See* panleukopenia
typhoid, fowl, in chickens, 268

unconsciousness in dogs, 35
uremia in cats, 113
urinary diseases and disorders: in cats, 84, 111–113, 122; in dogs, 42, 56–57; in rodents, 226